Nursing Research:
A Qualitative Perspective

Nursing Research:
A Qualitative Perspective

Second Edition

Patricia L. Munhall
and
Carolyn Oiler Boyd

National League for Nursing Press • New York
Pub. No. 19-2535

Copyright © 1993
National League for Nursing Press
350 Hudson Street, New York, NY 10014

ISBN 0-88737-590-1

The views expressed in this publication represent the views of the authors and do not necessarily reflect the official views of the National League for Nursing Press.

Library of Congress Cataloging-in-Publication Data

Nursing research : a qualitative perspective / Patricia
  L. Munhall, Carolyn Oiler Boyd. — 2nd ed.
        p.   cm.
    Includes bibliographical references and index.
    ISBN 0-88737-590-1 : $35.95
    1. Nursing—Research.   I. Munhall, Patricia L.   II. Boyd, Carolyn
Oiler.
    [DNLM: 1. Nursing Research—methods.   WY 20.5 N9735 1993]
RT81.5.N866   1993
610.73'072—dc20
DNLM/DLC
for Library of Congress   93-20494
                                                              CIP

Printed in the United States of America

Contents

v

Contributors

Charles J. Beauchamp, PhD, RN
Associate Professor
Chairman
Department of Nursing
Colby-Sawyer College
New Hampshire

Nettie Birnbach, EdD, RN, FAAN
Professor and Director, Center for Nursing Research
State University of New York - Health Science Center at Brooklyn
Brooklyn, New York

Carolyn Oiler Boyd, EdD, RN
Associate Professor
College of Nursing
Villanova University
Villanova, Pennsylvania

Marlene Zichi Cohen, PhD, RN
Director, Office of Nursing Research
Assistant Professor
Department of Nursing and Norris Comprehensive Cancer Center
University of Southern California

M. Louise Fitzpatrick, EdD, RN, FAAN
Dean and Professor
College of Nursing
Villanova University
Villanova, Pennsylvania

Carol P. Germain, EdD, RN, FAAN
Associate Professor
Chairperson, Science and Role Development Division
School of Nursing
University of Pennsylvania
Philadelphia, Pennsylvania

Sally A. Hutchinson, PhD, RN, FAAN
Professor
College of Nursing
University of Florida Health Science Center
Jacksonville, Florida

Kathleen A. Knafl, PhD
Professor and Associate Dean for Research
College of Nursing
University of Illinois
Chicago, Illinois

Sarah Steen Lauterbach, EdD, RN
Assistant Professor
School of Nursing
LaSalle University
Philadelphia, Pennsylvania

Carla Mariano, EdD, RN
Associate Professor and Director, Advanced Education in Nursing Science
Master's Degree Program
Division of Nursing
New York University
New York, New York

Patricia L. Munhall, EdD, ARNP, PsyA, FAAN
Professor and Associate Dean of Graduate Programs
Director for the Center of Nursing Science
School of Nursing
Barry University
Miami, Florida

Zane Robinson Wolf, PhD, RN, FAAN
Professor
School of Nursing, LaSalle University, Philadelphia, Pennsylvania
Associate Director of Nursing for Research
Albert Einstein Medical Center
Philadelphia, Pennsylvania

Preface to Second Edition

*B*earing witness to and participating in nursing's turn toward the qualitative paradigm over the course of the past 15 years or so has been, and continues to be, renewing. The matter of qualitative research has gained nursing's national attention during the past decade, although its inception can be traced to the 1960s in the nursing literature. Qualitative research activity has gained sufficient momentum and prominence to necessitate an in-depth introduction to qualitative research approaches at least at the graduate level. Cursory overviews of the range of approaches that constitute the qualitative paradigm may be sufficient for a time for undergraduate students of nursing, but such treatments are clearly not adequate in the longer term even at this level. To be knowledgeable about nursing, one must have an acquaintance with multiple ways of knowing in their scientific sense.

The discussions about the merit of the qualitative paradigm, particularly in regard to our ideas about science and knowledge development, have subsided a bit; recent years have shown a turn toward mastering and perfecting qualitative research methods in the study of a wide variety of nursing phenomena. There is a growing acceptance of nursing science as a composite of different perspectives; there is now an established accommodation of multiple paradigms in nursing. In many ways, the evolution of qualitative research in nursing has barely begun. Nevertheless, the progress is startling, and the task of an introductory volume is transformed. In this revised second edition, we have maintained a position of advancing the qualitative paradigm in nursing through a thorough examination of leading qualitative approaches. Readers can continue to expect that, although introductory in nature, this text will provide detail in explication of the various methods, both through description of each method and through illustration in studies that implement the various methods.

Based on our use of the text and on the thoughtful comments and suggestions from others, all the methods presented in the first edition have been retained with the exception of philosophical inquiry. In its place is case study method, which is gaining the attention and interest of increasing numbers of qualitative researchers. Methods chapters have been updated and revised, and all chapters illustrating use of the methods are new studies. The value of studies published in the first edition remains, and readers are encouraged to consult these as well as the many qualitative studies published in recent years. In addition, several new chapters have been included in this second edition to reflect new understandings and new developments in qualitative research. These new chapters address ethical concerns, institutional review, formatting proposals and reports, and the issue of combining research approaches. Readers of the first edition will find that the grounding for the qualitative paradigm in Part One has been retained with some revision but with continuing attention to the philosophical underpinnings that establish the paradigm as a legitimate way of knowing in nursing. In view of the fact that the dominant paradigm in our culture is positivistic, this attention continues to be highly relevant.

This second edition represents progress, growth, and promise in redefining the nature of reality, truth, knowing, and science in nursing. It is offered not only to students of nursing science but also to colleagues who teach, guide, and do qualitative research. We are clearly in a different place now, and this edition is intended not only to achieve its original purpose of introduction to the qualitative paradigm but also to serve the needs of seasoned qualitative researchers for updates on thinking expressed years ago when the first edition was put together. The revisions will address that need for communication among those of us who are involved in focused exploration of one or another approach, but who wish to keep abreast generally of other paths being explored in other ways.

It is truly gratifying to be a part of the scholarship that is so capably shared with readers by authors in this volume. We learn as we teach, and rightfully credit our students and our colleagues with the extensions and refinements of thought expressed in this second edition. The original preface and prologue have been retained as a reference point for this growth as well as for their continuing function as an orientation to the radical shift of the qualitative paradigm. With that, let us continue the dialogue and the productivity of doing qualitative research.

Patricia L. Munhall
Carolyn Oiler Boyd

Preface

*T*he impetus for this book on qualitative research approaches grew, ironically, from our indoctrination to empirical method in nursing research. Concerned with questions of meaning in the world of nursing, we learned, experientially, the limitations of empirical method in the pursuit of such research interests as empathic communication in nursing and moral reasoning among nurses. There is, then, in this preference for qualitative approaches in nursing research, an active choice on our part among alternatives; a choice based on both a perspective on the nature of the nursing world and an appreciation of the variety of modes and styles of investigating that world. This book represents, above all, an effort to share our growth toward a qualitative perspective with the hope that others' preferences—whatever they might be—will emerge from choice rather than indoctrination.

There is in this effort both a hope to achieve a work of lasting value and the knowledge that we will produce only a beginning— an introductory, illustrative work that can serve simply to stimulate interest in learning more.

The qualitative approach in nursing research is a fertile field for development. We dare to explore it at this exciting time when few rules must be observed. At the risk of patent audacity, we aim to describe our early exploration and to present the work of qualitative nurse researchers who are also engaged in this project of discovering and testing new and borrowed research paradigms.

This is a text and reference work for nurse researchers and students of nursing. It is divided into three parts. In Part One, a rationale for the choice of qualitative method in nursing research is described. Readers are invited to reflect on the value system we choose to guide nursing, and to consider the implications of these values for not only our practice but also our research and theory development. A case for qualitative research in nursing is presented on the basis of this analysis of values, the congruence of nursing values with qualitative method, and an assessment of nursing's state of theory development.

The argument for qualitative approaches in nursing research is advanced by a presentation of a broad philosophical framework for qualitative inquiry. The recurring themes of phenomenological philosophy are described to explicate this framework, common to the qualitative approaches contained in this volume.

In Part Two, selected qualitative approaches are described in terms of their methods and techniques, and each is demonstrated in a presentation of a research study. Phenomenology as a research method, grounded theory, ethnography, historical research, and foundational inquiry are the approaches selected for this volume. These approaches are believed to be representative of the wealth in qualitative nursing research. Alternative interpretation of these approaches as well as other tested approaches and to-be-discovered approaches must be described in future volumes as nursing research evolves.

In Part Three, an overall summary of the nature of qualitative research is provided within the context of a framework that one might use for interpreting, writing about, and evaluating qualitative research.

This text is a complete work in the sense that it introduces the reader to a variety of research approaches, alternative to empirical method, and thereby broadens our collective research perspective. Certain of the value of qualitative approaches in nursing research, we are less certain of their destiny. In nursing's contemporary formative stage of development, this effort is offered to promote the scientific legitimacy of qualitative research in nursing.

Prologue

*I*n order to consider the qualitative perspective in nursing research, we are well advised to come to terms about the meaning of "science," "scientific," "humanistic," and "research." The mere fact that a text like this can be distinguished from other nursing research texts as *qualitative* testifies to the presence in our work of a massive dichotomy that finds expression in our practice experiences as well as our research endeavors.

Science, as it is customarily used, is sometimes posed as a threat to humanistic ideals because it is frequently promoted as the single true vision of reality and route to truth. Nursing's concern with developing a body of knowledge and assuming professional status in the health care arena has resulted in an identification with empirical science as the model for intellectual endeavor in the field. The isolation of parts suitable for scientific analysis in the empirical model discourages those who envision the acceptance of other ways of knowing, particularly ways of grasping wholes and complex meanings in nursing situations.

In commenting on positivistic assumptions and approaches in the sciences of man, Merleau-Ponty (1964) states: "All of us live in the natural attitude—that is, in the conviction that we are a part of the world and subject to its action on us, which we passively receive from the outside" (p. 56). The term "objective" refers in positivism to a reality independent of the observer, and the aim thus becomes one of eliminating as much observer bias as possible in order to arrive at the truth of objective reality. The scientific observer of the objective world is ideally a camera of the reality he or she studies. In this way, a dichotomy between the objective and subjective worlds has been created.

The tension resulting from this splitting of the world into objective and subjective realities has been acknowledged and described by nurses striving to express and share what they know about nursing. This has been particularly apparent in nurses' writings during the 1960s about such skills as listening and touching. Travelbee, for example, developed an argument that sympathy and compassion are nursing assets in response to a growing effort to become more objective in nursing assessment (1964). Other nurse authors found support in existential philosophy for their development of subjective themes in nursing. (See Arnold, 1970; Black, 1968; Clemence, 1966; Ferlic, 1968; Raymond, 1968.) Either vestiges of our prescientific era or reactionaries to a rapidly growing observance of scientific mores in nursing practice, these nurses' ideas did gradually disappear from the nursing literature.

The significance of such subjective experience in nursing as nurses' attitudes, their empathetic awareness, their emotional responses to clients, continues to be recognized. What remains unresolved, however, is the tension they constitute in a discipline striving to establish itself as a scientifically based profession. Science, as we have come to understand it, demands that these subjective experiences be operationalized in terms of those objective manifestations that attest to their reality. Apart from this, there is no basis for knowing whether or not they are real. The problem arising from this demand, of course, is that of locating such evidence in measurable terms.

This latter realization serves to explain why nursing's pursuit of truth through empirical methodology warrants a critical examination for its fit with nursing reality. Davis (1968) argues that "the nature of the scientific method has not been and is not now a fixed, established datum" (p. 216). Further, Davis cites that research in nursing as well as nursing itself are social acts, and that social science is not qualitatively continuous with natural science. It is the social nature of nursing that lends credence to the idea that the observer exists in the world, and that reality is the observer's interpreted experience. In this sense, there is no

ctive reality, apart from the observer's experience in the
d, to be captured by scientific methods.
ience is, by definition, both a process of coming to know, and
product of knowledge. It is also characterized by being system-
in nature. Strictly speaking, there is nothing in the term
nce" that excludes, for example, philosophical inquiry as a
ess of knowing; and philosophical insight, as knowledge. Yet,
science has come to assume a narrow meaning that does exclude
philosophy, intuition, and much of nursing. It is opposed in its
usage to belief, art, and other subjectively based knowledge.

It is well known that science referred initially to the process
and product of study of the natural, or physical world. Over time,
this process was refined and principles emerged to guide scientific inquiry and to serve as gatekeeper to the world of science.
What are the assumptions and principles of natural science as they
have come to disciplines like philosophy, sociology, education,
and nursing?

First, it is assumed that the universe is orderly. For every effect,
there is a cause. The social scientists recognize that the cause may
be complex. There may be, and often are, multiple causative factors in complex interaction; but nevertheless, human behavior is
understandable in stimulus–response terms. For these patterns,
the experimental design, which controls variables to isolate
cause–effect relationships, is sacrosanct.

Second, it is assumed that human reality is two-dimensional.
That there is no pure consciousness, void of the world. We are always conscious of something, in one way or another. The complex
modes of consciousness unique to man open up multiple realities,
no one less true than the others. This, then, is an alternative assumption about the world and reality from which scientific study
might proceed: objective reality is grounded in our subjective experience in the world.

*The whole universe of science is built upon the world as di-
rectly experienced, and if we want to subject science itself to
rigorous scrutiny and arrive at a precise assessment of its
meaning and scope, we must begin by reawakening the basic
experience of the world of which science is the second-order*

expression. Science has not and never will have, by its na-
ture, the same significance qua form of being as the world
which we perceive, for the simple reason that it is a ratio-
nale or explanation of that world. (Merleau-Ponty, 1962,
p. viii)

Adherents of the scientific method in nursing recognize, of
course, the limitations of research findings vis-à-vis the complexities of nursing situations. Further, understanding is for all nurse
researchers, regardless of their methods, the ultimate aim of study.
Merleau-Ponty's statements, however, draw attention to several
significant considerations.

First, the scientific attitude is but one view of the world, rather
than the means to a grasp of a single reality. Further, that view
is one of commenting on lived reality as it appears from the
dictates and limitations of its methods. Secondly, this characteristic of science as a commentator on reality negates the idea that
scientific knowledge is equivalent to reality itself. In the qualitative researcher's view, the human experience underlies conceptual understanding, and needs to be reawakened in the
researcher. The more sedimented this original experience is in
the researcher's inquiry, the less meaning scientific expressions
will possess. Conversely, the observer's awareness of his or her
position in the world, which grounds inquiries in subjective experience, enhances the significance of one's scientific description as a presentation of reality. Scientific description in this
view is recognized as a presentation of the observer's reality as it
appears in the context of the position he or she has taken up in
the world.

Qualitative researchers suggest that lived reality serve as the focus of inquiry, toward the end that subjective and objective realities merge or unify in a closer alliance between lived reality and
our knowledge of it. Since the perceived world, or lived reality,
underlies scientific explanation, and since human experience is
the focus of concern in nursing practice, some means of describing lived experience in nursing situations is a paramount need
in nursing research. In the view of the qualitative researcher,

subjective experience is not merely a private, inner world; but rather, inextricably bound with objective reality, and the basis from which scientific knowledge is derived.

Subjective involvement in the objective world, then, is the origin of inquiry for researchers interested in contributing to a body of knowledge concerned with the variety of human experiences in nursing practice. Nurse researchers can profit from study of the methods and techniques qualitative researchers have developed in other disciplines; notably, philosophy, psychology, sociology, and anthropology. They may also be stimulated to discover new methods and techniques in this research perspective which is characterized by an openness to the search for access to human experience. Nurse researchers will find a congruence between nursing's philosophical embrace of humanism and holism and qualitative methodologies.

Not every research interest can be accommodated by the qualitative perspective, nor should nursing, in our view, adopt a single method for developing knowledge about our wonderfully complex, multi-dimensional nursing world. To do so is to impose a conformity in nursing that is inconsistent with the variety of roles, settings, goals and styles that comprise a societal service that is comprehensive, flexible, dynamic.

Qualitative research is, like empirical method, a tool of science. Each qualitative approach is structured by principles and methods which endow it with the systematic, disciplined quality that is requisite to science as opposed to superstition, propaganda, tradition or prejudice. Like empirical method, each qualitative approach requires certain steps, in a certain order, according to certain rules, and is thus subject to certain measures of the value of the research findings.

Qualitative approaches are scientific; they are legitimate members of the realm of science; and they lead to knowledge about the world. Readers are invited to consider them first, in the context of how they compare with the more familiar quantitative approach on a philosophical level; and secondly, in a more detailed examination of selected qualitative approaches in nursing inquiries.

REFERENCES

Arnold, H. (1970). I-thou. *American Journal of Nursing, 70,* 2554–2556.

Black, Sr. K. (1968). An existential model for psychiatric nursing. *Perspectives in Psychiatric Care, 6,* 178–184.

Clemence, Sr. M. (1966). Existentialism: A philosophy of commitment. *American Journal of Nursing, 66,* 500–505.

Davis, A. (1973). The phenomenological approach in nursing research. In E. Garrison (Ed.), *Doctoral preparation for nurses.* San Francisco: University of California Press.

Ferlic, A. (1968). Existential approach in nursing. *Nursing Outlook, 16,* 30–33.

Merleau-Ponty, M. (1962). *Phenomenology of perception* (C. Smith, Trans.). New York: Humanities Press.

Merleau-Ponty, M. (1964). *The primacy of perception* (J. Edie, Trans.). Evanston, IL: Northwestern University Press.

Raymond, Sr. M. (1968). Existentialism and the psychiatric nurse. *Perspectives in Psychiatric Care, 6,* 185–187.

Travelbee, J. (1964). What do we mean by rapport? *American Journal of Nursing, 63,* 725–728.

Part One

Language, Epistemology, and the Qualitative Paradigm

In the first three chapters of this volume, a cumulative discussion supports the foundation of qualitative methods as tools for nursing science. Chapter 1 invites us to reflect on our language system as it reveals our underlying philosophical structures of beliefs and values. This reflection, in keeping with an important theme of qualitative research, is embedded within context. We see the weaving of a tapestry that has the threads of our history, our early preparation of nurse researchers, our paradigmatic transitions, and the influence of theory derivation on our developing nursing science.

Building on these considerations, Chapter 2 describes the epistemological basis of nursing. Fundamental questions as to the purpose of science, research paradigms and traditions, and our epistemological interests are discussed. Qualitative and quantitative methods are presented as representing first- and second-order activities of science: qualitative methods are associated with the processes of discovery and clarification, and quantitative methods, with validation and verification. A cyclical continuum is proposed.

Chapter 3 extends the rationale for qualitative methods of research and provides an explicit philosophical framework for qualitative studies. In this chapter, phenomenological philosophy is introduced through the articulation of themes that guide the qualitative research project. Through a grounding in the qualitative paradigm of these first three chapters, we are prepared to read about methods with understanding, appreciation, and the critical stance so essential to scholarship.

Language and Nursing Research

Patricia L. Munhall

Discussing or talking is the way in which we articulate significantly the intelligibility of Being-in-the-world.
The way in which discourse gets expressed is language.
Heidegger (1962, p. 204)

*B*eing in the world, for those nurse researchers who embark on the path of discovery through qualitative research designs or methods, has many challenges. One of these challenges has to do with the limits and power of language. Our world is defined and organized through language. Language is one way we communicate meaning. In the very way we give definition to the particulars of our context, social and cultural agendas are set. So too in our research language; values, beliefs, and aims are communicated.

For many years, nurse researchers and theorists have engaged in a lively and enlightening dialogue of various paradigms, the two most common being the logical positivist or empirical-analytic paradigm and the contrasting one, phenomenology. This dialogue was prompted by many nurse researchers who initiated what was to become an "interpretive turn" in nursing research (Munhall, 1989). These nurse theorists and researchers began to raise these questions:

- Was nursing a natural science, like that of chemistry and biology, and therefore based on similar linguistic assumptions?
- Was nursing a human science based on differing linguistic assumptions?
- Was nursing research ready for a poststructuralist perspective (Dzurec, 1989)?

The purpose of this chapter is to place in context the words and definitions that have given rise to these discussions. Nursing language is both concealing and revealing of the stances and perspective we pose to nursing as we interact with the phenomenon of concern. For some nurse researchers, this discussion will be historical because they have chosen one paradigm over another for various reasons. For other nurse researchers, it will also be historical because they see a poststructuralist perspective of multiple research paradigms as not only acceptable but essential. (This is further discussed in Chapter 17 of this volume.) For purposes of this discussion, the logical positivist paradigm yields to quantitative research methods and designs and the phenomenological paradigm yields to qualitative research.

In this chapter, we will see, in the form of contrasting systems of language, competing articulations—in other fields as well as our own—that are reflective of various philosophical orientations. This particular focus on philosophical analysis is further elucidated in Chapter 3 and again in Chapter 17.

Research in nursing will be at the center of this linguistic exploration. Methods of doing research interestingly have been divided into two purportedly ideological (and thus far considered conflicting) schools of thought with two distinct language systems. These schools of thought have been categorized as the qualitative and quantitative approaches to research. By quantitative methods of research we mean the traditional scientific methods as presented in most of the contemporary nursing research textbooks. The methods are characterized by deductive reasoning, objectivity, quasi-experiments, statistical techniques, and control. In contrast, the qualitative methods, many of which are described within this text, are characterized by inductive reasoning, subjectivity, discovery, description, and process orienting (Reichardt & Cook, 1979).

We will explore this qualitative–quantitative dichotomy and perhaps will appear culpable of unnecessary polarization. This we do for the pedagogical advantage of clearly revealing the possible differences between these two research traditions. We also absolve ourselves of this polarization as the second chapter of this volume opens! In that chapter we suggest an "alliance of evidence" (Light & Pillemer, 1982, p. 19) that finds its origins in qualitative research and its validation in quantitative research.

The present chapter begins with a discussion on the living aspect of language, then progresses to a contextual analysis of nursing research so that we may ferret out the meanings of our linguistic expressions, their origins, and subsequent propulsions. This motion of transition from an earlier identification with medicine is representative of a broad worldview transition or paradigmatic shift. Nursing research and the quest for nursing theory development are discussed from the perspective of language development and language usage as we seek out the pattern and process of our articulation of meaning and experience. The chapter ends on a thematic note similar to the one expressed by West (1983) in *The World is Made of Glass:* "There is a pattern in all this which I begin slowly to understand and which I am trying to codify. The problem is that I lack the vocabulary" (p. 47).

LANGUAGE AND LIVED EXPERIENCE

Long before children speak actual words, they have learned effectively to express their physical, mental, and emotional states of being. Very early in our childhood we learn that laughing, crying, pouting, and looking quizzical stimulate a response from those who are "significant others." We are indeed beginning to learn the power of expressive language.

Eventually, we begin to develop a vocabulary and, interestingly, by the time we are 2 years of age or so, we have learned to treasure the word "no." Individuation, assertiveness, posturing, and a continuing desire for power in our environment render this one of the most important words in any language. People have written entire books on how, when, and where to say "no" effectively.

Nursing as a profession, concomitantly with women as a social force, is still very much involved in those processes of individuation, assertiveness, posturing, and claiming power in our environment. Like the significance of the word "no," our language and the use of specific sets of words simultaneously reveal and conceal who we are, both to ourselves and the world at large.

Thus, in our quest for individuation—and, we should mention, our autonomy (*auto-no-my*)—we are in the process of developing an original language system. This focus on autonomy correlates well with the point of the revelatory and concealing power of language and the exemplary word "no." Nursing has claimed the power to say "no" through the Greek word *autonomous,* meaning self-ruling. Thus, we see language alive in a word that says, "I have a right to be self-determined." The living of autonomy expresses the position of a profession and, in nursing, has called attention to our transition from the physician's handmaiden (just look at that word!) to an independent self-ruling practitioner. This posturing of ourselves is consistently illustrated in our transition from the primary usage of medical language to our concerted efforts to develop a nursing language, taxonomy, nomenclature, and nursing diagnostic system.[1]

The moment-to-moment language we choose reflects the posture or stance we assume in the space we believe is ours in the health care _____ (fill in the blank):

[1] There is considerable discussion within the profession about the usage of the term "nursing diagnosis." Many view this term (and activity) as an example of a continued imitation of medicine.

1. System
2. Arena
3. Delivery system
4. Field

For example, in the above multiple-choice option, we find it most interesting to study such words in their starkness for their literal or metaphorical meaning. Is health care "delivered"? Is there a "system" of health care? The word "arena," which is frequently used with health care, is a word that is often associated with a circus or sports. (The temptation is too great to resist pointing out how that word, with its noted association, may be the most apt description of the present so-called health care system.)

As noted, nursing language, like that of other professions, is revelatory of the stance and perspective we suppose as we interact with the phenomena of our experience. The symbols we choose as expressions either implicitly or explicitly lay open our assertions, propositions, assumptions, beliefs, values, and priorities. The significance of such expressions is centered in our emergence: our expressions bring us into existence. The noumenal or "thing in itself" depends on the phenomenal for its expression. This will be further explained.

DeVries (1983) succinctly and humorously illustrated the noumenal emerging from felt obscurity into shared, understood experience in the following passage:

In the beginning was the word. Once terms like identity doubts and midlife crisis become current, the reported cases of them increase by leaps and bounds, affecting people unaware there is anything wrong with them until they have got a load of the coinages. You too may have an acquaintance or even a relative with a block about paper hanging or dog grooming, a high flown form of stagnation trickled down from writers and artists. Once my poor dear mother confided to me in a hollow whisper, "I have an identity crisis." I says, "How do you mean?" and she says, "I no longer understand your father." Now we have burnout, and having heard tell of it on television or read about it in a magazine, your plumber doubts he can any longer hack it as a pipefitter, while a glossary adopted by his wife has turned him overnight into . . . a male chauvinist pig, something she would never have suspected before. (p. 4)

Though satirized, we can identify readily in the foregoing what is referred to as a concept development. The "thing itself" (the noumenal) existed, was felt; yet we needed the description and language of shared experience to connect us within the world and provide a way of perceiving the phenomenon. There are other recent contemporary phenomena that we have developed into abstractions of concrete events or, from some intuitive sense, into empirically expressed concepts and words that are commonly used to express our or others' positions/posture/stance in the world. Thus, we have codependency, women who love too much, deficit spending, premenstrual syndrome (PMS), and "control freaks"! The proliferation of support groups for various conditions of life as well as the many twelve-step programs speak also to our need for shared language to connect us within the world with one another.

Our language development will, as with all disciplines, bring us into emergence. We need to recognize and articulate our points of contact in a pluralistic world, and we need our language with the referent of nursing phenomena to have a recognized place in that world. These are among the first steps of nursing research: discovery, description, and concept clarification (Norris, 1982).

The word "undeveloped," describing Third World countries, was judged to be a pejorative adjective and was discontinued. The word "emerging" was used instead, to reflect optimism. Our emergence, like that of children and emerging countries, will depend on our ability to express ourselves clearly within the context of this pluralistic world. Let us look at the lived experience of nursing through a contextual analysis of our language development.

THE CONTEXT OF NURSING RESEARCH

Meshler (1979) argued that there *is no meaning* (italics added) without context dependence. So it appears appropriate, especially in a text on qualitative research that readily acknowledges and embodies its search within the context of "things," that we begin this exploration of language in nursing research by attending to the context in which it has occurred and is continuing to evolve.

Context is defined as "that which leads up to and follows and often specifies the meaning of a particular expression" and "the circumstances in which a particular event occurs" (*American Heritage Dictionary*, 1969). We believe that within this definition of context the following three antecedents and their evolutionary concurrent factors should be acknowledged with the contiguous expressions. They are:

1. Research in nursing evolved predominantly when nursing was in transition between broad philosophical worldviews.
2. Researchers in nursing were (are) being prepared in fields other than nursing.
3. Derivation and/or deduction for nursing research was (is) being drawn from disciplines other than nursing.

Each factor will be presently explored from the perspective of its contributions to our nursing research language.

Transition in Worldviews of Nursing

During the 1950s, as an outgrowth of the development and acceptance of new theoretical approaches to understanding physical and human phenomena emerging from other fields (approaches such as systems perspectives, quantum physics, adaptation, and ecological views), nurse scholars began questioning the prevalent acceptance and alignment of the medical model as the basis for nursing practice. At the same time, nurse scholars were acknowledging the need for our own distinct body of knowledge, a benchmark of a profession, and had begun in earnest to embark on this monumental endeavor of developing nursing theory.

These two factors, the acknowledgment of a major scientific revolution in other disciplines and the desire to attain a level of professionalism where we base practice on a distinct body of nursing knowledge, led to a perceptual shift in the way we spoke about nursing phenomena and simultaneously led to the scientific investigation of nursing phenomena.[2] It seemed, though, that the way we spoke about nursing and the way we investigated nursing phenomena often reflected assumptions, propositions, beliefs, and priorities of two different worldviews, one reflecting the new worldview and the other reflecting the old worldview. We will see shortly that this is a characteristic of paradigmatic shift within a discipline.

The spoken language in nursing began to change, reflecting this perceptual shift from the medical, atomistic, causal model to a distinct nursing, holistic, interactive model. This represented a paradigmatic innovation for nursing. The way phenomena were viewed in the world was changing in a way that is considered by some to be irrevocably conflictual in its basic premises and assumptions with the medical model.

This shift, which is well recognized in the discipline of physics, has begun to permeate the language of other fields as well as nursing. The change is representative of a transition from a mechanistic to an organismic perspective, from a philosophical perspective of realism to idealism (Filstead, 1979), and from the received view to a nonreceived view (Watson, 1981).

Illumination of the differences between and among these worldviews or paradigms can be demonstrated in the scrutiny of the respective language systems. It seems appropriate, though, to be clear at this point as to what a worldview or paradigm is. Patton (1978), in terms consistent with Kuhn (1970), defined a paradigm as:

> *A worldview, a general perspective, a way of breaking down the complexity of the real world. As such, paradigms are deeply embedded in the socialization of adherents and*

---

[2] For a more detailed explanation of the scientific revolution that eclipsed determinism and objectivism, the reader is referred to works on quantum physics, Heisenberg's principle of uncertainty, and Bohr's principle of complementarity. In Floyd Matson's *The Broken Image*, a most readable discourse can be found, and Larry Dossy's *Space, Time and Medicine* is wonderfully explicit and enjoyable reading on this topic.

practitioners: paradigms tell them what is important, legiti-
mate and reasonable. (p. 203)

If we accept the premise that things come into being through language, the language paradigm of a discipline will tell the practitioner what is important, legitimate, and reasonable. Kuhn (1970) suggested that a paradigm is a discipline's specific method of solving a puzzle, of viewing human experience, and of structuring reality. It is a worldview, a way of viewing phenomena in the world.

Laudan (1977), in a similar vein, used the phrase "research tradition" to communicate the same theme:

A research tradition . . . is a set of assumptions about the
basic kinds of entities in the world, assumptions about how
these entities interact, assumptions about the proper meth-
ods to use for constructing and testing theories about these
entities. (p. 97)

Morgan (1983) called our attention to the significance of these assumptions. He stated: "Assumptions make messes researchable, often at the cost of great simplification, and in a way that is highly problematic" (p. 377).

This reference about assumptions becomes more powerful when, as Morgan suggested, researchers choose their own assumptions on which to base their study. One could then say that this latitude or freedom gives the means for achieving what the researcher values. In the paradigms introduced in this chapter are assumptions about the world, believed in some way to be true, though they are actually the "taken for granted" views of human scientists. In a fundamental sense, then, researchers choose the values and "truths" on which they base their research endeavors.

Another way of expressing this shift was the idea that nursing was a human science. Nursing seems to be philosophically expressed through language to be compatible with the ideas and concepts of a human science. German philosopher–historian Wilhelm Dilthey (1926; as translated in Atwood & Stolorow, 1984) held these assumptions about a human science:

The natural sciences investigate objects from the outside whereas the human sciences rely on a perspective from the inside. (p. 2)

The supreme category of the human sciences is meaning. (p. 2)

The central emphasis in the natural sciences is upon causal explanation: The task of inquiry in the human sciences is interpretation and understanding. (p. 2)

Our transition in worldviews then seems to have moved from a narrowly defined type of science to a much broader connection of what constitutes science. In particular, as seen here, one now could ask: Are there different sciences—natural science and human science?

THE LANGUAGE OF WORLDVIEWS

What follows now are expressions belonging to different ways of viewing phenomena (worldviews). The language reveals different assumptions, beliefs, and values concerning human and physical reality. In essence, the paradigm or research tradition is a philosophy: it conceptualizes fundamental beliefs. It is for this reason that the research paradigm as a puzzle-solving method should be congruent with the discipline's larger paradigm, that is, the paradigm of nursing or nursing's philosophy.

Although this idea of congruency is not held as essential by all researchers, the most sophisticated or reasonable response to any either–or discussion would be to choose a dialectic approach (Moccia, 1988; Morgan, 1983). This approach, as Morgan (1983) stated, "also accepts the diversity of assumption and knowledge claims as an inevitable future of research and attempts to use the competing perspectives as a means of constructing new modes of understanding" (p. 379).

Each of the five tables (Tables 1-1 through 1-5) of paradigmatic-type language presents two contrasting belief systems. The language of the systems in the left columns is often the same language or, if not literally the same, it is at least consistent in syntax and meaning, reflecting the underlying continuity of beliefs, values, and assumptions. The same continuity in language will be observed in the systems presented in the right columns of the tables. The observations are important when we take into account that it is the paradigm that preserves and perpetuates the disciplinary matrix of a field (Kuhn, 1970).

A major premise that this volume suggests is that the language expressed within the left columns and found within the paradigms of the mechanistic, the realists, the received view, the medical model, and behaviorism is consistent with the scientific method or quantitative research. In contrast, the language expressed in the right columns reflects the paradigms of the organismic, the idealists, the nonreceived view, humanism, and many nursing models and is consistent with qualitative research methods.

We know well that there are more cultures than the two described by C. P. Snow in *The Two Cultures and the Scientific Revolution* (1959). Today, there are hundreds, and there are disciplines and subdisciplines of those disciplines. Often, the subdisciplines of a discipline speak in foreign tongues to one another. For this reason, it is important to understand the overall fundamental differences so that we may intelligently see what Kirby (1983) called "the points of contact in a plural world." Illustrating the plurality of worldviews, he optimistically stated that "there could be an underlying unity . . . and thus a single earth-centered perspective from which all problems may be viewed" (p. 25).

That is a stance with which we are in consort, yet we believe it is essential to understand the differences in worldviews and the language of the contrasting systems of thought. Only then will we be able to see the points of contact and propose an alliance where all sorts of evidence contribute to the richness of our comprehension and our ability to make sense of the world around us.

Paradigms in Psychology. It has been said that all contemporary psychological systems are derivative of either the mechanistic or the organismic paradigms (Table 1-1) (Looft, 1973). Many philosophers and psychologists argue that the assumptions of each are unbridgeable. Either humans are reactive organisms, as Skinner (1953) would have them, or individuals are active organisms, as

Table 1–1
Paradigms in Psychology

Mechanistic	Organismic
Human reacts and responds to the environment	Human acts upon and creates the meaning of an experience
Predictable response sets from humans can be determined	Understanding from individual human perspective—variable responses
Static reality—can be held constant	Dynamic reality—always changing
Control	Fluidity
Behavior—can be prescribed	Behavior—many possibilities

Piaget (1970) would predicate. One lays before us a thesis; the other, an antithesis.

The reader is asked to contemplate the differences in meaning as expressed in the descriptive language of the mechanistic and the organismic paradigms of psychology (Table 1-1).

Are the perspectives unbridgeable? With these paradigms, as well as the ones that follow, discussion about the bridgeability of these perspectives should prove lively and fruitful.

Paradigms in Philosophy. Filstead (1979, p. 34) stated that at the core of the distinction between the quantitative and qualitative methods of research lies the classical argument in philosophy between the schools of realism and idealism and their subsequent derivatives (Table 1-2). The Baconian reality of "seeing is believing" led to believing in the "real" as the only reality one could be

Table 1–2
Paradigms in Philosophy

Realism	Idealism
Static conception of world	Evolving conception of world
Seeing is believing	There is more than what meets the eye
Logical positivism	Dynamic
Social world as given	Social world as created
Independent physical reality	Reality is mentally perceived—sense perception

positive about. Hence, those who ascribed to that belief system were called "positivist." When reality could be held static, observations made, and experiments performed, science was done and the truth revealed. Those philosophers who questioned this positivist logic and method of science when it was applied to the understanding of human beings became known as "idealists" (Kneller, 1964).

Although the idealists acknowledged the existence of a physical reality, they argued that the mind was the creator and source of knowledge. In addition to the language expressed in Table 1-2 from the idealist school, the following short Zen parable is indicative of idealists' ideas and the place of human perception (Zen Buddhism, 1959):

> *One windy day two monks were arguing about the flapping banner. The first said, "I say the banner is moving, not the wind." The second said, "I say the wind is moving, not the banner." A third monk passed by and said, "The wind is not moving. The banner is not moving. Your minds are moving." (p. 52)*

Though briefly presented, inherent here is the great debate between the objective and subjective means of knowing. We are about to see now how research methods as worldviews are an inherent outgrowth of a philosophical worldview that precedes it and establishes its epistemological ways of coming to know about the world.

Subsequent Paradigms in Epistemology. Flowing from the paradigms of philosophy should be congruent paradigms or research traditions for the way in which each school of thought establishes how it comes to know about its particular account of the world. Epistemology is the branch of philosophy that concerns itself with the nature of knowledge. Each school of philosophy will have an epistemology. In other words, each belief system will have a congruent belief system about *coming to know* about the world and the nature of knowledge.

For our purposes, the realist philosophy is connected with the epistemological paradigm of the received view and the idealist is connected with the nonreceived view (Table 1-3). We must

Table 1–3
Paradigms in Epistemology

Received View	Nonreceived View
Logical positivism	Uncertainty
Materialism	Mental perception
Reductionism	Holism
Laws—quantification	Patterns—qualification
Predictions	Interpretations
Objectivity	Subjectivity
Neutrality	Human values
Operationalization	Context integration

acknowledge at this point or perhaps call attention to this very simplified version of what is most complex to philosophers. We are examining the gist of language differences, yet we strongly recommend further study in this area for those who are interested in greater in-depth knowledge. (Chapter 2 provides a further base to this aspect of the discussion.)

The expressions of the received view are those of the positivists and/or realists (Suppe, 1977; Watson, 1981). They are consistent with the scientific method[3] and are representative of expressions found most often in our present nursing research texts. The nonreceived view of coming to know about nursing phenomena is emerging, and those expressions are found in the language of qualitative epistemology as well as most nursing philosophies.

Paradigms in Education. The mechanistic and organismic paradigms are reflected in the field of education as behaviorism and humanism (Table 1–4). Learning theories emerging from these two paradigms are distinctively different, because they are reflective of differing beliefs, values, and assumptions about the world and the nature of human beings. The reader may find it interesting here to reflect on which paradigm is more prevalent in nursing education and discuss the relative merits of each and, again, the bridgeability or points of contact (Munhall, 1992a).

---

[3] As we have defined it in a traditional sense. All the methods presented in this text are considered scientific methods of research.

Table 1–4
Paradigms in Education

Behaviorism	Humanism
Homogeneous group	Heterogeneous group
Human reactiveness	Human activeness
Human malleability	Self-determination
Human passiveness	Unique interpretation of reality
Human objectivity	Subjectivity
Shaping concrete behavior	Changes in consciousness
Measurable outcomes	Hoped-for outcomes—variable
Preparation for specific roles	Preparation for world-at-large

Paradigms in the Health Professions. Table 1-5 seems to reflect nursing's congruity with the preceding paradigms of the organismic, the idealists, the nonreceived view, and humanism. In contrast, the language of medicine seems to have the same congruity with the mechanistic, the realists, the received view, and behaviorism. It seems important to note, then, that our language system is congruent with some paradigms and not logically consistent with other paradigms. This is particularly relevant when we acknowledge that each paradigm should have a compatible research paradigm or method. The relevance is demonstrated in the philosophical paradigms of the realistic and idealistic and

Table 1–5
Paradigms in Health Professions

Medicine	Nursing
Reductionism—treating the part	Holism—coming to the whole
Reactive human	Active human
Physical symptomatology	Integrated human
Linear causality	Multiple interaction
Closed system	Open system
Steady state	Dynamic
Objective	Subjective
Manipulation	Self-determination
Control	Choice
Paternalism	Advocacy

in the concomitant epistemological paradigms of the received view and nonreceived view, respectively. The languages of the medical model and most nursing models are readily distinguishable as to their perspectives, worldviews, tradition, or paradigms.

We believe it is important to return here to our first consideration: "Research in nursing evolved predominantly when nursing was in transition between broad philosophic worldviews."

The language represented in Table 1-5 as the language of medicine was for a long time that of nursing. When the worldview for nursing began changing, as reflected in proposed nursing models, the activity of nursing research concomitantly was underway. Ironically, the research activities that occurred in a parallel fashion often were not congruent with the premises of the nursing model. However, this is quite understandable when we review the second consideration in our language development: "Researchers in nursing were (are) being prepared in fields other than nursing."

Early Preparation of Nurse Researchers

Doctoral preparation in nursing is a relatively new occurrence. Doctoral preparation in disciplines other than nursing was pursued by nurses initially and preceded the development of doctoral-level education in nursing. Because this is the way our doctoral education evolved, we will proceed to examine its influence rather than discuss the merits and limitations of such evolution.

The outcome was the development of a community of nurse researchers who were educated in the better established disciplines and who subsequently developed a commitment to that discipline's research method (Chinn, 1983). Although this offered nursing a wide array of methods to choose from, it soon appeared evident that the scientific method, with its own language, was adopted to such an extent that, according to Watson (1981), "The scientific method is considered the one and only process for scientific discovery, experimental quantitative research methodology and design" (p. 414). Swanson and Chenitz (1982) stated: "While nursing exists almost exclusively in the empirical social world, the profession uses the laboratory method of the basic sciences in its research design" (p. 241).

Norris (1982) attributed this supremacy of the scientific method in part to nursing's "desperate attempt" to become a legitimate science by embracing the experimental research model as the way to proceed. Indeed, "science" and "scientific" cannot be considered neutral words (if there are such words!). In today's world, they are extensively value laden as expressing truth, goodness, worthwhileness, and legitimacy. Kaplan (1964) emphasized this legitimacy point:

> *There are behavioral scientists who in their desperate search for* scientific status, *give the impression that they don't much care what they do if only they do it right: substance gives way to form. (p. 406)*

However, as Norris (1982) pointed out in a discussion of nursing's leap to experimental research, many nurse researchers are hampered by the lack of concept clarification, theory development, and descriptive methods of research, all of which are linked to qualitative research methods. Norris (1982) observed that, during the period from 1958 to 1975, nursing scholars made a concerted effort to develop a body of nursing knowledge without the necessary training in the methods of concept clarification, which are prerequisite to experimental research.

This "scientific" influence continues to exercise its exclusivity, as is evidenced in the following scenario (Tinkle & Beaton, 1983):

> *It was her first dissertation committee meeting. The topic of discussion was the proposed research methodology. Two of the committee members (well-known for their "hard" research) began to dialogue about the "softness" of the approach in the proposal before them—the lack of control, the lack of quantitative measurement, and the lack of manipulation of variables. Before long, the committee was in accord about the relatively low scientific merit of this type of research methodology as opposed to an experimental approach. The student found herself agreeing to shift her methodology to one involving experimental manipulation. (p. 27)*

Downs (1982), in response to a similar theme, observed: "This distorted value system rode in on the coattails of the idea that scientific method was equivalent to experimental research" (p. 4).

Bronowski (1965), with a broader conception of science, surpassed this narrow view of the scientific method and enlarged the aperture. Science, he said, is:

Nothing else than the search to discover unity in the world variety of nature or . . . in the variety of our experiences. Poetry, painting, the arts are the same search.

And yet, decades later, in a cogent argument for a poststructural perspective, Dzurec (1989) commented on the tenacity of logical positivist methodology in nursing:

The period beginning in the 1960's and stretching to today is perhaps the first in which the power relations in nursing and in human sciences in general, have allowed the recognition of logical positivism as a single philosophy of science rather than as science itself. (p. 74)

We now know that our worldview has opened to allow for other methods of research. Coming to know and coming to discover rather than verify have become acknowledged as essential to the base of nursing knowledge.

Watson (1981) attributed this increased acknowledgment to the same processes of scientific development that have taken place in other sciences. She stated that our commonality with other fields lies in the process of first adopting the received view idea and then undergoing processes of rejection of that particular paradigm. We would not advocate the abandonment of all the characteristics of the received view or the scientific method, but two important points need to be made about the early preparation of nurse researchers (and, to a large extent, the present preparation of nurse researchers). These points will lead us into the next contextual consideration. They are:

1. Nurse researchers predominantly use the scientific method of inquiry and that language system.

2. The scientific method is used in nursing prior to the description and understanding of the phenomenon within the nurse-client context. In other words, we take leaps to a step without the necessary conditions for that step. Most often, we take those leaps within the context of deduction and derivation from theories from other disciplines.

A third possible point here is that some of nursing research is research done by nurses but not research in nursing.

Deduction and Derivation from Theories

Walker and Avant (1983, p. 163) defined theory derivation as "the process of using analogy to obtain explanations or predictions in another field." These authors make a good distinction between theory derivation and borrowing theory (p. 163), but, for our purpose here, we are speaking about a process in which the description and explanations of phenomena for the development of nursing theory were evolved from a discipline or field of knowledge other than nursing. Therefore, the language originates from a world other than the nurse-patient world. Nursing researchers identifying similarities from other fields believe a specific theory to be appropriate to a nursing or a patient situation and proceed to generate deductions and/or hypotheses from that theory. It is asserted that this theory derivation is useful when there are no available data or when the phenomenon is poorly understood (Walker & Avant, 1983). Thus, we have more than 25 years of nursing research and a collection of many based on theoretical frameworks that did not originate within a nursing or patient context.

It is not our intent here to debate the relative merits (or lack thereof) of this practice, although we will mention a few. Instead, we suggest other methods when approaching a situation where theory does not as yet exist and where the phenomenon under study has not yet been described, explained, or understood. That is, of course, what this book is all about in the main!

One point that we feel compelled to make at this juncture is that many borrowed and derived theories in nursing are based first on the natural and behavioral sciences and, with that, a mechanistic paradigm. Subsequently, the hypothesis deduced from such theories originated from how physical matter behaves, how people respond to forced choice questions, and, probably all too often, how college students respond to questionnaires and various experiments.

It amazes us that simple perusal of psychology texts reveals that one experiment after another, leading to the development of theory, has been performed on college students. In these many instances, theories evolved from a very specific age sample and then were generated to the population at large. The very specific sample has been for researchers of human behavior a real convenience sample, that is, their 19-year-old sophomore students.

Another potential problem with theory derivation and language development from other fields is the male bias inherent in many of our developmental theories (Belenky, Clinchy, Goldberg, & Taub, 1986; Chinn, 1985; Gilligan, 1978). Pinch (1981) proposed that we should critically examine theories of development generated by Freud, Piaget, Erickson, and Kohlberg to recognize how we have accepted worldviews as developed and evolved from a male perspective. When we apply a hypothesis derived from such theory to individuals who may be ill—whether the derivation is from a male perspective, a college student's perspective, a well person's perspective, and so on—we will always have problems of authenticity, validity, and, most important, contextual meaning.

Our wish and certainly part of our goal is that, at some point, examination of nursing textbooks would reveal that our research and subsequent theory development were derived from the thorough description and analysis of nursing phenomena derived from the original source: nurses' and clients' lived experiences in client situations.

In our history of knowledge development, Dickoff and James (1968) proposed a schema of four levels of theory (factor-isolating theories, factor-relating theories, situation-relating theories, and situation-producing theories), which dominated the development of nursing theory. We now need to evaluate how well we have proceeded with each of the four levels of theory. Often, when borrowing or deriving from theories from other fields, we proceed directly to situation-producing theories, sacrificing meaning and true significance to expedience. Dickoff and James (1968) cited this lack of attention to the beginning levels of theory development as being detrimental to the development of nursing theory. Wald and Leonard (1964) suggested that nurses develop their own concepts for nursing theory from inductive analysis of nursing experience rather than from deductive analysis from others' experiences. Perusal of many of the nursing research articles published today still indicates dependence on deducting hypotheses from unrelated contexts or populations.

Diers (1979), in a context correlative to the work of Dickoff and James, provided us with another classification of levels of theory (Table 1-6). Germain (see Chapter 8 of this volume) demonstrates how the qualitative method of ethnography fits into the factor-searching level of inquiry proposed by Diers (1979, p. 54) and shown in Table 1-6.

Table 1–6
Levels of Inquiry and Study Design

Level of Inquiry	Kind of Question	Study Design	Kind of Answer (Theory)	Study Design
1	What is this?	Factor-searching	Factor-isolating (naming)	Exploratory Formulative Descriptive Situational control
2	What's happening here?	Relation-searching	Factor-relating (situation-depicting, situation-describing)	Exploratory Descriptive
3	What will happen if . . . ?	Association-testing	Situation-relating (predictive)	Correlational Survey design Nonexperimental Natural experiment Experimental Explanatory Predictive
4	How can I make . . . happen?	Prescription-testing	Situation-producing (prescriptive)	

From *Research in Nursing Practice*, (p. 54) by D. Diers. Philadelphia: Lippincott, 1979.

Indeed, all the qualitative methods of research presented herein seem essential to the beginning steps of theory development.

In the first and second levels of inquiry, the questions "What is this?" and "What's happening here?" are answered within our own nurse–client context. With qualitative research methods, theory is not derived, borrowed, or modified from other fields but rather springs from observation of and participation in an actual phenomenon. Norris (1982) believed that the phenomena with which nurses have the social prerogative and mandate to manage concern human health, illness, and comfort. Newman (1983) identified additional patient-nursing phenomena, such as reciprocities, patterns, configurations, rhythms, and composition, and emphasized context dependency.

The Social Policy Statement of the American Nurses' Association (1980) specified that the phenomena of concern to nurses are human responses to actual or potential health problems. All are phenomena researchable through qualitative methods and in the end may well stimulate the development of combined methods of research. The paradigmatic transition of which we believe we are presently a part may very well herald a new research paradigm for nursing, leaving behind the old dichotomies as historical curiosities.

A TRANSITION: NURSING WORLDVIEWS, NURSING RESEARCHERS, AND THEORY DEVELOPMENT

The purpose of this chapter is to explore nursing's coinages (language), its posture in the world, and how we choose to express ourselves. The foregoing discussion is our attempt to place in context our present posture in nursing research and to suggest the origin and evolution of how we have come to express ourselves and the language we use to bring nursing phenomena into being. We suggest that this volume on qualitative research methods is a natural outgrowth of this context. It is contemporary, evolutionary, and congruent with paradigmatic shifts. Expanding research horizons, acquiring new languages, and bringing phenomena into view represent a reconstructing process.

Transitions in worldviews or paradigms are a gradual process wherein beliefs, values, and practices of the old and the new overlap (Kuhn, 1970). This is a time when there may be conflict, incongruity, and confusion. It is, though, a wonderful time for self-reflection, self-consciousness, and clarification. Thesis, antithesis, and paradigmatic shifting are all parts of scientific revolutions or, in Laudan's (1977) terminology, the evolution of research traditions. They are the history and essence of science.

Returning now to the three identified factors that seem to influence most the context of nursing research, let us consider them from the perspective of Kuhn's language in an application to nursing research. Kuhn (1970) observed:

During the transition period [of worldviews] there will be a large but never complete overlap between the problems that can be solved by the old and by the new paradigm. But there will also be a decisive difference in the modes of solution. When the transition is complete, the profession will have changed its view of the field, its methods and goals. (p. 84)

Chapter 2 discusses epistemology in nursing and the qualitative and quantitative methods of knowing, but let us see here the role of transition.

Nursing Worldviews

Nursing has attempted to abandon the language of the medical model, and concomitantly, to reject the mechanistic paradigm the language expressed. Ironically, but to a lesser extent, medicine itself appears to be in transition from its own medical model to one that seems more aligned with some of the beliefs we have most recently been espousing. There is within that field an emerging language that focuses on holism, psychosomatic phenomena, and ecology.

Even though nursing has changed its verbal language, it often continues to retain the philosophical foundations of the medical model for research and to express its significance and importance in the symbols and practices that traditionally belong to medicine. We hope that readers will discuss some of these nonverbal symbolic forms of language that nursing continues to use and even seeks to acquire from the perspective of paradigmatic transition (Roberts, 1973).

In view of Kuhn's suggestion (1970, p. 84) that when "the transition is complete, the profession will have changed . . . its methods . . . ," we repeat a question raised in an article by Munhall (1982):

> *Could it be that when nursing abandoned the medical model and the language of that discipline, it retained the research paradigm that perpetuated what nursing was seeking to dissociate from? (p. 68)*

Because transitions are gradual and because of the aforementioned contextual variables, we are inclined to view this as characteristic of a trajectory of transition in worldviews. Things do not change at once; Kuhn's (1970) words were: "When the transition is *complete*, the profession will have changed . . . *its methods* . . ." (our italics). Our transition is apparently not complete. However, many nurse researchers are catalyzing the progress and process of this transition.

Nurse Researchers

Many of our nurse researchers, identified earlier as being socialized into the scientific method, are emerging strongly from their orientation (often meaning experimental research) and are contributing now to the logical shift in research paradigms that would be congruent with the shift in the larger philosophical worldview and new perspective of viewing phenomena. What seems to have occurred is that questions and problems of the profession with its new and unique nursing perspective (e.g., holism versus reductionism) cannot be answered or solved by the old methods, at least not at first.

Laudan (1977) reassured us with the following observation:

But there are times when two or more research traditions, far from mutually undermining one another, can be amalgamated, producing a synthesis which is progressive with respect to both the former research traditions. (p. 103)

As of this writing, this is an accurate description of the transition in nursing research. We have moved from what Norris (1982, p. 6) identified as "the occasional nurse who used the podium or the literature to support a descriptive route to knowledge [as] a 'voice crying in the wilderness'" to regular publication of the merits of qualitative research, the need for qualitative methods, research programs highlighting qualitative research, and, in general, the recognition of the advantages of a broadened repertoire of research methods.

We are examining not only the syntactical parallelism but also the contextual congruency of our larger philosophical paradigm with our most prevalent research method. The language we use in the expression of the two demonstrates for us the emergence of the new worldview and the residual of the old worldview.

The expressions in Table 1-7 are provided to demonstrate the transitional nature of our worldviews and research paradigms (Munhall, 1982, p. 177).

Table 1-7 illustrates the expressions of competing paradigms and Kuhn's overlap as we examine the contextual parallelism for logical syntax. This overlap has stimulated for many nurse researchers the proliferation of competing views, debates about methods, and discontent over the impact of nursing research on practice. Kuhn (1970) believed such debates are symptomatic of a "transition from normal to extraordinary research," but it is our hope that we will not become bogged down with long-winded debates of an either/or nature.

Although we offered initially the advantage to dichotomizing paradigms for the sake of conceptual clarity, we wish to build

Table 1–7
Expressions in Worldviews and Research Paradigms

Expressions of Contemporary Nursing Philosophy

Humanism	Uniqueness
Individualism	Relativism
Self-determinism	Autonomy
Active organism	Advocacy
Open system	Organismic
Holism	

Expressions of the Scientific Method

Reductionism	Theory for the average
Objectivity–positivism	Categorization
Delimited problems	Prediction
Reality reduced to the measurable	Control
Human and environmental passivity	Mechanistic
Manipulation	

Conceptual Parallelism

Nursing Philosophy	Nursing Research
Individualism	Commonalities
Uniqueness	Generalizations
Relativism	Categorization
Open system	Closed system
Holism	Reductionism
Individual interpretation	Statistical analysis
Active organism	Reactive organism
Organismic	Mechanistic
Self-determination	Control

From "Nursing Philosophy and Nursing Research: In Apposition or Opposition?" by P. Munhall, May–June 1982. *Nursing Research, 31* (3), p. 177.

bridges rather than erect walls. The bridge may well represent a transcendence of the two competing worldviews with the emergence of a research paradigm that either synthesizes the two views or goes beyond them. The bridge too, we would hope, would enrich and empower our concerted efforts for theory development.

Theory Development

The transition from one paradigm to another paradigm or to the inclusion of another paradigm will be reflected, as we have suggested, in our language and expressions. We mentioned previously the borrowed theoretical frameworks that are used so prevalently in nursing research. We borrow freely from physics, biology, physiology, psychology, and sociology. This practice often leads to the exclusion of nursing language and, in this context, the discovery of unique knowledge for nursing. While acknowledging disciplinary overlap, we believe it is essential for each discipline to develop its own essence, its own substance, its own reason for being, and its own meaning.

Paterson (1978) generated a list of nursing phenomena (Table 1-8) selected by practicing nurses as essential to nursing. We would ask the reader to compare these expressions with the expressions found in many of our contemporary research titles.

Table 1–8
The Quintessence of Nursing

Acceptance	Give and take
Authenticity	Laughing–crying
Awareness	Loneliness
Becoming	Openness
Caring	Patience
Charge	Readiness
Choice	Response
Commitment	Responsibility
Confirmation	Self-recognition
Confrontation	Sustaining
Dedication	Touching
Dying and death	Trust
Food—its meaning	Understanding
Freedom	Waiting
Frustration	

From "The Tortuous Way Toward Nursing Theory," in *Theory Development: What, Why and How?* (p. 65) by J. Paterson, 1978. New York: National League for Nursing.

Read, think about, and respond to these words as perhaps the quintessence of nursing. Could any of us argue that they do not constitute nursing phenomena?[4] Would we not want them to? In an answer to those who wonder why there is not adequate description of such experience in nursing literature, we believe the answer lies in the arguments for qualitative research. We eagerly anticipate the extraordinary research that Kuhn promises as the outcome of scientific revolutions.

LANGUAGE AND COMPREHENSIBILITY

The existential–ontological foundation of languages is discourse or talk. Heidegger (1962, p. 203)

Discourse is existentially language, because that entity whose disclosedness it articulates according to significations, has, as its kind of being, being-in-the-world and being which has been thrown and submitted to the world. Heidegger (1962, p. 204)

And where does a nurse researcher thrown and submitted to the world learn to speak? In the pedagogical world of research, a new language is learned. We noted earlier that this language is sometimes chosen freely, sometimes encouraged in one or another direction, and sometimes "raised" to such high levels of abstraction it becomes incomprehensible. From a qualitative perspective, language and the ability to express oneself to others is the only way we can bring experience into a form that creates in discourse a conversational relation (Van Manen, 1990).

Before bringing this chapter to a close, it seems essential to mention an obvious inherent component of language: listening. Discourse and conversing include keeping silent and hearing. The openness that is required for new ideas to penetrate into a belief system requires silence and hearing.

The language of human science or phenomenology may at first sound strange to individuals who are steeped in a natural science

---

[4] Additional phenomena are discussed in Chapter 2.

Table 1–9
Expressions of Qualitative Research Methods

Subjective experience	Closeness to the data
Intuition	Process-orientation
Variability	Dynamic reality
Communication	Open system
Individual perceptions	Time and space considerations
Shared language	Patterns
Interrelatedness	Configurations
Lived experience	Context-dependence
Holism	Complementarity
Naturalism	Human development
Nonmanipulated observation	

language. Paterson and Zderad's (1978) first attempts to introduce this language into nursing were often met with firm preconceptions and assumptions about being-in-the-world that were dramatically different. Now, in 1993, this reprinted second edition lays the groundwork in many curricula to assist students in the language of understanding the meaning of both being human and nursing.

At the same time, it is important to note that not all of nursing education, research, and/or practice areas are familiar with the meaning of the languages associated with qualitative research. Qualitative nurse researchers must take care to be comprehensible. This is further elaborated in Chapters 15 and 16 and in Munhall (1992b).

SUMMARY

The intent of this chapter can be summarized by borrowing Paterson's (1978) words:

For responsible, effective existence the professional requires language *[emphasis added] to relate authentically the purposes, beliefs, concerns, and events experienced continually in the nursing world. (p. 51)*

The noumenal exists in those phenomena listed by practicing nurses, but each seems to be a thing in itself—something waiting for description to bring it into our everyday awareness and to give it significance.

It is as though we need to assert these events as nursing's, articulate our authentic experience with patients, claim what we believe is paramount to health (i.e., good nursing), and conceptualize what is uniquely the abstract and the concrete, the enduring and the relevant meanings of shared human experience between patient and nurse.

We believe that qualitative research methods have much to offer as a research paradigm that is congruent with nursing's larger worldview, paradigm, or model. We close this chapter with Table 1-9, an illustration of the language of the qualitative research methods, and leave our readers to draw their own conclusions.

REFERENCES

American Heritage Dictionary. (1969). New York: American Heritage Publishing Co.

American Nurses' Association. (1980). *Nursing: A social policy statement.* Kansas City: American Nurses' Association.

Belenky, M., Clinchy, B., Goldberg, N., & Taub, J. (1986). *Women's ways of knowing. The development of self, voice and mind.* New York: Basic Books.

Bronowski, J. (1965). *Science and human values* (rev. ed.). New York: Harper & Row.

Chinn, P. (1983). Editorial. *Advances in Nursing Science, 5*(2), ix.

Chinn, P. (1985). Debunking myths in nursing theory and research. *Image: The Journal of Nursing Scholarship, 17*(2), 45-49.

DeVries, P. (1983). *Slouching towards Kalamazoo.* Boston: Little, Brown.

Dickoff, J., & James, P. (1968). A theory of theories: A position paper. *Nursing Research, 17,* 197-203.

Diers, D. (1979). *Research in nursing practice.* Philadelphia: Lippincott.

Dilthey, W. (1926). *Meaning in history.* London: Allen & Unwin. [Cited in G. Atwood & R. Stolorow (1984). *Structures of subjectivity: Explorations in psychoanalytic phenomenology.* Hillsdale, NJ: Analytic Press.]

Downs, F. (1982). It's a great idea but it won't work. *Nursing Research, 31*(1), 4.

Dzurec, L. (1989). The necessity for and evolution of multiple paradigms for nursing research: A poststructuralist perspective. *Advances in Nursing Science, 11*(4), 69-77.

Filstead, W. (1979). Qualitative methods: A needed perspective in evaluation research. In C. Reichardt & T. Cook (Eds.), *Qualitative and quantitative methods in evaluation research.* Beverly Hills, CA: Sage.

Gilligan, C. (1978). In a different voice: Women's conception of self and of morality. *Harvard Education Review, 47,* 481-517.

Heidegger, M. (1962). *Being and time* (J. Macprairie & E. Robinson, Trans.). New York: Harper & Row.

Kaplan, A. (1964). *The conduct of inquiry.* Scranton, PA: Chandler.

Kirby, D. (1983). Seeing the points of contact in a plural world. *The Chronicle of Higher Education, 26*(7), 25.

Kneller, G. (1964). *Introduction to the philosophy of education.* New York: Wiley.

Kuhn, T. S. (Ed.). (1970). *The structure of scientific revolutions.* Chicago: University of Chicago Press.

Laudan, L. (1977). *Progress and its problems: Toward a theory of scientific growth.* Berkeley: University of California Press.

Light, R., & Pillemer, D. (1982). Numbers and narrative: Combining their strengths in research reviews. *Harvard Education Review, 51*(1), 1-23.

Looft, W. (1973). *Socialization and personality throughout the life span: An examination of contemporary psychological approaches.* In P. Baltes & K. Schaie (Eds.), *Life-span development psychology.* New York: Academic Press.

Meshler, E. (1979). Meaning in context: Is there any other kind? *Harvard Education Review, 49*(1), 1-19.

Moccia, P. (1988). A critique of compromise: Beyond the methods debate. *Advances in Nursing Science, 10*(4), 1-9.

Morgan, G. (1983). *Beyond method* (pp. 377-382). Newbury Park, CA: Sage.

Munhall, P. (1982a). Ethical juxtaposition in nursing research. *Topics in Clinical Nursing, 4*(1), 66-73.

Munhall, P. (1982b). Nursing philosophy and nursing research: In apposition or opposition? *Nursing Research, 31*(3), 176-177, 181.

Munhall, P. (1989). Philosophical pondering on qualitative research. *Nursing Science Quarterly, 2*(1), 20-28.

Munhall, P. (1992a). A new age ism: Beyond a toxic apple. *Nursing and Health Care, 13*(7), 370–375.

Munhall, P. (1992b). Holding the Mississippi River in place and other implications for qualitative research. *Nursing Outlook, 10*(6), 257–262.

Newman, M. A. (1983). Editorial. *Advances in Nursing Science, 5*(2), x–xi.

Norris, C. (1982). *Concept clarification in nursing.* Rockville, MD: Aspen.

Paterson, J. (1978). The tortuous way toward nursing theory. In *Theory development: What, why and how?* New York: National League for Nursing.

Paterson, J. A., & Zderad, L. J. (1988). *Humanistic nursing.* New York: National League for Nursing.

Patton, M. Q. (1978). *Utilization focused evaluation.* Beverly Hills, CA: Sage.

Piaget, J. (1970). *Structuralism.* New York: Basic Books.

Pinch, W. (1981). Feminine attributes in a masculine world. *Nursing Outlook, 12,* 29–36.

Reichardt, C., & Cook, T. (Eds.). (1979). *Qualitative and quantitative methods in evaluation research.* Beverly Hills, CA: Sage.

Roberts, S. (1973). Oppressed group behavior: Implications for nursing. *Advances in Nursing Science, 5*(4), 21–30.

Skinner, B. (1953). *Science and human behavior.* New York: Appleton-Century-Crofts.

Snow, C. P. (1959). *The two cultures and the scientific revolution.* Cambridge, England: Cambridge University Press.

Suppe, F. (Ed.). (1977). *The structure of scientific theories* (2nd ed.). Champaign: University of Illinois Press.

Swanson, J., & Chenitz, C. (1982). Why qualitative research in nursing? *Nursing Outlook, 30*(4), 241–245.

Tinkle, M., & Beaton, J. (1983). Toward a new view of science: Implications for nursing research. *Advances in Nursing Science, 5*(2), 27–36.

Van Manen, M. (1990). *Research lived experience: Human science for an action sensitive pedagogy.* New York: SUNY Press.

Wald, F., & Leonard, R. (1964). Towards development of nursing practice theory. *Nursing Research, 13,* 4–9.

Walker, L., & Avant, K. (1983). *Strategies for theory construction in nursing.* Norwalk, CT: Appleton-Century-Crofts.

Watson, J. (1981). Nursing's scientific quest. *Nursing Outlook, 29*(7), 413–416.

West, M. (1983). *The world is made of glass.* New York: Morrow.
Zen Buddhism. (1959). Mount Vernon, NY: Peter Pauper Press.

ADDITIONAL REFERENCES

Allen, D., Benner, P., and Diekelmann, N. (1985). Three paradigms for nursing research: Methodological implications (chap. 3) in P. Chinn (Eds.), *Nursing Research Methodology Issues and Implementation.* Rockville, MD: Aspen.

Baer, E. (1979). Philosophy provides the rationale for nursing's multiple research directions. *Image, 2*(3), 72-74.

Benoliel, J. (1984). Advancing nursing science: Qualitative approaches. *Western Journal of Nursing Research, 6*(3), 1-8.

Chenetz, W. C., & Swanson, J. M. (1986). *From practice to grounded theory: Qualitative research in nursing.* Menlo Park, CA: Addison Wesley.

Dossey, L. (1982). *Space, time and medicine.* Boulder, CO: Shambala.

Fawcett, J. (1983). Hallmarks of success in nursing theory development. In P. Chinn (Ed.), *Advances in Nursing Theory Development.* Rockville, MD: Aspen, Chap. 1.

Field, P., & Morse, J. (1985). *Nursing research: The application of qualitative approaches.* Rockville, MD: Aspen.

Gorenberg, B. (1983). The research tradition of nursing: An emerging issue. *Nursing Research, 32*(6), 347-349.

Johnson, J. (1991). Nursing science: Basic applied or practical implications for the art of nursing, *Nursing Research, 14*(1), 7-15.

Ludemann, R. (1979). The paradoxical nature of nursing research. *Image, 2*(1), 2-8.

Leininger, M. (1985). *Qualitative research methods in nursing.* New York: Grune & Stratton.

MacPherson, K. I. (1983). Feminists methods: A new paradigm for nursing research. *Advances in Nursing Science, 5,* 17-25.

Matson, F. (1964). *The broken image.* New York: George Brazillier.

Meleis, A. (1985). *Theoretical nursing: Development and progress.* Philadelphia: Lippincott.

Moccia, P. (Ed.) (1986). *New approaches in theory development.* New York: National League for Nursing.

Newman, M. A. (1979). *Theory development in nursing.* Philadelphia: Davis.

Newman, M. A. (1986). *Health as expanding consciousness.* St. Louis, MO: Mosby.

Oiler, C. (1982). The phenomenological approach in nursing research. *Nursing Research, 31*(3), 178-181.

Oiler, C. (1986). Qualitative methods: Phenomenology in P. Moccia (Ed.), *New approaches to theory development.* New York: National League for Nursing.

Omery, A. (1983). Phenomenology: A method for nursing research. *Advances in Nursing Science, 5*(2), 49-64.

Parse, R. R. (1985). *Nursing Research: Qualitative Methods.* Bowie, MD: Brady.

Reeder, J. (1987). The phenomenological movement. *Image, 19,* 150-152.

Sarter, B. (1988). Philosophical sources of nursing theory. *Nursing Science Quarterly, 1,* 52-59.

Silva, M. C. (1977). Philosophy, science, theory: Interrelationships and implications for nursing research. *Image, 9*(5), 59-63.

Watson, J. (1985). *Nursing: Human science and human care and theory of nursing.* Norwalk, CT: Appleton-Century-Crofts.

Epistemology in Nursing

Patricia L. Munhall

. . . since we have come to the understanding that science is not a description of "reality" but a metaphorical ordering of experiences, the new science does not impugn the old. It is not a question of which view is "true" in some ultimate sense. Rather, it is a matter of which picture is more useful in guiding human affairs.—Willis Harman

*W*e qualified in the preceding chapter that perhaps we might appear culpable of unnecessary polarization of worldviews but that we were indulging in such a practice for conceptual clarity and pedagogical purposes. Furthermore, we could not agree more with Gould (1984) when he observed:

Dichotomy is the usual pathway to vulgarization. We take a complex web of arguments and divide it into two polarized positions—them against us. We then portray "them" as a

foolish caricature of extremes in order to put "us" in a bet-
ter light. (p. 7)

However, complex webs are more stark when placed in contrasting systems; the differences between the systems become
more focused. Our intention is not to see one system as the truth
but to see each as different. As Harman (1977) stated, "It is not a
question of which view is true [but which] is more useful in guiding human affairs." This is our connectedness with the subject.

In this chapter, we propose an epistemology for nursing research that, as a whole, incorporates the qualitative and quantitative methods of research. This does not represent a conciliatory
effort at compromise but rather a belief in a cyclical continuum
that begins with discovery and moves toward verification. These
activities represent, respectively, the first- and second-order activities of science. We believe there are appropriate research methods
for different questions, and errors occur when a method is used
prematurely or contextually to answer a specific question or solve
a problem. As was suggested in Chapter 1, there are times when
both research traditions are amalgamated to produce a synthesis
that is progressive to both traditions (Laudan, 1977).

We will discuss paths to knowledge, the purpose of science, research paradigms, and research traditions. We will attempt to answer the questions "Knowing about what?" and "How do we get to
know?" and will then propose a qualitative–quantitative cyclical
continuum for knowing. Emphasis throughout is on qualitative research methods in response to a need identified by Johnson
(1978), who stated: "We are beginning at the wrong end . . .
engaging in experimental research before the variables significant
to that research have been determined" (p. 9). We see in the preceding quote the word "engaging." This chapter will further the
idea of research as engagement and, in so doing, will perhaps accomplish the goal stated by Morgan (1983):

To steer clear of the delusion that it is possible to know in an
absolute sense of "being right" and devote our energies to
the more constructive process of dealing with the implica-
tion of our different ways of knowing. (p. 18)

We also envision a poststructuralist perspective where the necessity for and evolution of multiple paradigms for nursing research will widen the operative of coming to know within the development of nursing knowledge (Dzurec, 1989).

This is the study of epistemology in nursing, that branch of philosophy that deals with knowledge and how we come to know about the world as we experience it.

PATHS TO KNOWLEDGE

Knowledge for nursing, about nursing, in nursing—where does this knowledge come from? In Chapter 1, we mentioned knowledge (theory) borrowed from related disciplines. Other disciplines are indeed one source of knowledge, perhaps more accurately stated from the perspective of Stevens's notion (1979, p. 85) of "shared knowledge": because disciplines have indistinct boundaries, there are areas "where the inquiries and answers of one field overlay those of another."

We noted this awareness in Chapter 1, where we cited the practice, among many nurse researchers, of identifying similarities from other disciplines and then utilizing those respective theoretical frameworks in order to derive hypotheses for nursing. We will return to this practice from the perspective of first- and second-order activities of science. However, let us acknowledge here that the first- and second-order activities are not from the same world or discipline and often will not be logically consistent or experientially valid. In other words, the first-order activities of coming to know or discovering come from another discipline and from that discipline's perspective. The second-order activities of validation and verification are then performed within the nursing discipline and from nursing's particular perspective. Before we go further, however, let us in a foundational manner discuss where knowledge generally comes from and some of the structures of knowing.

In a pedantic fashion, philosophers who study the way we come to know (epistemologists) have identified specific sources of knowledge, generally acceptable as structures of knowing. Among them are (Kneller, 1971):

1. Revealed knowledge: knowledge that God has disclosed. Revelations of truth are found in the Bible, the Koran, and the Bhagavad-Gita. We ponder why religion is not more prevalent in nursing research—for example, religion as a source of comfort and inspiration; belief as having curative power; and so on. We do know that from revealed knowledge comes the imperative to care for and about one another.

2. Intuitive knowledge: knowledge within a person, in the form of insight that becomes present in consciousness; an idea or thought produced by a long process of unconscious work. This process of discovery is nurtured through experience with the world.

3. Rational knowledge: knowledge from the exercise of reason. This knowledge takes the form of abstract reasoning and is exemplified in the principles of formal logic and mathematics.

4. Empirical knowledge: knowledge formed in accordance with observed or sensed facts and associated with scientific hypotheses that are tested by observation or experiments.

5. Authoritative knowledge: knowledge accepted in faith because it is vouched for by authorities in the field.

In the foregoing brief description of the sources of knowledge, the one least attended to, but the one holding much potential for nursing, is intuitive knowledge. The repudiation of intuition as a source of knowledge was one of the major themes when nursing moved toward establishing itself as a science. Intuition was unscientific; it was associated with women, who themselves were thought to be unscientific. More confident today, women of science—including nurses, of course—recognize the vitalness of intuition and have come to trust and value this important source of knowledge.

Belenky, Clinchy, Goldberg, and Taub (1986), in describing the different ways women come to know, have legitimized to a great extent the place of intuition, personal meanings, and the connection to ideas as means of knowing. Rather than focusing on "proof," these women scientists seek understanding. The work of Gilligan (1982), Belenky et al. (1986), and Freiri (1971) challenges us all to rethink our concepts about epistemology— the underlying assumptions and the critical consequences. Critical theory is one way to analyze the underlying structural and power relations inherent in the "sanctioned" ways of knowing (Allen, 1991).

Carper's (1978) framework of four fundamental patterns of knowing continues to be a way in which nursing identifies its epistemological interests. These patterns of knowing are described as follows:

1. Empirics: the science of nursing; emphasis is on the generation of theory and of research that is systematic and controllable by factual evidence. Within this pattern of knowing, there is a need for emphasis on knowledge about the empirical world, knowledge that will be organized into general laws and theories for the purpose of describing, explaining, and predicting phenomena of concern to nursing.

2. Esthetics: the art of nursing; emphasis is on expressiveness, subjective acquaintance, individual perceptions, and empathy. Rather than uniformity and general laws, there is a recognition of alternative modes of perceiving reality, which then clearly asks for a "many-different-ways" approach to designing and participating in nursing care.

3. Personal knowledge: the focus is on the importance of the interpersonal process and the "therapeutic use of self"; on knowing the self, knowing the other as a subject, and striving toward authentic personal relationships.

4. Ethics: the focus is on matters of obligation or what ought to be done. Knowledge within this domain requires understanding of ethical theories, conditions of society, conflicts between different value systems, and ethical principles.

All of the above are rich and essential sources of nursing knowledge that can be studied from various perspectives of science.

Munhall (1993) suggested a fifth pattern of knowing, while at the same time questioning the categorizing of knowledge in this way. The fifth pattern is one of "unknowing." "Knowing," in contrast to "unknowing," leads to a form of confidence that has the potential of a state of closure to alternatives and differences. "Unknowing," from an epistemological perspective, is a condition of openness and seems essential to the understanding of intersubjectivity and perspectivity. Kurtz (1989) stated:

> *[K]nowledge screens the sound the third ear hears, so we hear only what we know. (p. 6)*

We can become limited by our own belief systems. Often, once we believe something or think we "know" something, we cease further exploration or explanation.

Although the patterns of knowledge are presented as categories, we see them as mutually interdependent, not mutually exclusive. Intuiting in the empirical world while using one's personal knowledge embedded in an ethical context or founded on a philosophical perspective is a holistic approach to theory development.

We move now from general structures of knowing to the purpose of exploring those structures. Because nursing has identified itself as a science, let us review the purpose of science, or science in general. How does nursing conceptualize itself as a science?

PURPOSE OF SCIENCE

Laudan (1977), a philosopher, simply stated that the purpose of science is to solve problems, and theory tells us how! He further proposed that the rationality and progressiveness of a theory are not linked with its confirmation or its falsification but instead with its problem-solving effectiveness. This conception of science opens the windows and doors in the hallowed halls of science to include important nonempirical and even nonscientific knowing and provides a broader perspective that Laudan suggested was necessary to the "rational development" of science. Insight, spontaneity, accidental findings, mutability, vicissitude, and fortune all play a role in science.

Based on this conception of science and theory, it seems to us that all sources of knowledge and patterns of knowing are essential sources for problem solving. Nursing research, in its earliest years, began its quest to become a legitimate science with an almost unilateral pattern of knowing that can be categorized as empirics, logical empiricism, logical positivism, or, as described in most nursing research textbooks, "the scientific method."

Laudan (1977) set forth—in contrast or in explanation—a philosophy of science of historicism that incorporates the human elements of science; the study of scientific knowledge is often fostered by illogical and nonrational decision making. The two following quotes may illuminate this point:

> *That no major scientist ever has proceeded in his work along either Baconian or Catesian lines . . . has not prevented the* consecration of method *by these two powerful minds from exacting a dismal toll [our italics]. (Nesbitt, 1976, p. 14)*

> *Insight announces itself in mental images. Newton's conception of gravity and Einstein's notion of the constant speed of light came to them as perceptions, as images, not a hypothesis or conclusions drawn from logical deduction. Formal logic is secondary to insight via images, and is never the source of new knowledge. (Bohm, 1981, p. 444)*

Van Manen (1990), in contrast to Laudan's emphasis on problem solving, summarized what a phenomenological human science cannot do: "Phenomenology does not problem solve" (p. 23). Van Manen believed, from a research perspective, that phenomenological questions are "meaning" questions. However, one might wonder: If we did understand the meaning of specific phenomena, might we not have the basis for problem solving? Furthermore, might we also have understanding that could significantly contribute to the promotion of health and well-being? From his perspective, Van Manen stated:

> *[N]atural science studies objects of nature, "things," "natural events" and the way that objects behave. Human science, in contrast, studies "persons" or beings that have "consciousness" and that act purposefully in and on the*

*world by creating objects of "meaning" and that are expres-
sions of how human beings exist in the world. (p. 4)*

These ideas are not necessarily contradictory; rather, they seem
to be woven together as a whole. In addition, discussions about sciences and methods of science(s) often seem to lead us away from
concrete, lived experiences unless "that" lived experience is the
discussion of sciences. Researchers, we believe, need to be well-
grounded in the pedantics of the research enterprise but not at the
cost of creativity. We suggest to students that it is far more scientific to find a phenomenon that interests them, peaks their curiosity, and perhaps even fills them with passion, than to become
befuddled by method.[1] Substance should lead the way to form.

It is essential to understand the influence and power of research
paradigms and traditions in interweaving the ways of knowing and
shaping them into a body of knowledge. They can be restricting or
liberating, depending on their own ontology and supporting constituencies.

The critical nature embedded in research paradigms and traditions is found in the circumstance that they are rarely questioned
during the study of a discipline. It is a rare undergraduate or graduate student in any field who questions the research methods prevalent in that field. If most of us find guidelines helpful, and a
research tradition provides us with those guidelines—and if success within the field will be determined by how well one follows
those guidelines—the importance of those guidelines can hardly
be overstated! The next section describes the nature of research
paradigms and traditions connected with our discussion of paths to
knowledge and the purpose of science.

Paradigms and Research Traditions

Kuhn (1970) believed that a paradigm structures the questions to
be asked within a discipline and systematically eliminates those
kinds of questions that cannot be stated within the concepts and

---

[1] Van Manen's (1990) interpretation of why Gadamer's (1975) book *Truth
and Method* became popular in North America (p. 3) is relevant and recommended to readers.

tools supplied by the paradigm. This function then is enormously powerful. A paradigm can actually eliminate questions from being answered!

Laudan (1977), elaborating on his definition of a research tradition, wrote:

A research tradition is a set of general assumptions about the entities and processes in a domain of study, and about the appropriate methods to be used for investigating the problems and constructing the theories in that domain. (p. 81)

In both these ways, as suggested by Kuhn and by Laudan, the research paradigm and tradition will specify the domain of study, the legitimate modes, and the methods of inquiry open to a researcher within a discipline. This directedness is seldom questioned; in fact, complicity is usually required as well as rewarded.

Why one proceeds in this fashion is explained by Laudan's idea that we need to explore the scientists' work and their reasoning processes. Laudan suggested that scientific knowledge is often developed by illogical and nonrational decision making. Let us now tie together that idea with nursing's historical acceptance of the logical empiricist's worldview or, as stated, the large reliance on logic and empirics as our primary paths to theory development.[2]

We discussed in Chapter 1 the preparation of many nurse researchers in fields where the research tradition was one of logical empiricism. Let us look for evidence that supports the further use of this tradition and that may exemplify the nonrational or illogical side of science. This evidence is not always negative, but let us reflect on nursing research and on the subtle and not so subtle ways in which this paradigm or tradition has been perpetuated and still prevails today to a large extent.

The answers to the following questions, which were asked in the first edition of the book (1986), demonstrate how the values of

[2] Silva and Rothbart (1984) have written a most readable and highly recommended work synthesizing this material. Dzurec (1989), presenting a poststructural perspective, should also be considered.

scientists and their practices influence the general account of human nature. We believe it is quite significant that the same questions are relevant seven years later. Munhall (1992) attempted an explanation as to the reason for their relevance, in a discussion of life world fittingness:

1. If you were to request a research grant from the Division of Nursing of the Department of Health and Human Services or the Center for Nursing Research, what research method do you believe would be viewed most favorably?
2. If you wanted guidelines for doing research and consulted the most prevalent nursing research textbooks, which research method would seemingly be the only one available? What is the research method most taught in our research classes?
3. If you wish to submit an abstract of research for a research conference, what research method is represented in the format for the abstract?
4. If you wanted to critique a research study, what method is most represented under criteria for evaluation?

We believe that the purpose of nurse researchers who are questioning the general acceptance of the answers to those questions is to enlarge the lens, to broaden the scope, to widen the perspective. Furthermore, the answers to these questions demonstrate the subjectivity of the entire research enterprise. Humans determine which paths to explore. We need to explore all the paths to knowledge, all the patterns of knowing, because in some intuitive way we would then be celebrating the whole of the human condition.

Capra (1982) stated our need a decade ago:

What we need, then, is a new vision of reality: a fundamental change in our thoughts, perceptions and values. The beginnings of this change, of the shift from the mechanistic to the holistic conception of reality are already visible in all fields and are likely to dominate the entire decade. (p. ix)

Our endeavor here, built upon the works of many nursing scholars, among them the contributors to this volume, is to encourage this vision, to incorporate the qualitative and quantitative methods of research as representative of an epistemology of wholeness, to respect and reward all patterns of knowing. Let us move now to consideration of an epistemological question: "What is it we want to know about?"

EPISTEMOLOGICAL INTERESTS OF NURSING

As stated earlier, the purpose of science is to solve problems, and the subsequent theory development involves the solution of problems (Laudan, 1977). In this section, we explore schemata that have been developed by nurses in an effort to focus nursing research on nursing phenomena.

The schemata presented are not all-inclusive; rather, the purpose is to reflect on the extent to which these phenomena have been studied by nurse investigators at a descriptive, explanatory level from nursing's perspective and while using the essential qualitative tools of science. In Chapter 1, we cited Norris's belief (1982) that nurses should concern themselves with the phenomena of human health, illness, and comfort. We also cited Newman's (1983) direction to reciprocities, patterns, configurations, rhythms, composition, and context dependency as patient phenomena on which nurse researchers should focus.

In this section, five nursing perspectives are summarized in an effort to identify our epistemological interests. They are presented chronologically and may demonstrate consistency, overlap, complementarity, and/or much variation. Although they may sometimes seem to represent different perspectives and one can debate the merits or lack of merits of the various perspectives, each does answer the question "What do nurses study?" We will look at the ideas of Paterson and Zderad (1976), Donaldson and Crowley (1978), The American Nurses' Association's Social Policy Statement (1980), Fawcett's (1984) metaparadigm for nursing, and the emphasis on care (Newman, Sime, & Corcoran-Perry, 1991; Watson, 1985), in an effort to identify various nursing perspectives that will express the essence of the phenomena of concern to nurses and nurse investigators.

Paterson and Zderad (1976), to the question "What do nurses study?" (or "What should nurses study?"), might reply in this manner. Because the act of nursing is "the intersubjective transactional relation, a dialogue experience, lived in concert between persons where comfort and nurturance produce mutual human unfolding," nurses would do well to study the following situations (Paterson, 1978, p. 51):

1. Comfort—persons being all they can be in particular life situations.
2. Nurturance—promoting growth through relating.
3. Clinical—presence in the health situation, reflected and acted upon.
4. Empathy—imaginative moving toward oneness with another, sharing his or her being in a situation, resulting in an insightful knowledge of another's perspective.
5. All-at-once awareness of living many concepts, emotions, desires, and beliefs in a particular instance.

From these situations, the phenomenon of concern to nurses is one in need of quality nursing descriptions of those experiences inherent in the above situations and suggested in Table 1-7. Paterson and Zderad (1976) called our attention to existential, humanistic, phenomenological phenomena that should be our epistemological interests.

Widely cited, Donaldson and Crowley (1978) identified three major themes of nursing:

1. Concern with the principles and laws that govern the life processes, well-being, and optimum functioning of human beings, sick or well.
2. Concern with the patterning of human behavior in interaction with the environment in critical life situations.
3. Concern with the processes by which positive changes in health status are affected.

Concepts within the nurse-client world that relate to the above themes need to be discovered, and the methods of the first order of scientific activity, the qualitative methods of science, are essential to this process. Within this volume, an effort is made to demonstrate this basic activity of discovering what is there, naming it, understanding it, and explaining it. We can then give examples of what is meant and what is the potential within the scope of these themes.

The American Nurses' Association has consistently revised its definition of nursing according to society's needs and has focused nurse researchers' perspective on human responses within the following context: "Nursing is the diagnosis and treatment of human responses to actual or potential health problems" (1980, p. 9). Possible phenomena that bear investigation from this perspective of nursing are further suggested. They include:

1. Self-care limitations
2. Impaired functioning—physiological needs
3. Pain and discomfort
4. Emotional problems, such as anxiety, loss, loneliness, and grief
5. Distortion of symbolic functions
6. Deficiencies in decision making
7. Self-image changes
8. Dysfunctional perceptual orientations
9. Strains related to life processes
10. Problematic affiliative relationships

Readers familiar with the works of Rogers (1970), Roy (1976), Johnson (1980), Orem (1980), King (1981), Watson (1985), and other nursing theorists can readily see the influence of these theorists on the various phenomena that would constitute human responses.

Fawcett (1984) has identified a metaparadigm for nursing in pursuit of establishing boundaries within which the purview of nursing can be delineated. She has proposed that the metaparadigm comprises the central concepts and themes that represent the phenomena of interest to the discipline. Paradigms then are the conceptual models that provide "distinctive contexts for the metaparadigm concepts and themes" (p. 2).

The metaparadigm of nursing that has evolved, according to Fawcett (1984, p. 2), consists of four major concepts: person, environment, health, and nursing. These central concepts are defined as:

1. Person—the recipient of care.
2. Environment—significant others and the surroundings of the recipient of care; the setting in which nursing care occurs.
3. Health—the wellness or illness state of the recipient at the time when nursing occurs.
4. Nursing—actions taken by nurses on behalf of or in conjunction with the recipient of care.

Fawcett (1984) added the themes explicated by Donaldson and Crowley, presented earlier, to the metaparadigm of nursing by indicating the central concepts and the themes that should represent the phenomena of interest to nurse investigators. She then suggested that the four patterns of knowledge, as discussed by Carper (1978), link the concepts and themes.

With these varying perspectives have come articles that call for a focus of the discipline of nursing. Newman et al. (1991) pointed out that a discipline is distinguished by its domain of inquiry. As is readily apparent in the foregoing paragraph, nursing has a rather large domain of inquiry. Newman et al. suggested that nursing should have a focus statement. They pointed out that, from the time of Florence Nightingale to the present era of Leininger (1984), Watson (1988), and Benner and Wrubel (1989), health and caring have been linked. Incorporating Pender's (1982) use of the term "health experience," their focus statement is:

Nursing is the study of caring in the human health experience. (p. 3)

Nursing's domain of inquiry is then stated as "caring in the human health experience" (p. 3).

Perhaps we can enjoy the complexity of our profession because it affords us the opportunity to study and research an almost infinite variety of human and environmental phenomena. Some say we are "all over the place"; in actuality, nurses themselves are all over the place—in every developmental phase of an individual's life, in health and in crisis, in private practice, in schools, in hospitals, in foreign countries, and in the homes of patients. They are practitioners, educators, administrators, writers, researchers, and politicians.

We do not intend here to subscribe to one of the schemata but would rather stimulate reflection on the extent to which any of these phenomena have been studied on a descriptive level. However, to the question "What do nurses study?," we can identify the overlay from the five cited perspectives, add the ten or so conceptual models for nursing that are extant, and understand perhaps why there may be some confusion in the area of our epistemological interests.

If they need to be narrowed down to one broad aim that might encompass the intent of the foregoing discussion, our epistemological interests should be able to answer affirmatively the following question: "Does this research have potential to assist individuals and groups in achieving their freely chosen experience of health and being?"

EPISTEMOLOGICAL METHODS

In the foregoing discussion, we presented five perspectives or views of what nurses might investigate. Their broad scope reflects the expansiveness of the profession of nursing. Discussions among theorists and researchers often revolve around narrowing this scope, perhaps by adopting one model or accepting, for equally good reasons, a multiple-perspective approach. For our purposes here, we are gladly going to avoid written commitment on that issue and move instead to methods of investigation of nursing phenomena as presented. At the start of Chapter 1, we defined quantitative methods of research as:

The traditional scientific method as presented in most of the contemporary nursing research textbooks, characterized by deductive reasoning, objectivity, quasi-experiments, statistical techniques, and control.

In contrast, we defined the qualitative methods, many of which are described within this text, as "characterized by inductive reasoning, subjectivity, discovery, description, and process orienting" (Reichardt & Cook, 1979). We can view these two approaches from a historical perspective. During the seventeenth century, empiricism, as the scientific method, reigned supreme. That form of empiricism proceeds through sense knowledge, and that which connects with our senses is matter. This often is the origin of conceived objectivity, in which the physical world can be seen, touched, or measured. The hold that matter (materialism) has on us is connected with the simple fact that we think we can get hold of matter and control it. Thus, we have the controlled experiment with validation, significance, and the premise of confidence. As has been suggested, nursing research has, to a large extent, aligned itself with this positivistic and materialistic view of science.

With a giant leap, we come to a postpositivistic perspective articulated by Polkinghorne (1983), who cited recognition and acceptance of the following factors as enlarging the scope of science:

1. Different language systems reflect different perceptions of the same reality (as was illustrated in Chapter 1).
2. The essential study of complex wholes is through system theory, and human beings are complex wholes.
3. The ideas of purposive and intentional activity explain human action.
4. All knowledge, instead of being truth, is an expression of interpretation.

Such beliefs and assumptions have contributed to the acceptance of the worthiness and credibility of methods of knowing other than the positivistic worldview. Additionally, there was growing acceptance and recognition of the differences between the material and the experiential nature of human behavior and relationships. Benoliel (1984) cited some of these differences as follows:

1. *Social life is the shared creativity of individuals and their* perceptions *[emphasis added]*.

2. *The character of the social world is* dynamic *and* changing *[emphasis added]*.

3. *There are* multiple realities *and frameworks for viewing the world: the world is not independent of mankind and objectively identifiable [emphasis added]*.

4. *Human beings are active agents who* construct *their own realities [emphasis added]*.

5. *There are not any response sets that are highly predictable. (p. 4)*

To recount an orthodox point of view, there are those in science who believe that the quantitative (the traditional scientific method) and qualitative methods are philosophically unbridgeable in their paradigmatic worldviews. Benoliel (1984) stated that, rather than a continuum or a possible bridgeability:

> *Qualitative approaches in science are distinct modes of inquiry oriented toward understanding the unique nature of human thoughts, behaviors, negotiations and institutions under different sets of historical and environmental circumstances. (p. 7)*

Benoliel seems to take issue here with the fact that some nursing literature on qualitative research suggests that qualitative research is subsidiary to quantitative approaches.

We have taken this antecedent–sequence position not because we are able to substantiate the compatibility of the two worldviews but because the two worldviews both can be substantiated, not in truth per se but in understanding and problem solving according to the task at hand. Thus, for theory building in nursing, we see the need for the first-order activities of science, that is, the model building and discovery within our own patient–nurse context. These qualitative methods will help us to discover what is in that world, to name it, and to grasp at some meanings and understandings. These methods, as will be described and demonstrated within this text, will provide critical descriptive explorations and articulations of the events that are experienced continually in the nursing world. As in Diers's scheme (1979), we can answer such questions as "What is this?" or "What's happening here?" There may not be any other kind of question at the time, and surely there may not be an identified problem. Intuitively, one may believe there is a problem, but only research will lead to the identification of that problem and to further questions to be asked.

We believe that, in stating a problem at the outset of an investigation, one can often be led down the wrong path. An example serves as a rationale for the first-order activities of science (discovery; "What's happening here?") and qualitative methods of science.

A graduate student noted that the clientele of a certain nursing home appeared depressed. She validated her observation with a measurement scale. She then decided to see what effect remotivational therapy would have on this group of individuals. Within six treatment sessions, her sample was significantly less depressed, according to the scale. Thus, she tentatively concluded that remotivational therapy was effective. The student questioned her findings in light of a possible Hawthorne effect. Although an actual remotivational program was provided, inherent in the program were social interaction, attention, understanding, and caring. By reviewing her findings within the scope of an operationalized variable (remotivational therapy) instead of holistically, the student was limited in her perspective and should have examined, as she did afterward, an alternative perspective (Munhall, 1982).

It may very well be that individuals otherwise ignored or neglected will thrive if responded to, attended to, recognized, and brought together for social interaction. Using a naturalistic approach of dwelling in the environment (ethnography) and asking "What's going on here?," as Germain explains in Chapter 8, the researcher may find that the situation has little to do with lack of motivation on the part of the staff, limited visiting hours, limited staff, an absence of planned programs, and unspoken punitive sanctions for noise and expression. What happens then, when our nurse researcher leaves, if all those factors in the distance are left unaltered?

We start with qualitative methods, discovery: "What is going on in this environment?" What does it mean? What shall we call it? How shall we describe it and what can we do about it? Now that we know what sometimes goes on in a practice setting such as the one described by Zane Wolfe (Chapter 9), we come to understand the meaning of the vital content of nursing practices and procedures. If a staff is found to be unmotivated, "What can be done?" becomes the problem identified through an exploratory study. Table 2-1 illustrates some of the methods for the pursuit of this discovery.

By discovering what the experience and/or problems are from within the context, the researcher is able to form a hypothesis from a descriptive level of theory and can test to validate whether a hypothesis is supported (moving toward quantitative research), as illustrated in Table 2-1 and Figure 2-1.

We believe that we cannot overstate the importance of this first-level activity, for it is within this activity that we avoid what is referred to as a Type III error—solving the wrong problem (remotivating the wrong group of people!). Type III is called the "fallacy of misplaced precision"; the investigator obtains statistical significance versus epistemological relevance (Light & Pillemer, 1982). By going from first-level to second-level activities of science, we

Table 2–1
Epistemological Methods

Methods of Discovery
First Level of Activity of Science—Qualitative

    Phenomenology
    Grounded theory
    Ethnography
    History
    Analytic philosophy—foundational inquiry
    Case study

Methods of Validation
Second Level of Activity of Science—Quantitative

    Correlation
    Hypothesis testing
    Prescription testing

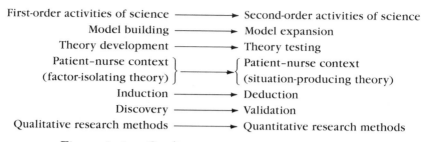

Figure 2–1.   Qualitative–quantitative continuum.

would be establishing a qualitative-quantitative continuum, which is illustrated in Figure 2-1.

Light and Pillemer (1982) proposed an alternative scheme. They believed that words and numbers are different languages; we have also presented that as the case. They suggested that investigators build an "alliance of evidence" that would include both descriptive and quantitative elements in the same review while maintaining the integrity of each.

Rather than one continuum, as proposed in Figure 2-1, Light and Pillemer's scheme appears as depicted in Figure 2-2.

Both types of evidence are viewed separately, yet in synchrony; they offer different information, different forms of evidence, which taken together can lead to important insights. The different types of evidence are complementary. If they should yield conflicting results, this is considered valuable information.

In Figure 2-2, each method is evaluated separately and, although not visualized, the pair can be reported together as an alliance of evidence. Light and Pillemer (1982) believed it was essential to

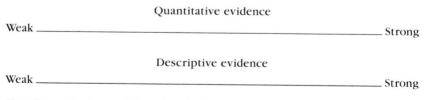

Note: From "Numbers and Narrative: Combining Their Strengths in Research Reviews," by R. Light and D. Pillemer, 1982, *Harvard Education Review,* 52(1).

Figure 2–2.   An alliance of evidence.

keep the two perspectives separate because of the economics involved in policy making. Percentages, averages, medians, significant differences among groups—all contribute to policy making, protocol, cost containment, and other decisions that are in a world of limited resources, often based on the pragmatism and utilitarianism of quantitative research.

However, we believe it would be premature to embrace wholeheartedly the proposed alliance of evidence, regardless of how rational it may sound (remember Laudan), at our stage of theory development. We quote Campbell (1975) to support this view:

After all, man in his ordinary way, is a very competent knower, and qualitative common sense is not replaced by quantitative knowing. Rather quantitative knowing has to trust and build on the qualitative, including ordinary perception. We methodologists must achieve an applied epistemology which integrates both. (p. 191)

Bolster (1983) also commented on the qualitative–quantitative linkage as we see it: "Thick, critical description is loaded with concrete detail . . . identifying salient patterns of events" and generating propositions that explain their interrelationship" (p. 304).

Once a number of such descriptions become available in the field as first-order activities of science, it becomes "possible to cross-compare their results in order to identify potentially significant variables whose validity and reliability could then be verified by experimental research" (Bolster, 1983, p. 307). Our book introduces readers to qualitative ways of coming to know and obtaining those "thick, critical" descriptions. After the "how to" chapter, a subsequent expository chapter will provide readers with such descriptions.

At this point in our thinking, we would like to propose a nonlinear schema where qualitative descriptions would lead to a quantitative analysis (when that is appropriate) and, from that analysis, nuances for further qualitative study would be identified. For example, many studies statistically support the proposition that preoperative teaching reduces anxiety for the majority of preoperative patients. There are some patients, however, in whom such teaching increases anxiety. This is a nuance and calls us back to a qualitative study: "What about those patients?" We need now to discriminate further within our populations. Theories always need re-evaluating, and the nuances or the exceptions often alert us to alternative or evolving ways of viewing phenomena. Thus, the qualitative–quantitative cyclical continuum represents the dynamic and changing world. Our linkages of the qualitative–quantitative methods are circular, as shown in Figure 2–3.

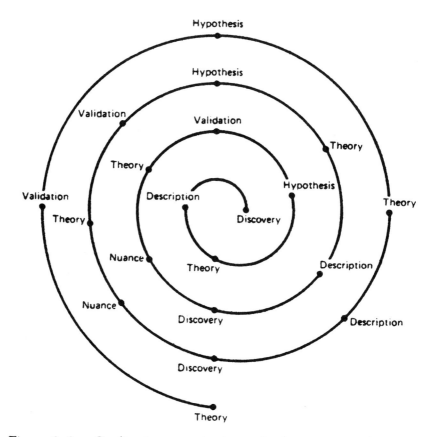

Figure 2–3. Qualitative–quantitative cyclical continuum. A nuance is defined here as a variation or a subtle aspect or quality.

READING THE FOLLOWING CHAPTERS

Up to this point, we are sure our readers are aware of and, we hope, share our belief in the potential that qualitative methods of research offer to our theory development. We have attempted to provide the background necessary to understand the differences in language, the philosophical perspectives, and the contexts in which nursing research developed. Additionally, we have attempted to explicate patterns of knowing, the purpose of science, what it is we want to know about, and how we go about knowing.

As we move on to Chapter 3, the final chapter of Part I, the qualitative tradition will be explored in more depth and breadth. We will then be ready to read specifically how one goes about knowing from a qualitative perspective. Readers will become aware of similarities among the methods as well as variations in carrying out the methods. The term "degrees of freedom" is not associated with qualitative research, but there is a freedom about qualitative research, a flexibility, room to move about in, room to explore. Our contributors exemplify the courage often necessary to deal with such freedom.

There are similarities and congruencies, yet there are differences. As this chapter opened, we quoted Harman in his belief that it matters less which view is true than what will be most helpful in guiding us in theory development.

The studies reported here as examples of qualitative research seem to us excellent examples of the organismic, humanistic perspective that embraces the philosophy of nursing. They are descriptive of experience at the very core of human caring, loving, and response.

Chapter 4 describes phenomenology as a research approach and Sarah Lauterbach uses this perspective to help us understand what it means for a mother to experience prenatal death of a wished-for baby. This sensitive study demonstrates the depth of understanding that is available to us: the mothers were encouraged to speak from their own interpretive reality.

Sally Hutchinson, in Chapter 6, introduces us to the grounded theory approach, another qualitative research method. Hutchinson then demonstrates the method in her study of people with bipolar disorder. We come to understand these people's problems and processes and what they most need and want.

Carol Germain describes the method of ethnography in Chapter 8. Zane Wolf, in Chapter 9, brings us into the rooms of nursing practice so that we might understand the culture of our rituals and, possibly, why we practice the way we often do.

New in this edition is the case study method (Chapter 10), described by Carla Mariano. We believe this method holds great potential for understanding nurse–patient interaction. Charles Beauchamp (Chapter 11), in a case study, prompts us to understand what is central to caring.

The historical method of research is discussed by M. Louise Fitzpatrick in Chapter 12 and demonstrated in a fascinating historical study by Nettie Birnbach in Chapter 13 that will help in understanding the evolution of our profession.

The chapters that describe the "doing of" a specific method and follow-up with an example of that method constitute Part II of this book.

Part III discusses various aspects of qualitative research more explicitly for those readers who will be doing or evaluating qualitative research.

In Chapter 14, ethical considerations are discussed. Chapter 15 offers suggestions that might be helpful in guiding a qualitative study through the institutional review process. Chapter 16 also attempts to help the researcher by providing a format or guide to organizing qualitative research proposals and reports. Chapter 17 discusses the combination of qualitative and quantitative approaches and elucidates the concerns expressed about such combinations. The last chapter, by Kathleen Knafl and Marlene Zichi Cohen, has to do with the always important consideration of evaluation of qualitative research.

We recommend that readers pursue further study in those more explicit areas as well as the ones introduced here. We believe that the most critical aspect of this book is its presentation of the epistemological relevance of the methods and the studies presented. The centrality of care, being there, questing for equanimity, nursing rituals, our professional history—all are phenomena that describe activities of concern to nursing. These chapters are rich in their detail, their descriptions, and their human centeredness.

REFERENCES

Allen, D. (1991). Applying critical social theory to nursing education. In N. Greenleaf (Ed.), *Curriculum revolution: Redefining the student-teacher relationship.* New York: National League for Nursing.

American Nurses' Association. (1980). *Nursing: A social policy statement.* Kansas City: American Nurses' Association.

Belenky, M., Clinchy, B., Goldberg, N., & Taub, J. (1986). *Women's ways of knowing.* New York: Basic Books.

Benner, P., & Wrubel, J. (1989). *The primacy of caring.* Menlo Park, CA: Addison-Wesley.

Benoliel, J. (1984, March). Advancing nursing science: Qualitative approaches. *Western Journal of Nursing Research in Nursing and Health, 7*(1), 1–8.

Bohm, D. (1981). Cited in H. Smith, Beyond the modern western mind set. *Teachers College Record* (Columbia University), *82*(3), 444.

Bolster, A. (1983). Toward a more effective model of research on teaching. *Harvard Education Review, 53*(3), 294–308.

Campbell, D. J. (1975). Degrees of freedom and the case study. *Comparative Political Studies, 8,* 178–193.

Capra, Z. (1982). Foreword. In L. Dossey (Ed.), *Space, time and medicine* (p. ix). Boulder, CO: Shanibhala.

Carper, B. A. (1978, October). Fundamental patterns of knowing in nursing. *Advances in Nursing Science, 1*(1), 13–23.

Diers, D. (1979). *Research in nursing practice.* Philadelphia: Lippincott.

Donaldson, S. K., & Crowley, D. M. (1978). The discipline of nursing. *Nursing Outlook, 26,* 113–120.

Dzurec, L. (1989). The necessity for and evolution of multiple paradigms for nursing research: A poststructural perspective. *Advances in Nursing Science, 11*(4), 69–77.

Fawcett, J. (1984, October). Hallmarks of success in nursing research. *Advances in Nursing Science, 7,* 1.

Freiri, P. (1971). *Pedagogy of the oppressed.* New York: Seaver.

Gilligan, C. (1982). *In a different voice: Psychological theory and women's development.* Cambridge, MA: Harvard University Press.

Gould, S. J. (1984, August 12). Science and gender. *The New York Times Book Review* (book review).

Harman, W. (1977). *Symposium and consciousness.* New York: Penguin.

Johnson, D. E. (1978). State of the art of theory development. In *Theory development: What, why, how?* (p. 9). New York: National League for Nursing.

Johnson, D. E. (1980). The behavioral system model for nursing. In J. P. Riehl & C. Roy (Eds.), *Conceptual models for nursing practice* (2nd ed.). Norwalk, CT: Appleton-Century-Crofts.

King, I. M. (1981). *A theory for nursing: Systems, concepts, process.* New York: Wiley.

Kneller, G. (1971). *Introduction to the philosophy of education.* New York: Wiley.

Kuhn, T. S. (Ed.). (1970). *The structure of scientific revolutions.* Chicago: University of Chicago Press.

Laudan, L. (1977). *Progress and its problems: Toward a theory of scientific growth.* Berkeley: University of California Press.

Leininger, M. (Ed.). (1984). *Care: The essence of nursing and health.* Thorofare, NJ: Slack.

Light, R., & Pillemer, D. (1982). Numbers and narrative: Combining their strengths in research reviews. *Harvard Education Review, 52*(1), 1-23.

Morgan, G. (1983). *Beyond method.* Newbury Park, CA: Sage.

Munhall, P. (1982, April). Ethical juxtapositions in nursing research. *Topics in Clinical Nursing, 4*(1), 66-73.

Munhall, P. (1992). Holding the Mississippi River in place and other implications for qualitative research. *Nursing Outlook, 10*(6), 257-262.

Munhall, P. (1993). Unknowing: Toward another pattern of knowing. *Nursing Outlook.*

Munhall, P., & Oiler, C. (1986). *Nursing research: A qualitative perspective.* Norwalk, CT: Appleton-Lange.

Nesbitt, R. (1976). *Sociology as an art form.* New York: Oxford University Press.

Newman, M. (1983, January). Editorial. *Advances in Nursing Science, 5*(2), x-xi.

Newman, M., Sime, A., & Cocoran-Perry, (1991). The focus of the discipline of nursing. *Advances in Nursing Science, 14*(1), 1-5.

Norris, C. (1982). *Concept clarification in nursing.* Rockville, MD: Aspen.

Orem, D. E. (1980). *Nursing: Concepts of practice* (2nd ed.). New York: McGraw-Hill.

Paterson, J. (1978). The tortuous way toward nursing theory. In *Theory development: What, why and how?* New York: National League for Nursing.

Paterson, J., & Zderad, L. (1976). *Humanistic nursing.* New York: Wiley.

Pender, N. J. (1987). *Health promotion in nursing practice.* Norwalk, CT: Appleton-Lange.

Polkinghorne, D. (1983). *Methodology for the human sciences.* Albany: SUNY Press.

Reichardt, C., & Cook, T. (Eds.). (1979). *Qualitative and quantitative methods in evaluation research* (pp. 33–48). Beverly Hills, CA: Sage.

Rogers, M. E. (1970). *An introduction to the theoretical basis of nursing.* Philadelphia: Davis.

Roy, C., Sr. (1976). *Introduction to nursing: An adaptation model.* Englewood Cliffs, NJ: Prentice-Hall.

Silva, M., & Rothbart, D. (1984, January). An analysis of changing trends in philosophies of science on nursing theory development and testing. *Advances in Nursing Science, 6*(2).

Stevens, B. J. (1979). *Nursing theory: Analysis, application, evaluation.* Boston: Little, Brown.

Van Manen, M. (1990). *Research on lived experience: Human science for action-sensitive pedagogy.* New York: SUNY Press.

Watson, J. (1985). *Nursing: The philosophy and science of caring.* Boulder: Colorado Associated University Press.

Watson, J. (1988). New dimensions of human caring theory. *Nursing Science, 1*(4), 175–181.

Wilson, L., & Fitzpatrick, J. (1984, January). Dialectic thinking as a means of understanding systems in development: Relevance to Rogers' principles. *Advances in Nursing Science, 6*(2), 41.

3

Philosophical Foundations of Qualitative Research

Carolyn Oiler Boyd

*T*he tension between our science and our practice serves as the primary impetus for qualitative research in nursing. The growing interest among nurse researchers in qualitative research represents a reaction against the prevailing view of subjectivity and the nature of reality that is established as premise in the positivist tradition. It is a reaction against a focus on an external reality, an existence of things and others independent of a subject who experiences them. In the quantitative paradigm, the dichotomization of reality as objective and subjective has propagated rather than resolved tensions in nursing practice between the technological and the humanistic aspects of that practice. Doing research in the dominant paradigm, nurse researchers have been led to view subjectivity as a private and personal reading of reality, given to error. For the researcher who identifies with and has allegiance to nursing practice, such a view is often contrary to the lived reality of nursing practice.

The idea of *client* subjectivity, however, is valued in two ways within the quantitative paradigm: as a data source and as an outcome variable in nursing. In keeping with a split vision of reality, many nurse practitioners and researchers focus on external reality, directing their observations to the world as object, including the patient's subjectivity. For many of us, basic inconsistencies arise from the premises concerning the nature of reality in the quantitative paradigm. Conflict is generated for us in several ways:

- Recognition of the nurse–client relationship as the medium of care conflicts with scientific devaluing of nurse subjectivity in the caring process.
- Nurses suffer the tension of a scientifically polarized reality, which drives subjective experience underground and deprives nurses of control over their realities.
- Awareness of nurses' realities is narrowly confined in the requirements of the professional role, and a gap emerges between their realities as lived and facts about these realities offered in scientific comment.
- A narrow vision of what happens in experience leaves nurses with unexplained dimensions of reality.
- To preserve objective detachment in nursing situations and some sense of integrity for themselves, nurses withdraw from and deny their awareness. This deflects us from values that center nursing as a humanizing influence in the health care system.
- The cumulative effect of these tensions in distancing nurses from their experiences renders them inarticulate, and the development of nursing knowledge is thus hindered in the gap between experiential and theoretical knowledge.
- A heightened sensitivity to some of the implications of a science that aims for prediction and control in view of a growing appreciation for the importance of the valuing of self-determination in health care has contributed to an unrest about our emerging science and to unsettling questions concerning our future development.

The prevailing views about subjectivity and reality in nursing establish a need to explore other ways of thinking about what is real, so that more in nursing might be considered real and true in a scientific sense. In this chapter, the tensions and conflicts generated by incompatibilities between nursing philosophy and practice and nursing science are the background for a discussion of the philosophical foundations for qualitative research. The aim is to resolve these tensions and conflicts through a research paradigm that coincides with nursing beliefs, values, and aims. Although the interest is in the nexus of philosophy with research methods, there is also a need to focus on the nexus with nursing practice and nursing education. The larger context for the discussion will not be addressed here, but its relevance is critical. (See, for example, National League for Nursing, 1988.)

Traditional nursing beliefs and values that shape and give expression to nursing in our society may change (or may already have changed), and this would certainly alter the arguments for qualitative research in this volume. In a sense, the strivings of qualitative researchers represent an effort not only to maintain nursing's humanistic current in its present form, but also to establish it more soundly as a grounding for our practice and our science (Paterson & Zderad, 1976, pp. 3–9). This goal is not shared by all; in what seems at times to be a denial of the tensions between science and humanism and, at other times, a turn toward beliefs, values and perspectives that are severed from nursing's traditional humanistic stance in health care. The intentions of qualitative researchers are thus important in distinguishing their work as part of the qualitative paradigm rather than an opportunistic use of some of the techniques and strategies associated with qualitative research.

This chapter limits its concern to the features of the qualitative paradigm, fully recognizing that some who do qualitative research may not attend to these features as grounding for their work. Nevertheless, the view presented here about philosophical foundations is essentially congruent with other presentations in the literature and has broad implications for nursing practice as well as for research. Each qualitative approach (ethnography, grounded theory, phenomenology, case study, historical research) discussed in this text carries its own orientation or perspective, draws on its own selection of theorists, methodologists, and philosophers, and reflects the parent discipline for that approach. Nevertheless, common premises link the various qualitative approaches in a tradition or a paradigm. The aim of this chapter is to relate some of these common premises to common characteristics of qualitative research and thereby to articulate the philosophical foundations or framework of the qualitative paradigm. Such a philosophical grounding provides both direction and rationale for research design and method.

WHAT IS QUALITATIVE RESEARCH?

Definition

The very general term "qualitative research" encompasses a variety of designs and methods. Nevertheless, the various designs generally share the following features:

- *A holistic approach to questions—a recognition that human realities are complex.* Research questions tend to be very broad. Some examples are: What are the birth experiences of women in foreign cultures (Sharts-Engel, 1989)? What is comforting? What is it like to feel lonely when hospitalized (Copel, 1984)?
- *The focus is on human experience.* This is a turn toward subjectivities or people's realities.
- *The research strategies used generally feature sustained contact with people in settings where those people normally spend their time.* There is careful attention to the contexts of human behavior.
- *There is typically a high level of researcher involvement with subjects; strategies of participant observation and in-depth, unstructured interviews are often used.*
- *The data produced provide a description, usually narrative, of people living through events in situations.*

A definition of qualitative research may be stated, then, as involving broadly stated questions about human experiences and realities, studied through sustained contact with persons in their natural environments, and producing rich, descriptive data that help us to understand those persons' experiences. The emphasis is on achieving understanding that will, in turn, open up new options for action and new perspectives that can change people's worlds.

Purposes

Knafl and Howard (1986) have classified the purposes of qualitative research as fourfold: instrumentation, illustration, sensitization, and conceptualization. For example, to serve the purpose of instrumentation, a researcher might use in-depth, unstructured interviews of wheelchair-bound adults to learn what it's like to live with impaired mobility. The information these adults provide the researcher could then be used to construct an instrument that includes categories based on their actual experiences rather than what we imagine them to be.

The purpose of illustration was served in Kramer's classic study of young baccalaureate graduate nurses' reality shock (1968). In this study, Kramer used qualitative interview data and subjects' journal entries to illustrate her quantitative findings about their role orientations. The purpose of sensitization is served by all qualitative studies to the extent that they effectively communicate insights about experiences we need to understand vicariously. Learning of these findings functions to sensitize research consumers to their patients and thereby to contribute to the quality of care. The researched may also profit from the heightened awareness and meaning that emerge in the research process. Lastly, qualitative studies may be undertaken to serve the purpose of conceptualization or theory development. For example, Hutchinson (1986) used the grounded-theory method to learn more about what it is like to be a nurse in a neonatal intensive care unit. After a protracted period of in-depth observation, participation, and interviews, Hutchinson constructed a theory descriptive of these nurses' coping strategies.

This classification of qualitative research purposes reveals the very broad interpretation of the term "qualitative research" in contemporary usages. On the one hand, qualitative research is seen as a precursor to quantitative study. Researchers whose purpose is instrumentation use qualitative strategies without necessarily adopting the beliefs, values, and orientation of the philosophical foundations or the set of features (outlined above) commonly associated with the qualitative paradigm. When the purpose is illustration, there may be a similar commitment to the positivist tradition rather than to the qualitative paradigm. The purposes of sensitization and conceptualization are more strictly in keeping with the qualitative paradigm.

Another way to think about the purpose of qualitative research is in terms of establishing a phenomenological baseline that would be a thorough description of the life-worlds of patients, families, and nurses as they are experienced by participants (Oiler, 1986, pp. 99–102). It would provide fully developed nursing concepts that are faithful to the real world of lived nursing/patient experience. The theory constructed on such descriptions would possess a greater relevance in their comments about nursing/patient phenomena because they would adhere more closely to participants' lived experiences. Establishing a phenomenological baseline, a coherent and accurate description of lived experience, will be accomplished through qualitative studies. The qualitative process is one of theory development; that of empirical studies is one of second-order comment.

Qualitative researchers strive to suspend foundations in our views that support second-order comment on experiences rather than insight into those experiences. Nursing management of dependency in the nursing situation, for example, may suffer from a lack of attention to the meanings of dependency in various nursing situations. We might consider how being bathed might facilitate recovery through a mechanism such as therapeutic touch. Or, how uncontrolled diabetes facilitates another goal by maintaining the noncompliant diabetic patient's relationship with a visiting nurse. Or, how ministering to clients makes it possible for nurses to be emotionally available to them. In this example of dependency, the phenomenological baseline for practice and research would provide a thorough description of human dependency in nursing situations. We would ask such questions as: "Dependent on whom, for what, with what consequences? What are the alternatives, and how does being dependent relate to health, to striving toward and achieving one's goals in one's world?" The baseline would provide us with the understanding needed for a clarified concept of dependency. This would be a nursing concept—one that might vary from the perspective in psychology or in sociology. On the other hand, when thoroughly grounded in lived experience, a nursing concept of dependency might be instructive to other disciplines. Establishing a phenomenological baseline for nursing knowledge is, from this point of view, the single overriding purpose for qualitative research.

As reflected in the working definition of qualitative research, the position taken here is that the mere use of qualitative strategies such as unstructured interviewing does not place a study in the qualitative tradition. Research that *does* belong in the qualitative tradition is characterized by a commitment to a philosophical grounding that orients us to particular views on the nature of being human and the nature of reality; in nursing research, this grounding includes particular views on the nature of health and nursing as well. This position directs the discussion in this chapter.

History of the Qualitative Tradition

Bogdan and Biklen (1982) provided a description of the historical context of qualitative research, noting that, although its recognition as a tool of science is relatively recent, its long and rich tradition in the United States began during the late 1800s. At that time, qualitative strategies were used to disclose the rapidly developing social problems in cities pursuant to industrialization, urbanization, and mass immigration. Qualitative descriptions encouraged social change by making urban problems visible to the public. The Pittsburgh survey, for example, provided statistics about the urban poor, but also gave us detailed accounts of urban life, conveyed through photographs, charcoal portraits, and interviews. The statistics were thus cast in human terms by the qualitative data (Bogdan & Biklen, 1982, pp. 3–8).

Concurrent with the productivity of social surveys at the turn of the century, anthropological field research methods were being developed and taught in universities. The anthropological strategy of participant observation migrated to sociology, where it was used along with the case study method to study social problems in communities from a social interaction perspective. During the 1920s and 1930s, sociologists used qualitative strategies extensively to study such social phenomena as race relations, ethnicity, and delinquency. From the 1930s through the 1950s, qualitative research waned as worthy scientific endeavor came to be defined in accord with the growing expectation that quantitative methods were the most promising means to solutions. Taking the lead primarily from medicine, public health, and sociology, nursing subscribed to this view; our short history of research activity meshed with the dominant quantitative paradigm in the scientific world (Bogdan & Biklen, 1982, pp. 8-18).

The 1960s, however, disrupted the scientific world's unquestioning faith in the promise of quantitative methods. A variety of social minority groups clamored to be heard, and there was a renewed interest in the power of qualitative methods to provide us with better understanding of minorities' views and circumstances. During this period, the grounded-theory method was developed (Glaser & Strauss, 1967). In nursing, this method was used to study nurses' and patients' experiences with death and dying (Quint, 1967). However, this kind of early work did not flourish nationally. Nurse researchers tended to focus their talents and energies on mastering quantitative methods.

Nevertheless, the social unrest of the 1960s, including the feminist movement, stimulated methodological debates in other fields. Education, sociology, and psychology in particular turned toward qualitative methods with renewed interest during the 1970s. These debates surfaced in the literature, in university courses, and at national conferences, and gradually engaged nurses in a serious consideration of the merit and prospects of qualitative research (Bogdan & Biklen, 1982, pp. 18-26). Paterson and Zderad (1976) introduced phenomenology to nursing in a work that intrigued some, but puzzled others. Nursing debates concerning the merit of qualitative research approaches took off in the early 1980s. (See, for example, Munhall, 1982; Oiler, 1982; Tinkle & Beaton, 1983.) Today, we are in a period of exploring qualitative methods and developing our expertise in their use. Although we continue to rely heavily on direction from other disciplines that have created qualitative approaches for their concerns, we are on the move and can look forward to increasing experimentation with new qualitative methods for the investigation of nursing problems. (See, for example, Newman, 1990; Parse, 1990; Paterson & Zderad, 1976.)

Structure and Characteristics

When qualitative researchers speak of subjectivity, they are referring to the ways in which people make sense of their experiences and lives. In nursing, this concern with subjectivity is one with meanings or "sense making" in situations. To understand the sense that a given situation bears for a person is to grasp something of that person's reality—to see what is true from his or her point of view. We have accumulated many facts, for example, about menopause, osteoporosis, and pain. However, these facts do not add up to an understanding of what it's like to live through menopause, or to have osteoporosis, or to suffer. Qualitative researchers are most interested in subjective meanings rather than facts alone. If a patient's experience is one of suffering, it matters little whether the facts about the patient's condition coincide with his or her experience from some other person's point of view (reality). In nursing, we have always attended as best we can to patients' experiences. To refer to their experiences as subjective is quite superfluous and quite dismissive, as if patients' subjectivities were erroneous. All realities are subjective if one means that the person interprets, lends meaning to, and makes sense of the facts of the world. The objective view of health care providers is simply *one* way of interpreting, forming meaning, and making sense of things. We worry when patients take on this kind of perspective, in recognition of its limited usefulness for them.

In order to construct methods that disclose subjectivity, qualitative researchers recognize that people construct meanings in relation to the world in which they exist. This is the second leading characteristic of qualitative methods: the natural settings in which people under study live, work, learn, and play are sought for the conduct of the study. The researcher strives to collect data descriptive of the person–environment relation, in the belief that human behavior is best understood in the context in which it occurs. If a researcher wants to learn about what it is like to ambulate in a wheelchair, for example, the natural setting would be subjects' everyday lives. The study design would involve finding ways to be with subjects for a period of time in their lives. A questionnaire, in contrast, would lift subjects away from their natural setting and experiencing and would obscure such data as their struggles with stairs and doors, their solicitation or rejection of assistance, and their myriad ways of accommodating a world of forms designed for ambulating via use of the lower extremities. Many qualitative studies rely heavily, if not exclusively, on interview data rather than on joining subjects in the course of their day-to-day lives. The distinguishing feature of a qualitative approach in interviewing, however, is the researcher's and the researched's turn toward the researched's day-to-day life. The interview is less structured and more intimate, akin to an initial therapeutic interview when the focus is also on understanding the patient's reality.

Because the aim is to disclose subjectivity, the qualitative researcher strives to locate and collect data that serve to describe the experience under study. Words, in the form of field observation notes and transcripts of interviews, are the most common form of qualitative data. However, photographs, videotapes, and the researcher's perceptions of sounds, tastes, and smells are sometimes included as data. Similarly, diaries, memos, letters, and art might be included if they contribute to presenting and understanding the human experience under study. The end product—the findings—represent the researcher's best effort to organize and present an accurate picture of what has been learned by going to people in their natural settings and being with them for a time in order to gain as much insight as possible about their lives.

The pictures that qualitative research produces are distillations of large amounts of various kinds of data that are tracked down by maintaining a research focus on human processes. For example, a quantitative researcher might study whether nursing home residents are lonely, and to what extent, by using a scale that measures loneliness. Facts are thus produced: yes, they are lonely (in the main); furthermore, the loneliness is extreme. The qualitative researcher, on the other hand, would pursue the question of *how* nursing home residents experience loneliness. Understanding is thus produced: loneliness as it is lived through is brought into focus. Other process-oriented questions are: "What is it like to work in an NICU?" (Hutchinson, 1986); "How are attitudes about women expressed in the physician–nurse relationship?" (Katzman & Roberts, 1988); "What happens to families when there is sudden death of a member?" Such process-oriented questions guide the qualitative researcher in a rigorous search for elusive data that helps to disclose complex human experiences that often defy attempts simply to report them in interviews or on questionnaires.

The organization and distillation of data that the researcher performs in order to present a picture of the experience under study constitute an essentially inductive process. Many instances of an event, process, or perception are grouped together to generate a characteristic that is then represented in the picture the researcher provides in the report of the findings. This inductive approach to building knowledge is sometimes referred to as theory development from the bottom up. For example, in Copel's study of loneliness (1984), she identified "problems with relationships" as a component of loneliness. A few of the instances that were grouped together to form this component were patients' statements of feeling unloved, isolated, and secluded and of having a sense of loss and lack of support.

A PHENOMENOLOGICAL PERSPECTIVE AS PHILOSOPHICAL FRAMEWORK

Leading themes of phenomenological philosophy offer a perspective on the nature of human reality that supports qualitative research efforts. Some qualitative methodologists draw directly from phenomenology to articulate a rationale and grounding for social science methods. Others make no reference to phenomenology as such. Yet, despite the fact that various qualitative methodologists have been inspired by thinkers who are not categorized as phenomenological thinkers, phenomenological themes can be discerned and are one of the leading influences. Patton (1980) noted that qualitative methods derive from a variety of philosophical, epistemological, and methodological traditions but that, generally, the qualitative paradigm is based on perspectives developed in phenomenology, symbolic interactionism, naturalistic behaviorism, ethnomethodology, and ecological psychology. The integrating theme of these perspectives is the idea of *verstehen:*

> *The advocate of some version of the* verstehen *doctrine will claim that human beings can be understood in a manner that other objects cannot. Men have purposes and emotions, they make plans, construct cultures, and hold certain values, and their behavior is influenced by such values, plans, and purposes. . . . The* verstehen *tradition stresses understanding that focuses on the meaning of human behavior, the context of social interaction, an empathetic understanding based on subjective experience, and the connections between subjective states and behavior. (Patton, 1980, pp. 44-45)*

Bogdan and Taylor (1975), writing about qualitative research in its general sense, credited phenomenology with the inspiration that the *verstehen* idea lends to the qualitative paradigm:

> *The phenomenologist is concerned with understanding human behavior from the actor's own frame of reference. . . . The phenomenologist examines how the world is experienced. For him or her the important reality is what people imagine it to be. (Bogdan & Taylor, 1975, p. 2)*

Bogdan and Biklen (1982) acknowledged that the word "phenomenology" is used in many ways, but, in its most general sense, "[A]ll qualitative researchers in some way reflect a phenomenological perspective" (p. 31). Not all qualitative researchers would classify themselves as phenomenologists, yet the idea of the *verstehen* would be readily recognized as a central tenet in their work.

The relevance of phenomenological philosophy to the qualitative paradigm is thus established in this discussion of philosophical foundations. The variety of qualitative designs that spring from the philosophy attests to the openness of the philosophy; it inspires and encourages extrapolations to both practice and research methods and processes. What is important to keep in mind, however, is that (because of our youth as an emerging science) the qualitative designs of grounded theory, ethnography, and phenomenology-as-method were extrapolations within other disciplines. They bear the perspectives of those disciplines, which do not coincide perfectly with the perspectives of the nursing discipline. To do grounded theory in a way that is faithful to the ideas of the methodologists (Glaser & Strauss, 1967, for example), a nurse researcher cannot be knowledgeable about the phenomenological roots alone—there is also symbolic interactionism to take into account.

On the other hand, when we borrow theory from other disciplines, we should be adapting it in the context of the nursing discipline. Paterson and Zderad (1976) and Parse (1990) provided examples of this kind of adaptation for phenomenologic method in nursing, but, to date, there is still a great deal of work to do in creating nursing methodologies for research. An embrace of a philosophical foundation for qualitative research will enable us to carry the qualitative tradition forward in nursing without risk of losing sight of the intentions of the turn away from the positivist paradigm. We clearly do not need to introduce new research methods that will divide and repress us further, and a sound grounding in the philosophical foundation will reduce this risk. For this reason, qualitative researchers need to be knowledgeable about and committed to the philosophy that grounds the designs, methods, and strategies of the qualitative tradition. It bears mentioning, however, that for such well-established designs as grounded theory, ethnography, and historical research, the leading methodologists may be sufficient for rationale and direction, particularly when acceptance and recognition of the scientific merit of such studies constitute the issue at hand. The grounded theory method of Glaser and Strauss, for example, is suffused with a philosophical grounding. Adopting their grounded theory methodology may satisfy any challenge to using a qualitative approach that may be encountered, without necessarily articulating that grounding. However, in a concern for scholarship and for a commitment to foundational beliefs and valuing, a grasp of the approach in a simplistic, technical way is not satisfactory. One can usually recognize qualitative studies that are not well-grounded in philosophy; they tend to take on a positivist flavor, to be plagued with incongruencies from design through discussion of findings, and to fall short of being compelling reading.

The Nature of Reality

In a simple turn of preference, qualitative researchers direct their attention to human realities as opposed to the concrete realities of objects. The distinctive valuing of and respect for people in qualitative research do not allow for their objectification as featured in quantitative research. People are thus centered in qualitative research in recognition that reality is constituted in human perspectives. There are always multiple realities (perspectives) to consider when a full grasp of a situation is sought. A question such as "What is treatment in an intensive care unit like?" may be considered from a number of perspectives—that of the patient, the family, the nurse, and the physician, each of which is decidedly unique and in some ways contradictory to the others. Further, each research participant's experience may be understood variously by him or her from a number of perspectives. Yet, each is equally "true"; each is equally real. The concrete objective reality of the intensive care environment is experienced differently by each of these people, creating different realities.

Human involvement in the world is, then, of primary concern to the qualitative researcher who, by choice, focuses on human realities. Schutz (1973) wrote:

> *The origin of all reality is subjective; whatever excites and stimulates our interest is real. To call a thing real means that this thing stands in a certain relation to ourselves.* (p. 207)

A focus on human realities must therefore take into account not only the "thing" but also the relation it bears to the experiencing person. The facts of the world—what we may customarily think of as objective reality—and the facts of human consciousness coincide in this focus. The very meaning of objectivity and subjectivity changes in this view of the nature of reality.

Merleau-Ponty (1962) reasoned that subjectivity as inner existence is false on the grounds that existence (or consciousness) is possible because we are present within the world. The world is assumed; experience in it and knowledge of it, however, are always through the subjectivity of presence in the world. There are not two views of reality; the view is always the subjective one of this presence. Reality as it can be known to us is thus unidimensional in this sense. The appearance of phenomena expresses this welded relationship of subject and object and is the first or fundamental reality on which our sciences and understandings are built.

The body is one's natural access to the world. Sensation, sexuality, language, and speech are all expressions of our existence, and all are constituted concretely in a bodily reaching toward the world around us. Even in the experience of feeling alone and lonely, one's reference is paradoxically to others in the world. Merleau-Ponty (1962, p. 70) regarded the body as one's point of view on the world; the body as access to the world produces for the subject what he referred to as one's gaze. He explained that existence is expressed in a particular manner of approach to the world, and the approach, or gaze, is brought into being by one's bodily existence in the world:

> *Even if I know nothing of rods and cones, I should realize that it is necessary to put the surroundings in abeyance the better to see the object and to lose in background what one gains in focal figure, because to look at the object is to plunge into it, and because objects form a system in which one cannot show itself without concealing others. . . . The object-horizon structure, or the perspective, is no obstacle to me when I want to see the object; for just as it is the means whereby objects are distinguished from each other, it is also the means whereby they are disclosed (Merleau-Ponty, 1962, p. 67).*

Concretely, we are able to experience the world through our bodies: we assume a position in the world, which in turn determines the object-horizon structure, both spatially and temporally, available to us. We are able to focus, to be conscious of one object over others in a figure–ground relationship of our choosing.

The human gaze reveals just that aspect of the object accessible through one's bodily involvement in the world in space and in time. Human experience and human reality are always perspectival in this sense. It is important to recognize here, however, that the subject's biography, past experience, knowledge of the world, and whatever social and political facticities may hold true are all qualifications of gaze. Merleau-Ponty (1962) described these qualifications, using a common experience:

> *When I look at the lamp on my table, I attribute to it not only the qualities visible from where I am, but also those which the chimney, the walls, the table can "see"; but back of my lamp is nothing but the face which it "shows" to the chimney. I can therefore see an object insofar as objects form a system or a world, and insofar as each one treats the others round it as spectators of its hidden aspects and as guarantee of the permanence of those aspects. (p. 68)*

In this way, a perspective on the world is formed. It is not pure experience but an interpreted experience that constitutes reality.

In what Schutz (1973) called the "natural attitude of daily life," consciousness is expressed within and on the world. The reality of experience is taken for granted and shifting perspectives are assumed as dictated by one's biography and by the practical need to achieve chosen purposes in the world. In the natural attitude, the world as experienced and interpreted by our predecessors is handed down to our own experience and interpretation. In the fashion of layers, a current experience is shaped by a stock of previous experiences and interpretations—one's own and those of one's parents and teachers. The natural attitude, a type of mode of consciousness, presents us with interpreted experience.

The natural attitude characterizes most of our existence. We assume that the meanings brought to the world coincide with an absolute, objective reality. Other realities (arising from other modes of consciousness) and different attentions to life (presenting other meanings) are incompatible. Merleau-Ponty explained that, in interpreted experience, positing an object makes us go beyond the limits of actual experience. He discussed the phenomenon of the phantom limb to demonstrate the inescapable relation of subject and object, which he referred to as being "situated":

> *What it is in us which refuses mutilation and disablement is an I committed to a certain physical and inter-human world, who continues to tend towards his world despite handicaps and amputations and who, to this extent, does not recognize them de jure. (1962, p. 81)*

Rejecting physiological and psychological explanations as inadequate, Merleau-Ponty acknowledged that the phantom limb can be related to both. The difficulty in these explanations resides in the experience of presence of a limb:

> *The man with one leg feels the missing limb in the same way as I feel keenly the existence of a friend who is, nevertheless, not before my eyes; he has not lost it because he continues to allow for it. . . . The phantom arm is not a representation of the arm, but the ambivalent presence of an arm. (p. 81)*

The body as a power is assumed at a preobjective level, and the amputated limb as a customary part of this being. The person with a phantom limb is living his body in the way to which he is accustomed.

This phenomenological view of the phantom limb is not a denial of physiological facts or of psychological explanations of memory, belief, or acceptance. Rather, it introduces a common ground for these facts—a situation for an existence. In an active engagement in present experiences, the person is committed to carrying through his intentions in the world. The patient with a phantom limb might try, for example, to reach for something with his amputated arm. In his lived body and in his attention to action, the reach makes perfect sense and is not simply a matter of psychological denial or physiological nerve transmission extension. Only when this engagement with the world in action is suspended can the patient consider the truth of the amputated limb and compensate for a lived body that may continue to press toward the world for some time.

The phantom limb is a transient phenomenon. The patient's perception ultimately is replaced with another perception from the new perspective given through his or her body. The amputated limb gives rise to experiences that, through time, direct attention to life in new ways. This is not accomplished by thinking about it but, rather, by living it over a span of time. "The world is not what I think, but what I live through" (Merleau-Ponty, 1962, p. xvii). It is not created by the subject's involvement with it; it is discovered through perception. Perception does not depend on external stimuli as if they were clear, defined, and unambiguous. Rather, stimuli are perceived in the context of the experience to which they belong:

> [T]o see is to have colours or lights, to hear is to have sounds, to sense is to have qualities. . . . But red and green are not sensations, they are the sensed, and quality is not an element of consciousness, but a property of the object. Instead of providing a simple means delimiting sensations, if we consider it in the experience itself which evinces it the quality is as rich and mysterious as the object, or indeed the whole spectacle, perceived (Merleau-Ponty, 1962, p. 4).

To clarify these statements, Merleau-Ponty explained that seeing a red patch on a carpet is contingent on shadows and lights, size, and the fabric of the carpet. This red would not be the same in the absence of these meanings which reside in it. It is not possible to perceive sensations, like the color red, without the overlays that form experience. Perception is awareness of the appearances of phenomena, and one must see the red patch on the carpet as it really is, with shadow, light, size, and fabric. From this totality, one is able to conceive of this particular red; that is, one lends an interpretation or gives meaning to one's experience—in this case, the experience of seeing a red patch on a carpet. Perception is open to an infinite variety of perspectives; they merge in a unique, individual style to define one's reality. Perception has the potential for access to meaning as it is discovered in living rather than as it is interpreted after-the-fact. Perception of an amputated limb as an ambivalent presence is not truth, but it is reality for the patient. It is this particular perspective that is taken up in qualitative research.

Modes of Awareness and Expression

Based on experience and perception, other human capacities for awareness enable us to bring meaning to our lives and world. Scientific awareness, for example, is one mode, one possible perspective, for interpreting experience. Like other modes of awareness, it posits what is figure and what is ground. In so doing, it provides a particular way of looking at things and yields a particular interpretation or reality while opening up future experiences as possibilities. Experience becomes known to us after-the-fact, when we reflect on it. To know an experience directly and immediately is not strictly possible. When we turn back to see it, we are then in a new experience: we are reflecting on an experience that has just passed. In other words, knowing what one is living through is interpreted experience, and the best we can do is to be aware of our awarenesses and recognize that knowledge is interpreted reality. Such self-consciousness expands awareness, confronts us with our freedom, and points us toward the necessity of choice and action. Qualitative research is not value-free, in other words. There is a reverence for life, for the individual, and for self-determination. Reflection and heightened awareness are accepted as instrumental in being free to choose among alternatives.

Values are brought into being through the meanings people attach to objects, events, or circumstances. People establish what is figure and what is ground, thereby bringing order out of chaos in the world. There are gaps between what is given and what is to be gained through human perspective, choice, and action; these gaps represent opportunities to perceive anew, to orient oneself in the world through choices, to construct one's own world.

The natural attitude described by Schutz (1970) is one possible perspective on experience. Reflection on experience, however, opens up other possible modes of awareness. As noted above, scientific awareness is one of these. Others include aesthetic awareness; empathic and intuitive awarenesses; imaginative, spiritual, and historical awarenesses. There are also the awarenesses of dreams and hallucinations and of belief and remembrance. Each mode of awareness presents us with a particular kind of evidence of the world. Expressions of these awarenesses are equally varied and are a rendering of awareness in behavior. Research, art, humor, worship, habit and ritual, acts of courage and of aggression—all are expressions of awareness of experience. They may be called consequences of the ways in which we make sense of our existence; they are sensible outcomes of perspectives taken up in the world.

Summary of Philosophical Themes

- To exist is to be conscious of something in the world. Reality and truth hinge on this fundamental relation of human existence in a concrete world of others, objects, events, circumstances, and situations. Human realities are thus interactive and transactional with the world.
- One is tied to the world in a perspective created by being bodily situated in the world in a particular way. Because human realities are contingent on one's turn of attention to the world in a perspective that comes into being by that turn, they are always subjective in nature.
- Experience refers to living through a situation, event, or circumstance in time. It can only be known reflectively.
- Perception refers to original awareness of the appearance of phenomena in experience and is constituted in one's perspective.
- Various modes of awareness characterize human capability and are superimposed on perception through reflection, providing various ways of interpreting/constituting meaning in experience. Awareness in a particular mode is a matter of taking up a perspective on experience.
- The range of human expression, or the ways to present one's awareness, strengthens one's links to the world through the effects of those expressions on the world and the constitution of perspective in awareness and expression. The scientific

mode of awareness and its various expressions constitute a perspective that, in turn, creates a particular way of involvement with things, others, and ourselves.

Lincoln and Guba (1985) provided an alternative summary or overview of what they referred to as axioms of the naturalistic paradigm. The axioms are as follows:

- There are multiple constructed realities that can be studied only holistically; inquiry into these multiple realities will inevitably diverge so that prediction and control are unlikely outcomes, although some level of understanding can be achieved.
- The inquirer and the object of inquiry are independent; the knower and the known constitute a discrete dualism—they are interactive and inseparable.
- The aim of inquiry is to develop an idiographic body of knowledge in the form of "working hypotheses" that describe the individual case. Only time- and context-bound hypotheses are possible.
- All entities are in a state of mutual, simultaneous shaping so that it is impossible to distinguish causes from effects.
- Inquiry is value-bound in at least five ways:

  1. By inquirer values as expressed in the choice and framing of the phenomenon to be studied;
  2. By the choice of research paradigm;
  3. By the choice of theory used to guide data collection, analysis, and interpretation;
  4. By values that inhere in the context;
  5. By value resonancy among problem, paradigm, theory, and context. (pp. 36–38)

Benner (1985) described the essential tenets of the philosophy that guided her work as follows:

1. *Human beings are self-interpreting and these interpretations are constitutive of the self.*

2. *Human beings take a position on the kinds of being they are.*

3. *The meanings available to an individual are constrained by the person's particular language, culture, and history. (p. 5)*

THE NEXUS OF PHILOSOPHY WITH RESEARCH PROCESS

The use of phenomenological philosophy to guide research methodology unquestionably modifies the researcher's involvement with his or her subject matter. In the recognition that researching is an experience for participants, there is a profound regard for how that experience might be perceived and interpreted. Stimuli that the researcher introduces include his or her observing, questioning, reacting presence. When a person agrees to be a participant, he or she has taken up a perspective that is oriented to the research and the researcher. Each question posed directs the participant's attention in certain ways, establishing a figure-ground relation and opening up possibilities for new meanings to emerge. The self-conscious concern for the individual and for the effects of the research on participants is a matter of valuing people in a certain way, and this provides direction for a wide variety of choices in selecting a research design and creating a method for the research.

The doctrine of naturalism in qualitative research is, in part, a methodological choice that defers to this understanding that realities are at the very least influenced by the research process. More to the point, the research process itself becomes part of the context of the phenomenon under study.

In a discussion of research as praxis, Newman (1990) stated:

The nurse researcher cannot stand outside the person being researched in a subject-object fashion. The researcher is part of the interaction pattern which is the process of pattern recognition and choice. (p. 40)

Drawing on critical social theory (see, for example, Allen, 1985; Lather, 1986), Newman explained that, in the course of her research on expanding consciousness, both the researcher and the researched were transformed:

> [W]e discovered that sharing our perception of the person's pattern with the person was meaningful to the participants and stimulated new insights regarding their lives. We discovered that our participation in the process made a difference in our own lives. We suspected that what we were doing in the name of research was nursing practice. (p. 37)

Not all qualitative researchers would embrace the idea that the research process is clinical nursing intervention, but the central message holds true. The aim of qualitative research in nursing arises from nursing's purposes and its intentions to intervene. Attending to patients' responses with an understanding of how realities are constituted enables us to introduce health care to them in ways that open up new perspectives for them, thereby perhaps expanding their choices and altering their realities.

Much of what makes nursing unique resides in our presence in people's lives when they are in crisis, as during illness and hospitalization, and when the nurse is the most qualified health professional available, as in some community-based practices. Nursing's ready access to clients' experiences is clearly a unique and fortunate twist for our qualitative researchers in several ways. Nurse researchers have clinical interviewing skills, for example, that transfer nicely in research interviews, and they may find that gaining access to informants is relatively easy, based on the general public's perceptions of nurses. Further, the nurse who combines his or her research with practice has the resource of different kinds of data that nurses and patients generate and use in the course of nursing care. The idea of combined purposes of clinical nursing and clinical research in the same situation has been opened up for exploration and is well worth the effort needed to address the ethical and logistical questions associated with the idea. Gadow (1977) described the nurse's range of awarenesses in the clinical situation; they include empathic and sympathetic, aesthetic and ethical, and scientific and objective awarenesses. Attending a patient through a night when he has pain and cannot sleep has the potential of yielding different and infinitely richer data than the most carefully executed qualitative interview. Benner (1983, 1985) has explicated the nurse's contextual knowledge in a number of patient care situations that illustrate how that knowledge is used in nursing practice. Her idea of "uncovering the knowledge embedded in clinical practice" refers to this understanding that meanings (1) inhere in situations and (2) both constitute and are constituted by those situations. Case studies in particular have been too infrequently used to aggrandize the nurse clinician's role in knowledge development.

The idea in qualitative research of researcher-as-instrument refers to several philosophical roots. Primarily, it refers to:

1. The tenet that humans are capable of exercising a variety of modes of awareness. Method is developed with this in mind, and strategies are used to maximize the researcher's range of modes of awareness.

2. The understanding that realities are constituted in a welded subject–object relation.

Qualitative researchers know that their findings are a function of the research context they create as well as the broader context of the phenomenon under study for the participant and for the researcher. In addition to searching for participant expressions that will help to disclose the phenomenon, the researcher plans strategies to track his or her subjectivity throughout the project. This contributes to the control of possible researcher distortions, but its greater value resides in "treating it as data to be analyzed for the information that it contains and contributes to the study" (Drew, 1989, p. 436).

When we request research subjects to tell us anything, we are requesting them to reflect on experience. Meanings are constituted in the particular perspective taken up in reflection. When we ask "What is it like for you when you become 'short of breath out-of-the-blue,' as you say?," the respondent looks back on the experience by taking on a mode of awareness that establishes a particular perspective. The respondent may, for example, regard the experience from a spiritual mode of awareness. The meaning that is constituted will be a function of that awareness, and the response to the question will be an expression shaped by the meaning. The fact that people often shift about from one mode of awareness to another will limit what can be learned from a single, short interview. An informant who is reflective by nature may have one thing to say today and another thing (perhaps contradictory) tomorrow.

When interviewing is used in qualitative research, in view of the task of grasping the complexity of another's reality, it can readily be seen that the success of the interview as an interpersonal dialogue has everything to do with how successfully the researcher obtains the desired data. Thus, a grasp of the elusiveness and complexity of human realities constitutes the philosophical root of the two qualitative features of collecting data (1) in subjects' natural settings and (2) over a protracted period of time. Merely interviewing people does not place a study in the qualitative paradigm. The nature of the relationship between researcher and researched and the process of the interview determine the data. As Newman stated, the process is the content (1990, p. 38).

SUMMARY

Although new and still emerging for us, qualitative research approaches have been receiving considerable attention for some time in other disciplines. Along with philosophical debates, there are debates about whether there needs to be a debate. On a philosophical level, there is irreconcilable conflict between the quantitative and qualitative paradigms. It is important to recognize this conflict, avoiding illogical compromise. Yet, proponents of each paradigm need to applaud both the existence of the other and the hybrid paradigms that inevitably are born of conflict. An apt beginning would be broader definitions of what constitutes science and research in nursing, eliminating the sense-organ bias that is so contrary to our philosophy for practice. This alone would provide qualitative nurse researchers with the sanction they need to progress in their exploration of various approaches to creating a science and a body of knowledge in, for, and about nursing practice.

In the chapters to follow, readers will be introduced to several qualitative research approaches. Each approach represents an interpretation of the qualitative paradigm in nursing research, grounded in the general perspective of phenomenological philosophy. This perspective focuses on phenomena as they appear and recognizes that reality is subjective and a matter of appearances for us in our social world. Subjectivity means that the world becomes real through our contact with it and acquires meaning through our interpretations of that contact. Truth, then, is a composite of realities, and access to truth is a problem of access to human subjectivity. This perspective guides the qualitative researcher in nursing to the subject matter of lived experiences, which are the original contacts with a world, and of the processes and content of interpretation—the meaning attributions that constitute realities and perspectives for a future of possibilities in the world. Other consequences of a phenomenological perspective in research include deliberate attention to the researcher's involvement in the study, engagement of multiple modes of awareness, and creative expression of findings. The product of efforts to establish a phenomenological baseline, a thorough and accurate description of nursing phenomena (a task that remains forever incomplete), will be clarified nursing concepts. If we encourage our qualitative nurse researchers, we can look forward to enhanced relevance in theoretical and empirical comments about nursing from studies guided by a mature nursing identity.

REFERENCES

Allen, D. (1985). Nursing research and social control: Alternative models of science that emphasize understanding and emancipation. *Image: The Journal of Nursing Scholarship, 17*(2), 58–64.

Benner, P. (1983). Uncovering the knowledge embedded in clinical practice. *Image: The Journal of Nursing Scholarship, 19*, 21–34.

Benner, P. (1985). Quality of life: A phenomenological perspective on explanation, prediction, and understanding in nursing science. *Advances in Nursing Science, 8*(1), 1–14.

Bogdan, R., & Biklen, S. (1982). *Qualitative research for education: An introduction to theory and methods.* Boston: Allyn & Bacon.

Bogdan, R., & Taylor, S. (1975). *Introduction to qualitative methods.* New York: Wiley.

Copel, L. (1984). *Loneliness: A clinical investigation.* Unpublished doctoral dissertation, Texas Woman's University, Denton.

Drew, N. (1989). The interviewer's experience as data in phenomenological research. *Western Journal of Nursing Research, 11*(4), 431–439.

Gadow, S. (1977, November 11). *Existential advocacy: Philosophical foundation of nursing.* Phase I Conference, Four-State Consortium on Nursing and the Humanities, Farmington, CT.

Glaser, B., & Strauss, A. (1967). *The discovery of grounded theory.* Chicago: Aldine.

Hutchinson, S. (1986). Creating meaning: Grounded theory of NICU nurses. In Chenitz & Swanson, *From practice to grounded theory* (pp. 191–204). Menlo Park, CA: Addison-Wesley.

Katzman, E., & Roberts, J. (1988). Nurse–physician conflicts as barriers to the enactment of nursing roles. *Western Journal of Nursing Research, 10*(5), 576–590.

Knafl, K., & Howard, M. (1986). Interpreting, reporting and evaluating qualitative research. In P. Munhall & C. Oiler, (Eds.). *Nursing research: A qualitative perspective.* Norwalk, CT: Appleton-Century-Crofts.

Kramer, M. (1968). Role models, role conception, and role deprivation. *Nursing Research, 17,* 115–120.

Lather, P. (1986). Research as praxis. *Harvard Educational Review, 56*(3), 257–277.

Lincoln, Y., & Guba, E. (1985). *Naturalistic inquiry.* Newbury, CA: Sage.

Merleau-Ponty, M. (1962). *Phenomenology of perception* (C. Smith, Trans.). New York: Humanities Press.

Munhall, P. (1982). Nursing philosophy and nursing research: In apposition or opposition? *Nursing Research, 31,* 176–177, 181.

National League for Nursing. (1988). *Curriculum revolution: Mandate for change.* New York: National League for Nursing.

Newman, M. (1990). Newman's theory of health as praxis. *Nursing Science Quarterly, 3*(1), 37–41.

Oiler, C. (1982). The phenomenological approach in nursing research. *Nursing Research, 31,* 178–181.

Oiler, C. (1986). Qualitative methods: Phenomenology. In P. Moccia (Ed.), *New approaches to theory development* (pp. 75–103). New York: National League for Nursing.

Parse, R. (1990). Parse's research methodology with an illustration of the lived experience of hope. *Nursing Science Quarterly, 3*(1), 9–17.

Paterson, J., & Zderad, L. (1976). *Humanistic nursing.* New York: Wiley.

Patton, M. (1980). *Qualitative evaluation methods.* Newbury, CA: Sage.

Quint, J. (1967). *The nurse and the dying patient.* New York: Macmillan.

Schutz, A. (1970). *On phenomenology and social relations* (H. Wagner, Ed.). Chicago: University of Chicago Press.

Schutz, A. (1973). *Collected papers I: The problem of social reality* (M. Natanson, Ed.). The Hague: Martinus Nijhoff.

Sharts-Engel, N. (1989). An American experience of pregnancy and childbirth in Japan. *Birth, 16*(2), 81–86.

Tinkle, M., & Beaton, J. (1983). Toward a new view of science: Implications for nursing research. *Advances in Nursing Science, 5,* 27–36.

ADDITIONAL REFERENCES

Oiler, C. (1983). Nursing reality as reflected in nurses' poetry. *Perspectives in Psychiatric Care 21*(3), 81–89.

Quint, J. (1966). Awareness of death and the nurse's composure. *Nursing Research, 15,* 49–55.

Part Two

Qualitative Approaches in Nursing Research

In the following chapters, the reader is invited to consider and enjoy the presentations of qualitative methods included in this volume. Many of the contributors are among those leaders who first ventured into uncharted territories where there were few maps or guidelines to interpret the methods in nursing. They undertook the challenge capably and have succeeded in establishing for nursing the significance and worth of qualitative study.

Part Two can be read from at least two perspectives. First, the method and illustration chapters are important and fascinating in themselves. Properly, they inform us about a wide range of topics. Second, aside from the wealth of information about patients, nurses, the research process as it is carried through, and the idea of nursing as a science, the chapters in Part Two clearly and in considerable detail provide an introduction to five important qualitative research methods.

From the second perspective, which is more aligned with the primary purpose of this text, the reader will grow to understand and to appreciate qualitative approaches to research. Nevertheless, the significance of the studies included in Part Two and the power of their findings are the best rationale for, at the very least, a profound respect for the work of qualitative researchers in nursing. The arrangement of a method chapter followed by an illustrative study provides an opportunity to witness the influence of the research purpose on design and style of reporting. The variety available to us in this volume creates an occasion to contemplate other possibilities in our efforts to produce and communicate research findings that illuminate the complexities of the nursing world. The grounding of the qualitative paradigm is thus realized through the presentation of accomplishments and the possibilities awakened by those accomplishments.

4

Phenomenology: The Method

Carolyn Oiler Boyd

*I*n this chapter, overviews of the various interpretations of phenomenological method in nursing will be presented with the expectation that readers who wish to make the method their own will follow through on leads to other writings and other thinkers, in order to acquire a thorough understanding of any one or more of these interpretations. Despite the many meanings of phenomenological method, an effort will be made to distinguish it as a method, in contrast to other qualitative approaches. These distinctions are the author's interpretations and are very much guided by a shared longer-range goal of making phenomenology work well for us in nursing research—that is, of extrapolating nursing research methodology from phenomenology. Phenomenology invites this kind of effort and insists on an openness that can protect us from reducing such ideas about method to dogma.

The discussion picks up where the presentation of phenomenological themes left off in the preceding chapter. Phenomenology will be defined first as a philosophical method with an emphasis on its defining characteristics. Overviews of selected modifications of phenomenology in social science will then be presented to acquaint the reader with the cluster of research approaches that may be properly referred to as phenomenologies in nursing.

WHAT IS PHENOMENOLOGY?

As noted in the preceding chapter, phenomenology is a word that is used in a wide variety of ways, obfuscating efforts to locate a clear response to the question, "What is phenomenology?" Merleau-Ponty, in a 1956 publication, acknowledged that phenomenology has not managed to define itself, and began his defining comments by noting:

> [P]henomenology was practiced and recognized as a manner or style, . . . it existed as a movement before arriving at a complete philosophical consciousness. It has been on the way for a long time, and its disciples find it everywhere: in Hegel and Kierkegaard certainly, but also in Marx, Nietzsche and Freud. . . . It is in ourselves that we will find the unity and true meaning of phenomenology. . . . Phenomenology is accessible only to a phenomenological method . . . . [Through a deliberate synthesis of phenomenological themes], [p]erhaps then we will understand why phenomenology has remained so long in a state of beginning, a task yet to be accomplished. (pp. 59-60)

Phenomenology has a long history as a general way of thinking among a number of theorists who had profound impact on Western culture. Almost as a kind of attitude or a set of predilections that produce a certain style, we can identify many ideas and ways of thinking about things that are phenomenological in spirit. It is first, then, a continuing intellectual movement, an attitude, a style of regarding the world that in itself has been pervasively influential in the social sciences. For overviews of phenomenology as a movement, Cohen (1987) and Reeder (1987) are excellent sources in the nursing literature. For a fuller account, Spiegelberg (1976, 1981, 1982), a phenomenologist and historian of phenomenology, is the most widely used reference.

Phenomenology is more than a general movement; it has arrived at a "complete philosophical consciousness." Merleau-Ponty directed readers who seek definition to the task of comprehending the themes of phenomenological philosophy. Simply, in order to know what phenomenology is, one must know the themes that constitute the philosophy. Some of these themes were identified in the preceding chapter as the philosophical foundations of the qualitative paradigm generally. Others, notably phenomenological description and bracketing and phenomenological reduction, will be discussed in this chapter. These themes speak directly to phenomenological method, and, as Merleau-Ponty stated, phenomenology is accessible only through its method. The grounding in phenomenology is, in other words, in its philosophy and its method. Readers are advised to take advantage of the various presentations of phenomenology in the nursing literature (Anderson, 1989; Benner, 1983, 1985; Davis, 1973; Oiler, 1982, 1986, 1988; Omery, 1983; Parse, Coyne, & Smith, 1985; Parse, 1990; Paterson & Zderad, 1976; Ray, 1985). It is important to recognize, however, that these nurse authors' efforts to present and explain are not substitutes for the readers' efforts to get inside the phenomenological framework and to see from there what becomes visible concerning those phenomena of interest in nursing. The process of struggling to see is, in other words, phenomenological method.

Social science modifications of phenomenological method aside, it is reasonable to question how relevant phenomenological method, in its strict philosophical sense, is to nursing research. This judgment does not hold for qualitative research in general; we need to turn heartily toward the qualitative paradigm not only in nursing research but also in nursing education and nursing practice. To the extent that the qualitative paradigm is assumed by the nursing profession, there will be phenomenological study in nursing, in accord with phenomenological method as philosophical method. However, these will be intimately related with other kinds of research (particularly those inspired by phenomenological philosophy) that are pursued in the interest of a variety of nursing practice aims. In other words, this optimistic view of a perfect world rewards us with a vision of coherence within the nursing discipline.

METHODOLOGICAL THEMES

In addition to the phenomenological themes presented in the preceding chapter as foundational to qualitative research, others will be described here to disclose common features across the variety of phenomenologies that collectively indicate something of the scope of phenomenology. Progress toward clarity in the definition will be made by narrowing the sense of the word if not by achieving precision for its use. Recurring ideas among authors delineate an area of consensus that will help us to establish some kind of boundary for what is to be considered phenomenological research in nursing as opposed to other qualitative research approaches. A particular boundary will be proposed, but in the spirit of continuing consideration of criteria for phenomenologies in nursing.

Aim: Phenomenological Description

Merleau-Ponty (1956, p. 59) stated that the whole effort of phenomenology is to describe experience as it is and to describe it directly, without considering the various causal explanations that social scientists may give. This seems simple enough, but the difficulty resides in the meaning of experience as consciousness or existence itself. Husserl (in a 1965 translation) argued for phenomenology as rigorous science and explained that the focus on experience in phenomenology does not coincide with a natural science about consciousness:

> [P]sychology is concerned with "empirical consciousness," with consciousness from the empirical point of view, as an empirical being in the ensemble of nature, whereas phenomenology is concerned with "pure" consciousness, i.e., consciousness from the phenomenological point of view. (p. 91)

Experience is "something psychical, a 'phenomenon' comes and goes; it retains no enduring, identical being that can be objectively determinable as such in the sense of natural science, e.g., as objectively divisible into components, 'analysable' in the proper sense." Experience "appears as itself through itself, in an absolute flow, as now and already 'fading away,' clearly recognizable as constantly sinking back into a 'having been'" (p. 107). Experience can be recalled, having been perceived at some point in time.

For Merleau-Ponty (1962), the world is not perceived through a combination of sensations and perspectives. Reality is not constituted by perceiving representations of reality. Coherence in the world is lived. Relation with the world is a living and nonirreducible impulse that is understandable only as a unified experience. It is not knowledge of the world such as posed by an analysis of sensation. Perception is original awareness of the appearances of phenomena in experience. It is defined as access to truth, the foundation of all knowledge. Perception gives one access to experience of the world as it is given prior to any analysis of it. "To perceive is to render oneself present to something through the body; all the while the thing keeps its place within the horizon of the world" (p. 42). The focus on experience in phenomenology is, then, a focus on human involvement in a world; the oft used term "lived experience" emphasizes this focus. Phenomenology recognizes that meanings are given in perception and modified in analysis. "By these words, 'primacy of perception,' we mean that the experience of perception is our presence at the moment when things, truths, values are constituted for us" (p. 25). Perception presents us with evidence of the world, not as it is thought but as it is lived. Perception of an amputated limb as an ambivalent presence is not truth, but it is reality. It is this evidence that is considered to be the foundation of science and knowledge. Beyond this, there is nothing to understand (p. 365).

In essence, phenomenologists hold that human existence is meaningful and of interest only in the sense that we are always conscious of something. Existence as being-in-the-world is a phenomenological phrase that acknowledges that people are tied to their worlds and are comprehensible only in their contexts. Human behavior occurs in the context of relationships to things, people, events, and situations, in what Merleau-Ponty refers to as embodiment. People, in all their subjectivity, are inseparably caught up in the physical world in such a way that the truth we search for in nursing research efforts will be grasped only by attending to the realities constituted in individual experiencing. Lived experience is, however, layered with meanings that are brought to the relation of being-in-the-world. This occurs through the attention to life taken up in experience, which is to take up a perspective in the world.

> *Man finds himself at any moment of his daily life in a biographically determined situation, that is, in a physical and sociocultural environment as defined by him, within which he has his position, not merely his position in terms of physical space and outer time or of his status and role within the social system but also his moral and ideological positions. (Schutz, 1970, p. 73)*

Seeing experience directly is thus not strictly possible, on two grounds: first, experiencing is living forward and, to be self-conscious, it must be suspended to yield to the experience of reflecting back on it; and second, to suspend one's biography is to lose one's tie to the world. We can, however, become more self-conscious in reflection and resist the ready-made interpretations offered up by our biography in order to see more clearly the ties we have to the world.

Farber (1966) noted that a purely descriptive method is an ideal with numerous obstacles:

> *It is the aim of description to give an account of all the pertinent facts; it cannot be an account of all the facts, because the facts are infinite in number. . . . There are not only the difficulties resulting from the individual or the group which conditions him, but also the problems caused by the facts themselves; and there is the necessity of weighing the evidence of events which continue to recede into the past. (pp. 45–46)*

We are limited by our "blinkers" and "spectacles"; that is, we see the world as an already interpreted phenomenon, the result of past scientific inquiry and fixed traditional conceptions. For Farber, the nature of perception and of other modes of experience is the proper theme of phenomenological inquiry (pp. 48–49). In contrast to the interpretations of phenomenology in the social sciences, this delineation of the aim of phenomenology limits it to philosophical inquiry into acts of consciousness themselves. Merleau-Ponty's (1962) phenomenology of perception is such an inquiry. Zderad's (1968) philosophical dissertation on empathy is another example. Other acts of consciousness that would be included in the realm of phenomenology from Farber's point of view are remembering, judging, intuiting, and valuing. The phenomenological questions concern how these ways of attending to the world are possible.

Merleau-Ponty (1956) stated that perception:

[I]s the basis from which every act issues and it is presupposed by them. The world is not an object the law of whose constitution I possess. It is the natural milieu and the field of all my thoughts and of all my explicit perceptions. Truth does not "dwell" only in the "interior man" for there is no interior man. Man is before himself in the world and it is in the world that he knows himself. When I turn upon myself from the dogmatism of common sense or the dogmatism of science, I find, not the dwelling place of intrinsic truth, but a subject committed to the world. (p. 62)

• • •

The evidence of perception is condemned to meaning. (p. 69)

All description of experience is thus inescapably interpretive. The various techniques that can be used in phenomenological method serve, in the unity of knower and known, to forward the project of seeing a phenomenon and the project of describing what has been seen. Phenomenological description is the final "step" of phenomenological method; in it, the other steps taken (and the degree of success with which they were accomplished) are reflected such that the process is the content. The nature of the task of description in phenomenology can thus be understood only through a grasp of antecedent steps of phenomenological method.

Bracketing and the Phenomenological Reduction

The process of recovering original awareness (perception) is called "reduction" in phenomenology. Phenomenological reduction is a particular manner of rigorous reflection, and bracketing is the leading methodological technique used in phenomenology to aid in this process. In order to describe lived experience, it must first be disclosed. Bracketing and phenomenological reduction are the means to this disclosure. Merleau-Ponty (1956) described the scope of this task:

> Our relation to the world is so profound and so intimate that the only way for us to notice it is to suspend its movements, to refuse it our complicity . . . or to render it inoperative. (p. 64)

He instructed us to make our presuppositions and common sense appear by deliberately abstaining from them. He advised us to be astonished before the world; in other words, to describe lived experience, we must set aside the natural attitude toward the world that our biography has given us. In astonishment, the layers of meaning given by interpretation, knowledge, and explanation are carefully preserved but laid aside. Our ties to the world in roles, knowledge, belief, habit, common sense, and the like are disrupted in order to make them apparent. Bracketing our presuppositions about the world is performed "not to deny them and even less to deny the link which binds us to the physical, social and cultural world" (Merleau-Ponty, 1964, p. 49). The reduction is performed in order to expose the link.

What is revealed in phenomenological reduction, then, is not "pure" experience; rather, it is experience constituted in one's ties to the world. Complete reduction is impossible because consciousness is engaged in a world. Phenomenological description is always contingent on the perspective given in experience and presented in perception. People are "always situated and always individuated" (Merleau-Ponty, 1964, p. 51). In the reflection of reduction, which strives to freeze time and suspend acts of consciousness, time nevertheless continues. There is always, in phenomenological description, then, the layer of this experience in time, the study of the experience that has just passed. "Our existence is too strictly caught up in the world to know itself as such at the moment when it is thrown forth upon the world" (Merleau-Ponty, 1956, p. 65). For this reason, phenomenological reduction and description will yield incomplete profiles of reality because "one never goes beyond time" (Merleau-Ponty, 1964, p. 49).

Schutz (1973) illuminated the complex idea of reduction by acknowledging that, although the technique of bracketing in reduction is extremely difficult, it is yet within human capability. In performing the reduction, one assumes an attitude of doubt toward the world:

What we have to put in brackets is not only the existence of an outer world, along with all the things in it, inanimate and animate, including fellow-men, cultural objects, society and its institutions. Also our belief in the validity of our statements about this world and its content, as conceived within the mundane sphere, has to be suspended. Consequently, not only our practical knowledge of the world but also the propositions of all the sciences dealing with the existence of the world, all natural and social sciences, psychology, logic and even geometry—all have to be brought within the brackets. (p. 105)

As the layers of meaning that give us interpreted experience are bracketed, the perceived world emerges. In the reduced sphere, objects appear in a figure–ground relation, with each object having a horizon that implicates other objects in a meaningful system of relations. This is the meaning of holism, and perception is the level at which holism occurs. Intuition figures prominently in grasping this meaningful system of relations as a mode of awareness that adheres closely to the perceived world.

Phenomenological reduction is a matter of refraining from judgments. Schutz's (1973) description of the natural attitude as layers of meaning helps us to understand that reduction is a process that can be used in degrees. Layers can be peeled away one at a time. Perception can be revealed relative to a painstaking effort to peel away some of our ready-made interpretations of experience:

> *Our knowledge of an object, at a certain given moment, is nothing else than the sediment of previous mental processes by which it has been constituted. It has its own history, and this history of its constitution can be found by questioning it. This is done by turning back from the seemingly ready-made object of our thought to the different activities of our mind in which and by which it has been constituted step by step. (p. 111)*

In its most important sense, phenomenological method is a call to reflective thoughtfulness of the most rigorous kind, at the most rigorous level. The point of the effort is to return to the natural attitude where insights gained within the reduced sphere can be put to use (Schutz, 1970, p. 59).

Essential Elements

In a description of the characteristic core in the various phenomenologies, Spiegelberg (1976) identified seven steps of phenomenological method. He noted that the first of these steps, investigating particular phenomena, is easily the most adoptable and has a completeness of its own. There are three operations in this step: intuiting, analyzing, and describing. Of the first operation, he wrote:

> *[Intuiting] is one of the most demanding operations, which requires utter concentration on the object intuited without*

*becoming absorbed in it to the point of no longer looking
critically. Nevertheless there is little that the beginning phenomenologist can be given by way of precise instructions
beyond such metaphoric phrases as "opening his eyes,"
"keeping them open," "not getting blinded," "looking and listening," etc. (pp. 659-660)*

Comparing and contrasting the phenomenon under investigation
with related phenomena, and studying phenomenologists' approaches to and accounts of phenomena are also offered as aids in
learning to perform the operation of intuiting a phenomenon.

The second operation of investigating particular phenomena,
phenomenological analyzing, involves identifying the structure of
the phenomenon under study. Anderson (1989) drew our attention
to the problem of knowing what is meant by the term "structure."
She argued that the problem is not so much knowing what the nature of structure is as it is identifying *whose* structures are being
described:

It is not as if the researcher is describing structures that are
out there and are independent of the researcher and informant. . . . *[W]hat needs to be made explicit is that the
structures described are those that one creates and imposes
on the world—these structures are embedded in the system
of relevances of the researcher;* which gets produced *as
knowledge results from the dialectical process between researcher and informant. (pp. 22-23)*

In her discussion, Anderson alluded to the difficulty introduced in
phenomenology when experience is studied vicariously, as is the
case in the social sciences. (Readers may wish to see Spiegelberg's
discussion of phenomenology through vicarious experience for
another treatment of this difficulty (1975, pp. 35-53).) Anderson
stressed that knowledge is created ideally in a joint project in
which the researcher and the researched are mutually committed
to describing the phenomenon under study. The structure that is
identified through phenomenological analyzing is, in the end, the
researcher's structure. It is an identification of the phenomenon's

elements and of the relations and connections of those elements to adjacent phenomena.

The third operation of investigating particular phenomena, phenomenological describing, is undertaken after phenomenological seeing has been accomplished through intuiting and analyzing the phenomenon.

> *Phenomenology begins in silence. Only he who has experienced genuine perplexity and frustration in the face of the phenomena when trying to find the proper description for them knows what phenomenological seeing really means. (Spiegelberg, 1976, p. 672)*

Spiegelberg cautioned that premature description is, in fact, one of the main pitfalls of phenomenology. The aim of this describing operation is to communicate: to guide the listener by giving distinctive guideposts to the phenomenon. The description serves to direct the listener to his own experience of the phenomenon, whether actual or potential:

> *Describing is based on a classification of the phenomena. A description, therefore, presupposes a framework of class names, and all it can do is to determine the location of the phenomenon with regard to an already developed system of classes. (p. 673)*

In the case of new phenomena or new aspects of familiar phenomena, there will not be any such existent framework to house the description. Spiegelberg advised that description by negation, metaphor, and analogy can then be used cautiously to indicate the phenomena in a suggestive manner. Phenomenological description is always necessarily selective and, as such, always represents a particular perspective or interpretation of the phenomenon under study.

To perform the reduction is to choose to perceive from another vantage point; one seizes experience and lives it through for oneself in phenomenological analyzing. Insight is communicated in the description. In performing the reduction, one suspends his or her preconceptions in order to explore the phenomenon not from what is known about it but from what might be so. Merleau-Ponty (1964) referred to this process as the imaginary free variation of certain facts:

> *In order to grasp an essence, we consider a concrete experience, and then we make it change in our thought, trying to imagine it as effectively modified in all respects. That which remains invariable through these changes is the essence of the phenomena in question. (p. 70)*

The task of phenomenological analyzing is a matter of identifying those elements of a phenomenon that entail a relation which, if omitted, would annihilate the phenomenon; that is, that which is essential for the phenomenon to *be* is isolated. This is a process akin to induction. Merleau-Ponty pointed out that the difference between induction and phenomenological reduction and description is a matter of degree. However incomplete phenomenological descriptions may be, to the extent that they succeed in disclosing experiences from some points of view, they bring us closer to understanding lived experiences.

Spiegelberg (1976) asserted that intuiting, analyzing, and describing particulars may be considered a common program for those who identify themselves as phenomenologists. The scope of phenomenology, however, goes beyond the study of particulars to include investigating general essences, essential relationships among essences, modes of appearing, and the constitution of phenomena in consciousness; suspending belief in the existence of phenomena; and interpreting the meaning of phenomena. Investigation of general essences and relationships among essences refers to looking at particulars as examples or instances to apprehend their natural affinity in a common pattern shared by particular phenomena that belong together in a natural grouping. Based on antecedent or simultaneous intuiting of particulars, this extension of phenomenology to a concern with essences draws on seeing particulars in their structural affinities. Their pattern or essence is the ground of those structural affinities (Spiegelberg, 1976, p. 678). When an essence is apprehended, the next step can be attempted:

a search for relationships within an essence or among several essences. Throughout, the operations of intuiting, analyzing, and describing must be performed. In the phenomenological steps of watching modes of appearing and exploring the constitution of phenomena in consciousness, phenomenology directs its attention not only to the sense of what appears, but also to the way in which things appear, establish themselves, and take shape in consciousness. The step of suspending belief is phenomenological reduction and has been discussed earlier. Lastly, the step of interpreting concealed meanings, refers to the attempt to interpret the sense of certain phenomena. Spiegelberg (1976) noted that this effort has been focused and developed in hermeneutic phenomenology, a particular type of phenomenology. In a sense, all of phenomenology is concerned with meaning and interpretation:

> For not only our purposive behavior but our whole cognitive and emotional life, as phenomenology sees it, is shot through with meaning and meaningful intentions. No description can leave them out, even though it may refrain from accepting them at face value. Thus hermeneutic phenomenology must aim at something different and more ambitious: its goal is the discovery of meanings which are not immediately manifest to our intuiting, analyzing, and describing. Hence the interpreter has to go beyond what is directly given. (p. 695)

The appearance of references to hermeneutic phenomenology in the nursing literature needs to be understood as one way in which to practice phenomenology (Allen & Jensen, 1990; Benner, 1985; Leonard, 1989; Parse et al., 1985). The common theme among the various phenomenologies is the concern for describing lived experience, which is understood to be a concern for human meanings and ultimately for interpreting those meanings so that they inform our practice and our science. The variations in accounts of phenomenology among nurse authors is best understood in terms of recognizing the many ways to phenomenology and the exercise of choice among these paths in the design and conduct of a phenomenological study.

CRITERIA FOR PHENOMENOLOGIES

The divergencies of the various phenomenologists in their interpretations and prescriptions for phenomenological method are further embellished in the various translations and modifications of phenomenology in social science; they have made phenomenology an increasingly broad approach with multiple paths. For both the observer and the learner of qualitative approaches, acquaintance with the common ground of phenomenology assists with consideration of interpretations of method. Spiegelberg (1975) proposed a set of seven criteria for distinguishing phenomenological inquiry from other approaches (pp. 10-12). These will be discussed briefly as a point of reference for consideration of selected interpretations of phenomenological method in nursing and for a closer look at some of the particulars associated with those interpretations. Although the criteria are not sacrosanct, they do at least establish a framework for considering phenomenological method in its many variations. Over time, as phenomenological methods are used in nursing, other criteria may emerge to designate more aptly what phenomenological method is for nursing.

Spiegelberg emphasized the aim of phenomenology as the premise for his comments on characteristics of phenomenologies: to give access to layers of our experience unprobed in our everyday living, thus providing deeper foundations for both science and life. The first characteristic of phenomenologies, then, is the focus on concretely experienced phenomena, as free as possible from conceptual presuppositions. The performance of phenomenological reduction to achieve a fresh approach to the study of experience distinguishes phenomenology clearly from the positivist tradition, but is less powerful in distinguishing it from other qualitative approaches. This is due, in part, to the influence of phenomenological method on aspects of other approaches to qualitative research. The notion of bracketing, for example, is featured in all qualitative research designs.

The second characteristic is the inclusion of nonsensuous data as well as sense experience. Nonsensuous data include relations, abstract entities, and values, for example, as long as they present themselves intuitively. An intuitive foundation and verification for all formal concepts is the third characteristic, and resistance to transforming the given in interpretation is the fourth. The central role of intuition in phenomenology presents a quandary for us. Little understood and thus suspect, intuition is associated with a lack of rigor. Nevertheless, it introduces to research a unique relation between researcher and researched. Figure 4-1 represents this by contrasting researcher (R) and subject (S) relations among quantitative, qualitative, and phenomenological approaches to inquiry. In phenomenology, researcher and subject join in reflection on the experience under study, creating the circumstances for the researcher's inclusion in the study. Two nursing studies come to mind as illustrations of this: Lynch-Sauer (1985) described the introduction of her diary entries as data in a study of postponed child-bearing; Drew (1989) described the use of her personal responses in the interviewing process as data in a study of patients' experiences with caregivers.

The fifth characteristic is attention to the distinctions of the phenomena reflected in shades of ordinary language without sole reliance on language as a basis for study. The sixth and seventh characteristics concern producing as faithful a description as possible with cautious objectification of experience and responsible generalization based on insight into the relations between concrete experiences and abstractions.

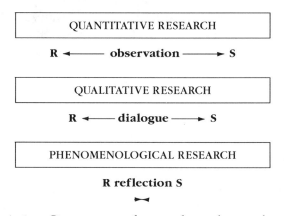

Figure 4-1.   Comparison of researcher-subject relationship.

PHENOMENOLOGICAL METHODS
FOR SOCIAL SCIENCE

An overview of selected interpretations of phenomenological method will be presented to extend its description and to indicate its openness to interpretation as well as, indirectly, to point out some of the difficulties with this research approach. All these interpretations have been influenced by hermeneutic phenomenology to varying extents; all bear unique modifications to accommodate the aims of social science.

The Search for Structure and Essence in Experience

Phenomenological psychology introduces several interpretations for method taken up by a number of qualitative nurse researchers. Van Kaam's (1959) study of "really feeling understood" focuses on a psychological phenomenon and seeks to disclose the core of this experience. The research process in van Kaam's phenomenology requires posing the research question to a large number of subjects who are asked to respond by writing descriptions of their experiences with regard to a select phenomenon. It is presumed that people can express lived experience in such a way, and that analysis of their descriptions will reveal an essential structure (core) of the human experience under study. Once the researcher obtains the descriptions from willing subjects, the analysis proceeds as follows:

1. Each expression (word or phrase) that describes some aspect of the experience is listed separately from the others.
2. Similar expressions are grouped together and labeled.
3. Irrelevant expressions are eliminated.
4. Groups of expressions that bear close relationship to one another are clustered together and labeled.
5. The identified core of common elements is checked against a random sample of original descriptions by subjects. Discrepancies at this point direct the researcher to start again with the analysis.

6. The steps of analysis (1–5) are performed independently by judges to check the reliability of the results.

The essential structure of really feeling understood was reported in the following statement:

> *The experience of really feeling understood is a perceptual-emotional gestalt: a subject, perceiving that a person co-experiences what things mean to the subject and accepts him, feels, initially, relief from experiential loneliness, and gradually, safe experiential communion with that person and with that which the subject perceives this person to represent. (van Kaam, 1959, p. 69)*

The full report of findings includes justification and explanation of each phrase of the description of the essential structure.

A number of published nursing studies have used van Kaam's approach to phenomenology, often with some modifications of the process. These modifications usually are reduced sample size and/or the substitution or addition of interview for the written description. Sandelowski and Pollock (1986), for example, interviewed 48 women to identify recurring themes in their experiences of infertility treatment. Those themes were ambiguity, temporality, and otherness. The description of the experience of infertility pivots around these three themes (elements) and includes elaboration on varying expressions of them by participants in the study (p. 142).

In Colaizzi's (1978) interpretation of the method, interview is the selected strategy for generating data. Often, lengthy and repeated interviews are necessary to facilitate subjects' descriptions of their experiences, thus accounting for there typically being fewer subjects in studies that use Colaizzi's approach. Haase (1987) used the Colaizzi method in her study of chronically ill adolescents' experiences of courage. She interviewed 9 chronically ill, hospitalized adolescents and analyzed transcripts of these interviews in a process similar to van Kaam's (described above). To illustrate this process of searching for themes in interview data, Haase (1987) reported the following example of abstractions from subjects' words:

Subject: "My mom just held my hand and talked to me. That made it better." Researcher's abstractions:
  1. *Mother holding hand and talking improved situation.*
  2. *Touch and verbal expressions of caring by mother decreased feelings of despair to a tolerable level. (p. 67)*

It can be seen from this example that the process of analysis is one of abstracting from subjects' words to formulate essential meanings in the experiences. Such meanings are grouped to constitute themes; themes are grouped into clusters; and clusters are grouped into categories. In Haase's study, 9 categories, 30 clusters, and an even larger number of descriptive themes within those clusters were identified. Figure 4-2 illustrates this inductive ordering of the data from the more concrete themes to the more abstract clusters and categories (Haase, 1987, pp. 77-78). This kind of inductive approach is a primary feature of both van Kaam's and Colaizzi's phenomenologies.

Perhaps because so much attention is given to analytic steps and because the data are formally limited to what people say in writing or in interview, both these phenomenologies appear to fall short of the criteria for phenomenologies described above. In Parse's

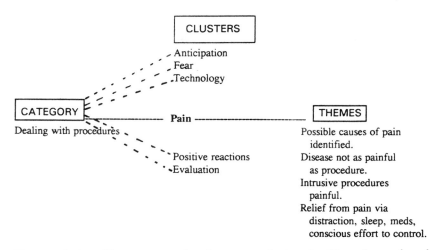

Figure 4-2. Illustration of inductive ordering in Haase's study of adolescent courage.

(1990) phenomenology, some of these shortcomings were addressed. Parse identified lived experiences of health such as feeling lonely and feeling joyful as the entities for study, and stated, as
the aim of phenomenology, understanding the structure of lived
experience. Four processes are used to accomplish this aim:

1. Participant selection to achieve redundancy in or saturation
   of the data. Two to ten participants are usually sufficient.
2. Dialogical engagement of researcher and participant in an
   unstructured discussion. The quality of this engagement is
   one of intersubjective "being with" the other.
3. Extraction–synthesis of the data so that descriptions given
   in participants' language are moved up to the level of abstraction of the language of science. This process involves
   attentive study of the transcribed discussions and creative
   conceptualization. Creative conceptualization in turn involves various operations of abstraction and synthesis of
   abstractions to generate a structure that identifies core concepts and their relationships to one another.
4. Heuristic interpretation of the finding of the study by relating it to Parse's man-living-health theory (pp. 10-12).

In a study of hope, Parse illustrated the use of her phenomenology. Ten patients were interviewed for 30 minutes or more while
receiving hemodialysis. The process of extraction–synthesis is illustrated below:

> Extracted essence: *While waiting for a 2nd kidney trans-
> plant, looks forward to his situation getting better as he re-
> members and wishes for a life without the machine.*
>
> Synthesized essence: *Anticipating is fostered by envisioning
> the was and will be as it is now.*
>
> Proposition: *The lived experience of hope is anticipating
> through envisioning the was and will be as it is now while
> engaging in activities that create harmony and unfold in a
> different perspective. (p. 13) Ten propositions were created;
> one for each participant. (p. 14)*

Extracted core concepts:

- *Anticipating possibilities through envisioning the not yet.*
- *Harmoniously living the comfort–discomfort of every-dayness.*
- *Unfolding a different perspective of an expanding view.*
  (p. 15)

The structure of the lived experience of hope, then, is: "Hope is anticipating possibilities through envisioning the not yet in harmoniously living the comfort–discomfort of everydayness while unfolding a different perspective of an expanding view" (p. 15). Each core concept is then interpreted in terms of Parse's principles: "Hope is the persistent picturing of possibles (imaging) while incarnating opportunities–limitations all at once (enabling-limiting) which unfolds in viewing the familiar in a new light (transforming)" (p. 16). Last came the conceptual interpretation: "Hope is imaging the enabling–limiting of transforming" (p. 16). Parse's man-living-health theory provides the overriding framework in her phenomenological method, a feature that is viewed by some as contributing to the grounding of phenomenological inquiry in a nursing perspective. For others, this feature bleeds the work of phenomenological reduction and, from this point of view, transgresses what is regarded as the hallmark of phenomenology.

The Search for Expanded Consciousness

In another style of the phenomenologies, the work of Paterson and Zderad (1976) and Benner (1983, 1985), and Van Manen's interpretation in education (1990), may be grouped loosely together in a contrast to the phenomenologies described above. In the author's view, these approaches are more closely aligned with phenomenological philosophy and with Spiegelberg's criteria for phenomenologies.

Phenomenology was first introduced to a wide nursing audience in Paterson and Zderad's *Humanistic Nursing* (1976), which by their own account was a collection of metatheoretical essays about the nature of nursing. The phases of their phenomenological method are:

1. *Preparation of the researcher:* The researcher needs to be an open, self-aware person. These qualities can be nurtured especially well by ongoing study in the humanities.

2. *Primary data collection:* Observations are made from *within* the situation under study. The researcher must therefore be a practicing nurse rather than an outside observer of nursing. Data will include firsthand observations inclusive of intuitive insights and empathic awarenesses.

3. *Scientific analysis:* The researcher conceptualizes and expresses understandings in a reflective turn toward the data collected from clinical experience.

4. *Scientific synthesis:* The researcher locates other related or similar situations (from past experience and in the literature) in order to compare and contrast the data with other known realities. This is an interpretive activity performed to sort and classify the data thematically.

5. *Abstraction:* The experience is finally conceptualized to account for its relatedness to other knowledge and its variations. Nursing knowledge is thus expanded, and the researcher as clinician is transformed in perspective. (pp. 76-81)

Paterson and Zderad's report of a study of comfort serves as an illustration of the use of their method for nursing research. Primary data were collected and recorded over several months from weekly interactions with 15 hospitalized psychiatric patients. Through reflective analysis and synthesis of these data, 12 nurse behaviors aimed toward patient comfort were identified, together with 4 criteria for estimating the degree of a patient's comfort and 52 items of knowledge needed by a nurse whose aim is to comfort (pp. 107-11, 123-129). The following theoretical construct of comfort emerged from this study:

Comfort is [a universal nursing] aim toward which persons' conditions of being move through relationship with others by internalizing freedom from painful controlling effects of the past. These effects have inhibited their self-control, realistic planning, and prevented them from being all that they could be in accordance with their potential at any particular time in any particular situation. (p. 111)

An outline of Paterson and Zderad's approach for conceptualization of nursing phenomena is presented in Figure 4-3. An intuitive grasp of a phenomenon is contingent on the researcher's openness to the phenomenon and encompasses the first two phases of the phenomenological method listed above (preparation

INTUITIVE GRASP	*Be Open to the Phenomenon* 1. Be aware of own view 2. Identify a priori notions and set aside 3. List different ways of looking at the phenomenon: • Objective–subjective • Passive–active 4. Be immersed in the arts and in evidences of the phenomenon wherever found 5. Observe from within the phenomenon
ANALYTIC EXAMINATION	*Consider Many Instances of Phenomenon* 1. Compare/contrast 2. Identify common elements/themes 3. Determine how elements are interrelated 4. Distinguish from and relate to similar phenomena
DESCRIPTION & SYNTHESIS	*Define, Describe, Construct* 1. Classify 2. Negate 3. Use metaphor 4. Use analogy 5. Isolate central characteristics 6. Synthesize

Note: Adapted from *Humanistic Nursing* (pp. 71-91) by J. Paterson and L. Zderad, 1976. New York: Wiley.

Figure 4–3. An approach for conceptualization of nursing phenomena.

of the researcher and primary data collection). The techniques listed as aids to an intuitive grasp reflect bracketing and the phenomenological reduction and use of the researcher's access to an array of modes of awareness. Analytic examination coincides with the third phase (scientific analysis) and directs the researcher to consider many instances of the phenomenon through techniques that have been noted in Spiegelberg's discussion of phenomenological analysis. Description and synthesis coincide with the fourth and fifth phases (scientific synthesis and abstraction). Again, the operation of phenomenological analysis is apparent in the techniques suggested to define, describe, and construct a conceptualization of the phenomenon under study. The overriding context for this phenomenology is the nursing situation; products of the inquiry speak directly to that context.

Benner (1985), Leonard (1989), and Allen and Jensen (1990) all provided presentations of hermeneutic phenomenology, one of the many possible groundings in phenomenology. The particular focus is on human nature as constituted by interpretive understanding (Leonard, 1989, p. 47), and the aim is understanding through interpretation of the phenomenon under study (Allen & Jensen, 1990, p. 242). Benner (1985) gave this overview:

> *The goal is to find exemplars or paradigm cases that embody the meanings of everyday practices. The data are participant observations, field notes, interviews, and unobtrusive samples of behavior and interaction in natural settings. Human behavior is treated as a text analogue and the task is to uncover the meanings in everyday practice in such a way that they are not destroyed, distorted, decontextualized, trivialized, or sentimentalized. (pp. 5-6)*

Familiar phenomenological themes ground the method. Lived human meanings are understood to constitute and to be constituted by one's experiences. Understanding human experience, then, requires attending to what Benner refers to as the transaction between the individual and the situation (p. 7).

Three phases of the research strategies of hermeneutic phenomenology were listed by Leonard (1989, pp. 53-55):

1. *Thematic analysis:* Interview material and observations are converted to text through transcription. A global analysis is performed to accomplish four tasks:

   a. Identify lines of inquiry from emerging themes and theoretical background of the study.

   b. Develop interpretive plan and coding protocol.

   c. Code the interviews.

   d. Identify general categories that form bases of study's findings.

2. *Analysis of exemplars:* An exemplar, by definition, is a "vignette or story of the particular transaction that captures the meaning in the situation" (Benner, 1985, p. 10) so that it is recognizable in other situations. It provides a presentation of the person in the context of his or her situation inclusive of "intentions of actors and meanings in the situation" (Benner, 1985, p. 10). In this phase, all aspects of a particular situation and the participant's responses to it are coded to capture the lived meanings of the participant's experiences.

3. *Identify paradigm cases:* A paradigm case, by definition, is a "strong instance of a particular pattern of meanings" (Benner, 1985, p. 10). In this phase of hermeneutics, analysis is carried forward to articulate both what the case depicts and why it stands out as an instance of a particular meaning. Paradigm cases are what Benner refers to as markers "so that once a paradigm case is recognized . . . other more subtle cases with similar global characteristics can be recognized" (p. 10). Presentation of a paradigm case provides the description necessary to understand how a person's actions and interpretations emerge from his or her situational context—that is, his or her concerns, practices, and background meanings. Beyond this, such a presentation provides what Leonard (1989, p. 54) referred to as a family resemblance between the paradigm case and a particular situation one is attempting to understand and explain.

Allen and Jensen (1990) illustrated the use of hermeneutics in a study of what it means to be visually impaired (pp. 246–249). In the context of interviews, these questions were addressed: What does it mean to have a visual impairment? How does the impairment affect day-to-day living? What changes have been made or will have to be made because of your visual impairment? What do you believe will happen in the future? Five major categories were identified to classify the data. These categories and the text as a whole were "used in a circular fashion to understand the meaning of visual impairment" (p. 247) in order to obtain a deeper awareness of participants' experiences. The identified categories served in this study to provide an organizational scheme for the narrative discussion of meanings associated with each category. The interpretive strategies of paradigm cases, exemplars, and thematic analysis served, as Benner noted, in the process of discovery of meaning as well as in the presentation of that meaning. They are distinct from grounded theory in that "the goal is not to extract theoretical terms or concepts at a higher level of abstraction" (Benner, 1985, p. 10); rather, the goal is to discover meaning and to achieve a deeper understanding of experience in the context of that meaning and the situation in which it occurs.

The last phenomenology to be considered here is Van Manen's human science (1990). Van Manen identified his phenomenology as hermeneutic, but the processes of inquiry were sufficiently different from those described above to warrant their separate presentation. The human science that Van Manen proposed:

> *[A]ims at explicating the meaning of human phenomena (such as in literary or historical studies of texts) and at understanding the lived structures of meanings (such as in phenomenological studies of the lifeworld). . . . The fundamental model of this approach is textual reflection on the lived experiences and practical actions of everyday life with the intent to increase one's thoughtfulness and practical resourcefulness or tact. Phenomenology describes how one orients to lived experience, hermeneutics describes how one interprets the "texts" of life, and semiotics is used here to develop a practical writing or linguistic approach to the method of phenomenology and hermeneutics. (p. 4)*

For Van Manen, doing phenomenology is a matter of questioning the ways that we experience the world, bound through the research project to the world in a particular perspective. Researcher involvement thus has a particularly prominent place in his phenomenology, accounting for its growing appeal to qualitative nurse researchers.

Figure 4-4 presents Lauterbach's outline (personal communication) of Van Manen's phenomenology, and is adapted from Van

Four concurrent procedural activities involving 11 steps

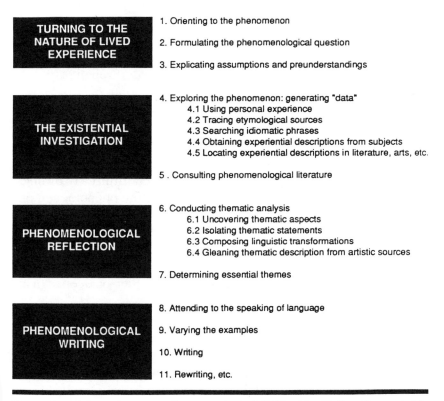

TURNING TO THE NATURE OF LIVED EXPERIENCE	1. Orienting to the phenomenon 2. Formulating the phenomenological question 3. Explicating assumptions and preunderstandings

THE EXISTENTIAL INVESTIGATION	4. Exploring the phenomenon: generating "data"
	    4.1 Using personal experience
	    4.2 Tracing etymological sources
	    4.3 Searching idiomatic phrases
	    4.4 Obtaining experiential descriptions from subjects
	    4.5 Locating experiential descriptions in literature, arts, etc.
	
	5 . Consulting phenomenological literature

PHENOMENOLOGICAL REFLECTION	6. Conducting thematic analysis
	    6.1 Uncovering thematic aspects
	    6.2 Isolating thematic statements
	    6.3 Composing linguistic transformations
	    6.4 Gleaning thematic description from artistic sources
	
	7. Determining essential themes

PHENOMENOLOGICAL WRITING	8. Attending to the speaking of language 9. Varying the examples 10. Writing 11. Rewriting, etc.

Note: Adapted from "Practicing Phenomenological Writing" by M. Van Manen, 1984, *Phenomenology and Pedagogy, 2*(1), p. 5.

Figure 4–4. Van Manen's method of phenomenology.

Manen's presentations (1984, 1990). Van Manen (1990, pp. 8–13) oriented us to his phenomenology through the eight summative statements that follow.

1. *Phenomenological research is the study of lived experience.* Phenomenological inquiry is concerned with questions of what this or that experience is like, and aims at understanding the meaning of the experience. The product of such inquiry is what Van Manen referred to as plausible insight that brings us in more direct contact with the world rather than theoretical explanations which, by superimposing abstractions, distance us from the world as lived.

2. *Phenomenological research is the explication of phenomena as they present themselves to consciousness.* The phenomenological theme of consciousness as existence through a bodily involvement in the world is affirmed in this statement. Van Manen noted that one cannot reflect on experience while living through it, and stressed that phenomenological reflection is retrospective in nature.

3. *Phenomenological research is the study of essences.* By definition, an essence is a universal that is grasped intuitively through study of the internal structure of instances of the phenomenon under study. Phenomenological method is designed to disclose and describe the internal-meaning structures of lived experience. "The essence or nature of an experience has been adequately described in language if the description reawakens or shows us the lived quality and significance of the experience in a fuller or deeper manner" (p. 10).

4. *Phenomenological research is the description of the experiential meanings we live as we live them.* In a focus on meanings, description is interpretive by nature. The product of phenomenological inquiry articulates meaning embedded in experience— meaning as it is lived through.

5. *Phenomenological research is the human scientific study of phenomena.* Phenomenology is, Van Manen stated, systematic, explicit, self-critical, and intersubjective—all characteristics of scientific ways of knowing. It is always characterized by its concern

for the subject matter of the structures of meaning of the lived human world.

6. *Phenomenological research is the attentive practice of thoughtfulness.* The impetus for doing research is the researcher's everyday practical concerns in his or her orientation as nurse, for example. Doing phenomenology, then, is "in the service of the mundane practice of [nursing]: it is a ministering of thoughtfulness" (p. 12). The use of phenomenological research for nurses is "knowing how to act tactfully in [nursing] situations on the basis of a carefully edified thoughtfulness" (p. 8).

7. *Phenomenological research is a search for what it means to be human.* Ultimately, the aim of phenomenological research is to fulfill human nature, to actualize more fully who we are.

> *For example, to understand what it means to be a woman in our present age is also to understand the pressures of the meaning structures that have come to restrict, widen, or question the nature and ground of womanhood. Hermeneutic phenomenological research is a search for the fullness of living, for the ways a woman possibly can experience the world as a woman, for what it is to be a woman. (p. 12)*

8. *Phenomenological research is a poetizing activity.* The presentation of phenomenological findings is characterized by the passion and aim that inspire the research process. The words that describe the experience are what Van Manen referred to as a primal telling, an original singing of the world. The language speaks the world rather than speaking of it.

> *And that is why, when you listen to a presentation of a phenomenological nature, you will listen in vain for the punchline, the latest information, or the big news. As in poetry, it is inappropriate to ask for a conclusion or a summary of a phenomenological study. To summarize a poem in order to present the result would destroy the result because the poem itself is the result. The poem is the thing. (p. 13)*

Phenomenological description is, then, characterized by inspirational insight won through reflective writing. Research and writing are thus closely related. The task is to bring to speech one's understanding of a phenomenon achieved through rigorous reflection. Such description differs from poetry and literature in a concern for explicating universal meanings.

Chapter 5 presents aspects of Lauterbach's phenomenological research, guided by Van Manen's phenomenological method.

SUMMARY

Anderson (1989) argued that the proper focus for phenomenological nurse researchers is working out the problems and dilemmas of doing phenomenology well, rather than pondering the possibilities of triangulated research. Among those problems are questions concerning how and when one "brackets," how the researcher's self is featured, and the issue of rigor in analysis of phenomenological data. In accord with this position, the overview of phenomenological method in this chapter reveals a need to continue development of a phenomenology that produces nursing knowledge to guide nursing practices. It has been proposed that the qualities and characteristics of the researcher–researched relationship are particularly important to reconsider.

The commonalities of the various phenomenologies that are engaging nurse researchers have been emphasized; their variations serve to raise methodological questions, redirecting us to yet another look at philosophical foundations for our science. The very subject matter of phenomenology is described variously. Some phenomenologies specify that the subject matter is such experiences as being in pain, doubting treatment, hoping to be well again, recovering from illness, or preparing for discharge. However, it may also be the mode of doubting or hoping, or it may be a focus on ways that it is possible to be in the world, such as what it is like to parent a child with a chronic illness, for example. The product of phenomenological inquiry, the description of experience, is inescapably interpretive, but the extent of the interpretation is another variability among the phenomenologies. However, to the extent that the description is an effective communication of insights into human experience, its relevance is immediate and direct.

As a particular qualitative approach in nursing research, phenomenology has the distinction of turning the researcher on the self, that is, on his or her own reflective and intuitive grasp of experience. The researcher's direct experience constitutes the data, whether immediate or vicarious. It also has the distinction of deliberate modification by nurses for its use in nursing. This is a fortuitous development well worth our attention as the qualitative paradigm in nursing continues to gain momentum in revolutionizing our science and our practice.

REFERENCES

Allen, M., & Jensen, L. (1990). Hermeneutical inquiry: Meaning and scope. *Western Journal of Nursing Research, 12*(2), 241-253.

Anderson, J. (1989). The phenomenological perspective. In J. Morse (Ed.), *Qualitative nursing research: A contemporary dialogue* (pp. 15-26). Rockville, MD: Aspen.

Benner, P. (1983). Uncovering the knowledge embedded in clinical practice. *Image: The Journal of Nursing Scholarship, 19,* 21-34.

Benner, P. (1985). Quality of life: A phenomenological perspective on explanation, prediction, and understanding in nursing science. *Advances in Nursing Science, 8*(1), 1-14.

Cohen, M. (1987). A historical overview of the phenomenological movement. *Image: The Journal of Nursing Scholarship, 19,* 31-34.

Colaizzi, P. (1978). Psychological research as the phenomenologist views it. In Valle and King (Eds.), *Existential phenomenological alternatives for psychology.* New York: Oxford University Press.

Davis, A. (1973). The phenomenological approach in nursing research. In E. Garrison (Ed.), *Doctoral preparation for nurses* (pp. 212-228). San Francisco: University of California.

Drew, N. (1989). The interviewer's experience as data in phenomenological research. *Western Journal of Nursing Research, 11*(4), 431-439.

Farber, M. (1966). *The aims of phenomenology.* New York: Harper & Row.

Haase, J. (1987). Components of courage in chronically ill adolescents: A phenomenological study. *Advances in Nursing Science, 9,* 64-80.

Husserl, E. (1965). *Phenomenology and the crisis of philosophy* (Q. Lauer, Trans.). New York: Harper & Row.

Leonard, V. (1989). A Heideggerian phenomenonologic perspective on the concept of the person. *Advances in Nursing Science, 11*(4), 40-55.

Lynch-Sauer, J. (1985). Using a phenomenological research method to study nursing phenomena. In M. Leininger, *Qualitative research methods in nursing* (pp. 93-107). Orlando, FL: Grune & Stratton.

Merleau-Ponty, M. (1956). What is phenomenology? *Cross Currents, 6,* 59-70.

Merleau-Ponty, M. (1962). *Phenomenology of perception* (C. Smith, Trans.). New York: Humanities Press.

Merleau-Ponty, M. (1964). *The primacy of perception* (J. Edie, Trans.). Evanston, IL: Northwestern University Press.

Oiler, C. (1982). A phenomenological approach in nursing research. *Nursing Research, 31,* 178-181.

Oiler, C. (1986). Qualitative methods: Phenomenology. In P. Moccia, *New approaches to theory development.* New York: National League for Nursing.

Oiler Boyd, C. (1988). Phenomenology: A foundation for nursing curriculum. In National League for Nursing, *Curriculum revolution: Mandate for change.* New York: National League for Nursing.

Omery, A. (1983). Phenomenology: A method for nursing research. *Advances in Nursing Science, 5*(2), 49-63.

Parse, R. (1990). Parse's research methodology with an illustration of the lived experience of hope. *Nursing Science Quarterly, 3*(1), 9-17.

Parse, R., Coyne, A., & Smith, M. (1985). *Nursing research: Qualitative methods.* Bowie, MD: Brady Communications.

Paterson, J., & Zderad, L. (1976). *Humanistic nursing.* New York: Wiley.

Ray, M. (1985). A philosophical method to study nursing phenomena. In M. Leininger, *Qualitative research methods in nursing.* Orlando, FL: Grune & Stratton.

Reeder, F. (1987). The phenomenological movement. *Image: The Journal of Nursing Scholarship, 19,* 150-152.

Sandelowski, M., & Pollock, C. (1986). Women's experiences of infertility. *Image: The Journal of Nursing Scholarship, 18,* 140-144.

Schutz, A. (1970). *On phenomenology and social relations.* Chicago: University of Chicago Press.

Schutz, A. (1973). *Collected papers I: The problem of social reality* (M. Natanson, Ed.). The Hague, Netherlands: Martinus Nijhoff.

Spiegelberg, H. (1975). *Doing phenomenology.* The Hague, Netherlands: Martinus Nijhoff.

Spiegelberg, H. (1976). *The phenomenological movement: Vols. I and II* (2nd ed.). The Hague, Netherlands: Martinus Nijhoff.

Spiegelberg, H. (1981). *The context of the phenomenological movement.* The Hague, Netherlands: Martinus Nijhoff.

Spiegelberg, H. (1982). *The phenomenological movement* (3rd ed.). The Hague, Netherlands: Martinus Nijhoff.

van Kaam, A. (1959). Phenomenal analysis: Exemplified by a study of the experience of "really feeling understood." *Journal of Individual Psychology, 15,* 66-72.

Van Manen, M. (1984). Practicing phenomenological writing. *Phenomenology and Pedagogy, 2*(1), 36-69.

Van Manen, M. (1990). *Researching lived experience: Human science for an action sensitive pedagogy.* Albany, NY: SUNY Press.

Zderad, L. (1968). *A concept of empathy.* Unpublished doctoral dissertation, Georgetown University, Washington, DC.

ADDITIONAL REFERENCES

Bergum, V. (1988). *Women to mother: A transformation.* S. Hadley, MA: Bergin & Garvey.

Bergum, V. (1989). Being a phenomenological researcher. In J. Morse (Ed.), *Qualitative Nursing Research: A Contemporary Dialogue,* Rockville, MD: Aspen Pub., Inc., pp. 43-57.

Bishop, A., & Scudder, J. (1990). *The practical, moral, and personal sense of nursing: A phenomenological philosophy of practice.* Albany: State University of New York Press.

Drew, N. (1986). Exclusion and confirmation: A phenomenology of patients' experiences with caregivers. *Image, 18,* 39-43.

Giorgi, A. (1970). *Psychology as a human science: A phenomenologically based approach.* New York: Harper and Row.

Knaack, P. (1984). Phenomenological research. *Western Journal of Nursing Research, 6,* 107-114.

Oiler, C. (1980). A phenomenological perspective in nursing. Unpublished doctoral dissertation, Teachers College, Columbia University, New York, NY.

Oiler, C. (1983). Nursing reality as reflected in nurses' poetry. *Perspectives in Psychiatric Care, 21,* 81-89.

Paige, S. (1980). *Alone into the alone: A phenomenological study of the experience of dying.* Unpublished doctoral dissertation, Boston University.

Paterson, J. (1971). From a philosophy of clinical nursing to a method of nursology. *Nursing Research, 20,* 143–146.

Psathas, G. (1973). *Phenomenological sociology: Issues and applications.* New York: John Wiley & Sons.

Riemen, D. (1986). The essential structure of a caring interaction: Doing phenomenology. In Munhall & Oiler, *Nursing Research: A Qualitative Perspective,* 1st ed., Norwalk, CT: Appleton-Century-Crofts.

Rose, J. (1990). Psychologic health of women: A phenomenologic study of women's inner strength. *Advances in Nursing Science, 12*(2), 56–70.

Stanley, T. (1978). The lived experience of hope: The isolation of discrete descriptive elements common to the experience of hope in healthy young adults. Unpublished doctoral dissertation, Catholic University of America, Washington, DC.

Strasser, S. (1963). *Phenomenology and the human sciences.* Pittsburg: Duquesne University Press.

Swanson-Kaufmann, K. (1988). Phenomenology. In B. Sarter (Ed.), *Paths to Knowledge: Innovative Research Methods for Nursing.* New York: National League for Nursing.

van Kaam, A. (1969). *Existential foundations of psychology.* New York: Doubleday.

Zaner, R. (1970). *The way of phenomenology.* Indianapolis: Pegasus.

5

In Another World: A Phenomenological Perspective and Discovery of Meaning in Mothers' Experience with Death of a Wished-for Baby: Doing Phenomenology*

Sarah Steen Lauterbach

Non ridere, non lugere, neque detestari, sed intelligere. (Not to laugh, not to lament, not to curse, but to understand.) Spinoza

* From S. Lauterbach (1992), unpublished doctoral dissertation, Teachers College, Columbia University, New York.

AIM OF STUDY

*U*sing a phenomenological perspective for inquiry, the aim of this research was to understand what it means for a mother to experience perinatal death of a wished-for baby. The inquiry focused on exploring and interpreting data of mothers' lived experience. Along with phenomenological reflection, a hermeneutic process, uncovering hidden as well as explicit meaning, was used in data analysis. The inquiry included the larger world of human experience, as depicted in the creative arts—painting, photography, memorial and mourning art, music, literature, and other art forms.

The phenomenological inquiry, as part of uncovering meaning, articulated "essences" of meaning in mothers' lived experiences when their wished-for babies died. Using the lens of the feminist perspective, the focus was on mothers' memories and their "living through" experience. This perspective facilitated breaking through the silence surrounding mothers' experiences; it assisted in articulating and amplifying mothers' memories and their stories of loss. Methods of inquiry included phenomenological reflection on data elicited by existential investigation of mothers' experiences, and investigation of the phenomenon in the creative arts.

PHENOMENON OF INTEREST

The phenomenon investigated was mothers' experiences of perinatal death of wished-for babies. Using a phenomenological perspective, the study attempted to uncover "originary" experience of the phenomenon by focusing on mothers' "secondary remembrance or recollection." Schutz (1967), quoting Bergson, stated that secondary memory is recalled in this way:

> *We accomplish it either by simply laying hold of what is recollected . . . or we accomplish it in a real, reproductive, recapitulative memory in which the temporal object is again completely built up in a continuum of presentifications, so*

that we seem to perceive it again, but only seemingly, as-if.
(p. 48)

The perinatal period, as defined in this study, included late-pregnancy loss. Mothers who participated had experienced fetal deaths after 24 weeks' gestation or up to 2 weeks following birth. Perinatal death, according to national perinatal mortality statistics (U.S. Department of Human and Health Services, 1990), usually refers to stillbirth and infant loss occurring between 28 weeks' gestation and 4 weeks following delivery.

JUSTIFICATION FOR QUALITATIVE STUDY OF PHENOMENON

From examining the literature surrounding the phenomenon and from listening to mothers' stories, one is struck by the discrepancy between what is known about the phenomenon and human care practice. The discrepancy provides existential validation for the need for qualitative research aimed at increasing understanding. The particular methodology selected addressed the discrepancy of understanding and sought to discover "essences" of meaning in mothers' experiences.

RESEARCHER ASSUMPTIONS AND BIASES

In the tradition of phenomenological research, researcher assumptions, biases, intuitions, and perceptions link the researcher to the research world. In qualitative research, the process of explicating researcher bias and a priori convictions enables biases to be held in abeyance. Assumptions are made explicit during proposal development and are carried through in data collection, analysis, and interpretation, and in writing. In bracketing personal knowledge and bias, the researcher attempts to experience and understand the phenomenon, as if looking at it for the first time. Biases explicated and bracketed in this study came from personal and professional experiences with perinatal loss.

SELECTED QUALITATIVE RESEARCH METHOD

Gaining an understanding of an experience, as if seeing the phenomenon for the first time, is the aim of phenomenological inquiry. According to Husserl (1952):

> It [phenomenology] has to place before its own eyes as instances certain pure conscious events, to bring these to complete clearness, and within this zone of clearness to subject them to analysis and the apprehension of their essence, to follow up the essential connections that can be clearly understood, to grasp what is momentarily perceived in faithful conceptual expressions, of which the meaning is prescribed purely by the object perceived or in some way transparently understood. (p. 174)

Phenomenology seeks to explicate personal meanings in experience and ultimately seeks to understand experience. As a research methodology, phenomenology is grounded in existential philosophy and seeks to uncover meaning and "essences" in experience so that understanding is facilitated. It focuses on lived experiences with human phenomena and lends itself to study phenomena and their transactional relationships.

In this inquiry, the discovery of meanings in mothers' experiences with perinatal death is intended to glean deeper understanding. Phenomenology guided this investigation of mothers' experiences with perinatal death and provided a structure for revealing the phenomenon to the researcher and to readers. The process has uncovered meanings as well as the "essences" of meaning in these experiences, in an effort to create understanding. As the phenomenological method evolved, it provided the researcher with many examples of human experiences with perinatal loss. Art, literature, the historical context of mourning expressed in art, cemeteries, changing funerary rituals, and stories passed on through generations of mothers—all provided a window through which phenomena of mothers' experiences with infant death were viewed and distilled.

Merleau-Ponty (1964) stated that "A successful work has the strange power to teach its own lesson" (p. 19) and that the meaning of a work, for the artist or for observers, cannot be stated except by the work itself. Neither the thought that created it nor the thought that receives it is completely its own master:

Expression is like a step taken in the fog—no one can say where, if anywhere, it will lead. (p. 3)

Merleau-Ponty (1964), noting that Cézanne wondered whether what came from his hands had any meaning and would be understood, observed:

So it is with the artist, researcher, or other creators. Cézanne won out against chance, and men, too, can win provided they will measure the dangers and the task. (p. 5)

When the present study was conceptualized, the extent of data recorded and "generated" through investigation of the phenomenon was essentially unknown to the researcher. In the world of art, music, photography, and literature, it lay waiting in silence, undiscovered. The phenomenological vantage directed the researcher toward the artistic and creative world. The varied human recording found there elucidated and illuminated the data. Phenomenology assisted in analyzing and conceptualizing the significance and meaning of these mothers' personal experiences.

ULTIMATE AIM OF INQUIRY

The ultimate aim of phenomenological inquiry is to facilitate the process of becoming more fully human. The findings from this research speak in mothers' voices about what it is like to be a mother and then live through the death of a wished-for baby. The mothers interviewed, in response to the opportunity offered by the research setting, discussed, reflected on, and remembered their experiences of living through pregnancies, births, deaths, and memorials. "It is the things themselves, from the depths of their silence, that it [phenomenology] wishes to bring to expression" (Merleau-Ponty, 1968, p. 4).

Sartre (1965) asserted that the goal of literature is to reveal the world and particularly to reveal man [sic] to other men [sic] so that the latter may assume full responsibility before the object which has been thus laid bare. (p. 18)

•   •   •

If you name the behavior of an individual, you reveal it to him; he sees himself. And since you are at the same time naming it to all others, he knows that he is seen at the moment he sees himself. (p. 16)

Greater understanding was voiced for mothers participating in the study. The willingness of mothers to participate in continuing research provides further existential validation for the phenomenological perspective and the human understanding facilitated by the method. Understanding will potentially be facilitated for the larger public audience of mothers and families, the social/public world, and professional audiences. With greater understanding, phenomena surrounding perinatal death may be resolved through research and caring connections rather than through continued silence.

Heidegger's (1962) writings on the concept of Being were found particularly relevant to the present inquiry's data analysis, phenomenological reflection, and hermeneutic interpretation of findings. For purposes of this study, the personal meaning of being-a-mother-to-a-baby-who-died was the focus.

This study also used a hermeneutic process for interpreting data yielded by the investigation. Spiegelberg (1965) identified hermeneutics as:

. . . a method for bringing out the normally hidden purposes of such goal-determined things-in-being as human beings. (p. 324)

Thus, a hermeneutic process uses a method that:

> *. . . goes beyond mere description of what is manifest and tries to uncover hidden meanings by anticipatory devices. (p. 324)*

The process of interpreting hidden meaning can be compared to psychoanalysis in that each attempts to uncover meaning. (The researcher's practice of and interest in psychotherapeutic nursing provided further support for hermeneutic analysis.) By uncovering and explicating hidden meaning, this inquiry promised the discovery of greater depth of meaning, thus contributing to understanding.

EVOLUTION OF STUDY

Historical Context of Study

As the study unfolded, the historical context surrounding the phenomenon gained increasing relevance. Death has been a topic of concern throughout human recorded history. Freud (1915) expressed his opinion that death was a central topic of human concern. In his Pulitzer Prize winning book, *The Denial of Death*, Ernest Becker (1973) provided a synthesis of theological and psychological insights about human efforts to escape the ultimate burden of life—death:

> *The hero was the man who could go into the spirit world, the world of the dead, and return alive. (p. 12)*

Becker noted that a revival of interest in death had piled up considerable literature in the field. However, infant death has been a hidden subject, even when other death topics are explored in-depth.

In an interview with Bill Moyers, Joseph Campbell pointed out that there was no evidence that humans had thought about death in a significant way until the Neanderthal period. Campbell (1964) said:

[We] do know that burials always involve the idea of the continued life beyond the visible one, of a plane of being that is behind the visible plane, and that is somehow supportive of the visible one to which we have to relate. (p. 90)

The belief that life is supported by an invisible plane is related to the current study and is elaborated in the mothers' narratives. Campbell also stated that the mythical world is full of reference to the connection between life and death, that "death is life, and life is death, . . ." (p. 134).

The exploration of myth validates a recurrent theme in the findings regarding to meaning of mothers' experiences when their babies die. The meaning of mothers' lives is intimately connected with the lives of their children. This somewhat mythical explanation was illuminated in the findings: mothers' experiences with infant death, when overlaid with life, served to enhance mothers' coping with their losses.

As the study evolved, it was found that changes in the societal mourning rituals surrounding infant death had increasing relevance. For example, in the late 1890s and early 1900s, the subject of death was gradually removed from public scrutiny, although interest in the phenomenon continued to exist in private.

Early infancy deaths of wished-for children have been viewed in the second half of the twentieth century as ultimate tragedies (Knapp, 1986). The disappearance of ceremony and ritual accompanying infant death, which occurred in the mid to late 1900s, is astounding. In contrast, nineteenth-century Americans mourned visibly, exhibiting what Pike and Armstrong (1981) called "sentimental concentration on death and dying":

[Their] fascination with the memorialization of the dead through elaborate mourning customs all seem excessive— even morbid—today. (p. 11)

Twentieth-century Americans appeared not to mourn their lost pregnancies, stillbirths, and babies who died shortly after birth. The absence of ceremony and of infant memorials, which had been common in the mid-1900s, reflected a seemingly prevailing denial of the significance of infant death, coupled with a perception voiced by some mothers that their experience of loss was invalidated.

In the early 1980s, as a result of attention focused on perinatal losses, hospital protocols for bereavement care included activities for families to build memories of the baby. However, from the mothers' stories of perinatal infant death told in this study, one is often struck by the seemingly uniformed care that is prevalent as the dawn of the twenty-first century approaches.

Experiential Context of Study

The researcher's interest in the phenomenon stems from the unanticipated death of a twin in her last pregnancy eleven years ago. This experience provided an access to perinatal support group networks and had impact on framing the study. The researcher was also brought to study the phenomenon through involvement with students, mothers, families and from an increased sensitivity to needs that the personal experience facilitated. Because of personal experience, knowledge about death, grief, and bereavement was bracketed to limit bias. Where personal experience underpinned the need and guided framing of the study, providing a view of the phenomenon from the inside out as well as from the outside in, it was coupled with bracketing. This is especially important with research that potentially will create new insights and understandings.

VAN MANEN'S METHOD OF "DOING" PHENOMENOLOGY

This study followed Van Manen's (1984) method for doing phenomenology, an eleven-step method with four concurrent processes detailed in the preceding chapter. Van Manen stated that phenomenology is the study of the life-world; the world of experience as actually lived rather than as conceptualized, categorized, or theorized. It is the study of "essences" of experience in an attempt to understand experience.

Van Manen (1984) stated, "Phenomenological research is the attentive practice of thoughtfulness" (p. 1). It is the search for what it means to be human,

> *of what it means to be in the world as a man, woman, a*
> *child, taking into account of the sociocultural and historical*
> *traditions which give meaning to our ways of being in the*
> *world. (p. 2)*

The ultimate aim of phenomenology is "to fulfill our human nature; to become more fully who we are" (p. 2).

Merleau-Ponty (1964) called phenomenology a language that "sings the world," so that in words, or in spite of them, we find memories that we never thought or felt before. Through eliciting and analyzing mothers' reminiscences, it was found that mothers' memories yielded greater understanding. The phenomenological method provided the use of concepts and language through which meaning was interpreted.

Van Manen (1984) stated that phenomenological research is unlike other research, describing it as a "poetizing activity,"

> *It tries an incantive, evocative speaking, a primal telling,*
> *wherein we aim to involve the voice into the original singing*
> *of the world. (p. 2)*

The eleven-step methodological outline for doing phenomenology involves an interplay of the four methodological themes. This research method-in-action is a reflective process. Each discovery is accompanied by phenomenological reflection, focusing and refocusing informed attention back on the phenomenon. The phenomenon is examined from many perspectives of human experience. Inquiry into the meaning of mothers' experience has included an existential investigation in art, music, creative literature, mourning and memorial art, and posthumous photography.

This study also used the perspective of Munhall (1992), outlined in Figure 5–1, which includes using the researchers' personal experience, journaling throughout the existential investigation. This

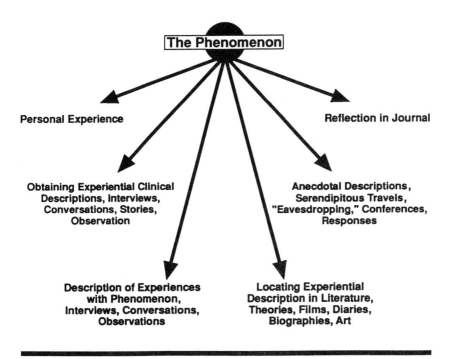

Figure 5–1. Munhall's (1992) model of existential investigation.

nursing perspective serves to expand Van Manen's model to include the temporal perspective of personal and nursing experience. Figure 5-2 combines the method of Van Manen (1984) and Munhall (1992) into a description of the four concurrent processes in this phenomenological inquiry. This method is viewed as an ongoing reflective process that includes continual discovery and phenomenological reflection. It involves a process of bending back attention to the phenomenon with each example of lived experience found.

As the research process-in-action developed and unfolded, the selection and contribution of Van Manen's method, coupled with Munhall's process of existential investigation, placed the researcher in a unique vantage point through which many lived human experiences with the phenomenon were viewed. The methods

Four concurrent steps:

#1   Turning to Phenomenon of Interest:
Mothers' Experiences of Perinatal Death of a Wished-for Baby

#2   Existential Investigation of Phenomenon:
     Researcher's Personal Experience
     Professional Clinical Experiences of Researcher
     Reflection Recorded in Researcher Journal
     Mothers' Descriptions of Experience:
         Interviews
         Stories
         Journals
         Writings
     Sharing Mothers' Memorabilia of Experience:
         Tapes
         Copies of Memorial Services
     Inquiry into Creative and Artistic Sources:
         Art and Painting
         Observation of Memorial Art in Cemeteries
         Mourning Art
         Mourning Photography
         Literature, Autobiography, Poetry
         Historical Literature
         Music
     Professional Literature
     Consultation of Phenomenology Literature

#3   Phenomenological Reflection on Phenomenon

#4   Phenomenological Writing and Rewriting of Discovery

Return to Phenomenon with Understanding of "Essences" of Meaning in Mothers' Experience and Continued Inquiry

Figure 5–2. Model of phenomenological perspective of inquiry.

guided "generating" data as well as understanding and interpreting data. The findings have implications and direct applicability to both nursing practice and nursing research methodology.

TURNING TO THE NATURE OF LIVED EXPERIENCE

To do a phenomenological study, Van Manen (1984) stated,

the experience must be recalled in such a way that the essential aspects, the meaning structure of this experience as lived through, are brought back, as it were, and in such a way that we recognize this description as a possible human experience, which means as a possible interpretation of that experience. (p. 7)

The phenomenological question that animated the inquiry was, "What are the meanings in mothers' experiences with perinatal death of a wished-for baby?" In this phase, the researcher must turn to and become oriented to the phenomenon. This phase included explicating researcher biases and assumptions and bracketing these, along with knowledge and preunderstandings. The use of a research journal, reflecting and writing ideas as generated, using broad open-ended questions and asking for clarification during interviews with mothers, also facilitated bracketing.

EXISTENTIAL INVESTIGATION

The second procedural activity in Van Manen's (1984) method has two steps: (1) exploring the phenomenon and (2) consulting phenomenological literature. Exploring the phenomenon, or generating data, consists of a thorough exploration of the scope of lived experience. Materials investigated and sought out to yield significant interpretive understandings were personal experiences, etymology of relevant terms, idiomatic phrases and expressions, other people's experiences, biographies and reconstructed life stories of mothers who participated, and experiential and existential explorations of examples of the phenomenon presented in art, music, and literature. Figure 5–3 describes sources pursued and discovered in "generating" data of lived experiences with perinatal death through existential investigation in this inquiry. Figure 5–3 is designed with lived experience of the phenomenon in the center, providing the focus for investigation. As data was discovered, the researcher reflected further and more deeply on the phenomenon

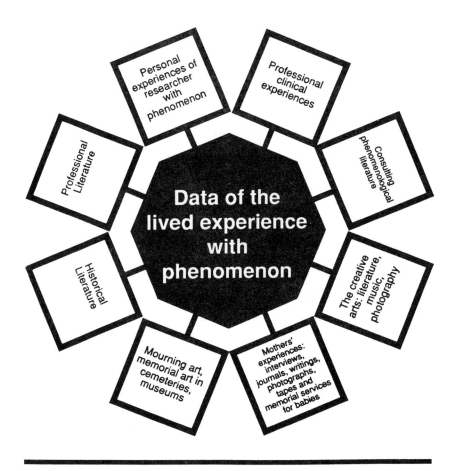

Figure 5–3.   The existential investigation of phenomenon: mothers' experience with death of a wished-for baby.

while pursuing other sources of data at the same time. Figure 5-4 outlines the discussion of findings in existential investigation.

The Phenomenon within the Literary Context

Grief fills up the room of my absent child
Lies in his bed, walks up and down with me,
Puts on his pretty looks, repeats his words,
Remembers me of all his gracious parts,
Stuffs out his vacant garments with his form:
Then have I reason to be fond of grief. Shakespeare.
(Enright, 1987, p. 288)

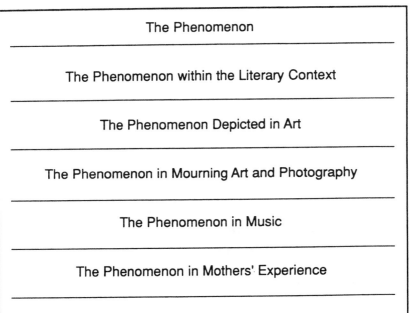

The Phenomenon

The Phenomenon within the Literary Context

The Phenomenon Depicted in Art

The Phenomenon in Mourning Art and Photography

The Phenomenon in Music

The Phenomenon in Mothers' Experience

Phenomenological Reflection on Phenomenon

Figure 5–4.   Existential investigation.

Many wonderful creative works of literature were discovered in existential investigation (Enright, 1987; Eliot, 1936, 1955; Lewis, 1961; Lindbergh, 1973; Linscott, 1932; Mason, 1970; Untermeyer, 1962) that included descriptions of lived experiences. The selected literature speaks about human phenomenon of perinatal death, thus continuing to establish it as a legitimate topic of inquiry.

The discovery of the ancient Sumerian verse narrative, *Gilgamesh,* a moving work of art, speaks with a voice similar to mothers in this study.

Like a hungry animal through empty lairs
In search of food. The only nourishment
He knew was grief, endless in its hidden source
Yet never ending hunger.

All that is left to one who grieves
Is convalescence. (Mason, 1970, p. 53)

Mothers described the existential experience in mourning "as the closest thing to being with the baby." They described their reluctance to move through grief hurriedly, but discovered early in mourning that their only choice was to move "through" grief. It was only after getting through it, that they learned to live with the reality of the baby's death.

A wonderful short story by Anton Chekhov was discovered in the public domain literature search entitled, *Grief* (Linscott, 1932), subtitled, *To Whom Shall I Tell My Grief?* Written in the late 1800s, Chekhov lived through the death of his brother to tuberculosis in 1889. The story is about Iona, a cabby who, after several attempts to share his grief after his son dies, finds that his little horse is the only willing listener.

The poet, Robert Frost (Untermeyer, 1962), stated that, "All an artist needs is samples. Without telling all, he suggests all" (p. 31). Frost said that, "The thing art does for life is to clean it up, to strip it to form" (p. 31). In his poem, "Home Burial," he speaks of differences in socialized responses of fathers and mothers, men and women, to the death of a child. Mothers described how they and their husbands, or intimates who were fathers, dealt differently with death.

The poem entitled, "Mother's Day," written by a participant mother provides a poignant description of the mother's lived experience with the death of her baby, delivered stillborn at twenty-eight weeks gestation. This, along with data from other journal entries of mothers in the study reflect the mothers' needs to articulate and write about their experiences. Mothers were, in general, happy to participate in the study and devoted much time and energy into thinking about their experiences and sharing experiences and memories stimulated by phenomenological interviews and sharing memorabilia. They hoped to gain greater personal understanding at the same time hoping to make a contribution to knowledge.

Mother's Day

On Sunday I was a mother for a little while.
With one final push the baby was out.
And everyone said how beautiful he was,
Perfectly shaped little fingers and toes.
They let me hold him, and he really was beautiful.
He lay there motionless, dark hair like his father's,
One eye opened slightly as I shifted his position,
And closed again.
They weighed him and finger printed him and took his picture.
They let me hold him again.
He seemed to be growing older and more wizened.
His arms and legs no longer felt warm to the touch.
They left us alone with him for a long time, and we sat and gazed at him.
Then they took him away.
Now I'm a mother no longer, left only with a brief moment, and an emptiness where I had felt full before.

The Phenomenon Depicted in Art

Art is another way of seeing. (Jean Erdman, WHYY, 1991)

The exploration of the phenomenon in art has taken several paths. Part of the historical exploration has focused on memorial art in cemeteries. Several famous, old Victorian and several newer cemeteries in the Philadelphia area and in northern Florida, where the researcher spent her childhood, were visited to observe graves of infants and children.

Many private collections of mourning memorabilia exist and are described in books (Pike & Armstrong, 1980; Schorsch, 1976) and housed in public and private collections and libraries. Two private museums containing collections of mourning art were visited by the researcher: one in a Philadelphia private cemetery; and one in a museum that contains the artifacts of its family business, a general store dating back to the 1800s in northern Florida.

A wonderful painting by Henriette Wyeth in 1935 entitled "Death and the Child," was discovered and hangs in a school in the Delaware Valley. The painting is a beautiful impressionistic painting, depicting a child being taken up to heaven by hands of a woman looking down in a loving manner.

The artist portrays prevailing sentiment regarding infant death in early 1900. In the painter's own words,

This child is being saved from all the loathsome disappointments and corruption of life. It's a saving grace. There are worse things than death. (Meryman, 1991, p. 96)

The theme of infant salvation, death being preferable to a life burdened with travesty, is consistent with the times as well as with current popular view regarding infant death.

The Phenomenon Discovered in Mourning Art and Photography

During nineteenth century America, it was a common custom to commission post-mortem portraits. According to Lloyd (1980) this practice provided the family a means of establishing continuity, using art to bridge the chasm between life and death. After the development of photography as a medium, often post-mortem portrait paintings were photographed and had the effect of restoring the dead to life-like images. These photographs were often the only images the family had of the deceased.

In the 1970s and early 1980s, post-mortem photography portraiture was introduced in hospitals as a therapeutic method of providing mourning care for families experiencing infant death. When seen in light of recent practice, the custom and use of mourning art in the nineteenth century establishes a social historical context for current use of mourning photography.

Mothers in this study kept and displayed pictures and other memorabilia of their babies in their scrapbooks and homes. Items shared and investigated during interviews with mothers were: pregnancy and birth pictures, birth certificates and baby footprints, hospital bracelets, audiotapes and copies of memorial services, and other memorabilia of experiences. Only one mother did not have pictures of her baby who was a stillborn baby girl delivered prematurely at twenty-four weeks gestation. The birth occurred before the hospital had a universal protocol for taking pictures of babies who died. One mother stated that her partner had taken the pictures of her holding her critically ill baby. At the time "it seemed like a strange thing to do," but in retrospect, she was happy to have the photographic record of the experience. Another mother regretted that she had not had her picture taken with her stillborn baby boy. She found that she needed to be within arm's reach of pictures of her baby for months, and that after three years, she continued to have periods when she needed to see and be close to her pictures.

Mourning art flourished in early nineteenth-century America. Inspired by the European custom of memorializing public figures, departed Americans were memorialized by their families in creative art; needlework, art, and photography. During the inquiry, several books were discovered to have pictorial representations of death, funerals, grief, and post-mortem mourning portraits (Burns, 1990; Pike & Armstrong, 1980; Schorsch, 1976).

The Phenomenon Discovered in Music

Musical gift and genius combined with a profound turmoil of spirit and rich life experience, Gustav Mahler (1860–1911) composed symphonies that depicted the composer's perception of the poignant transience of life and death (Greene, 1985). One such composition is *Kindertotenlieder* (Songs to Dead Children), completed in 1904. This symphony was composed to settings of five poems by German poet Ruckert, around the topic of child death. This collection was written at a time when many early deaths were due to diphtheria and other communicable diseases. Mahler's beloved oldest daughter died of scarlet fever. Themes of life and death run throughout Mahler's work.

The depiction of the phenomenon in music, with themes relating to death and life was seen recurrent within contexts of art, memorial and mourning art, music, poetry, literature, and validate findings from interviews with mothers to be discussed, giving further validity to study findings.

The Phenomenon Described in Mothers' Experiences

The study used multiple strategies for collection of data that described mothers' experiences. These included locating experiential descriptions in journals and writings of mothers and in interviews with mothers. The existential investigation "generated" a wealth of data of lived experiences and was interwoven and reflected on during ongoing analysis and interpretation. In addition, consultation of phenomenological literature was concurrent with existential investigation, assisted in interpreting and analyzing interviews, and was interwoven with writing and rewriting. Phenomenology literature enabled the researcher to reflect more deeply on interpreting experience of phenomena.

Participants. The participant mothers were a convenience sample of five mothers who had experienced perinatal death. Interviews were piloted by the researcher with a mother who experienced early pregnancy loss. The participant sample was solicited from the support group network.

Three audiotaped open-ended interviews were held with each participant over an eight-month period. The purpose of the first interview was to stimulate mothers' remembrances of experiences by asking them to describe their birth and perinatal death experiences. The interviews took place in mothers' homes, providing for privacy and convenience as well as comfort. The home setting facilitated easy access to mothers' memorabilia, writings, and pictures relating to the phenomenon. First interviews were lengthy, usually taking from one and one-half hours to three hours. Subsequently, second interviews were arranged from two or three weeks to within two months of first interviews. Third interviews took place some months later. All interviews were completed within eight months of consent.

In addition to interviews, participant mothers shared journals and writings. Two mothers kept detailed journals in the months following their baby's death and three mothers shared creative and professional writings. Three mothers shared copies of funerals and one mother shared an audiotape of the funeral.

Since the interview in this inquiry was acknowledged to be sensitive and potentially anxiety-producing for participants, an ongoing assessment of effects of research on mothers' mental health status was initiated before, during, and after each interview. Mothers in general wept when sharing painful memories. Personal experience of the researcher with perinatal death of a baby facilitated sharing. First interviews were generally more emotionally laden than second or third interviews and contained description of the lived experience in greater detail. Subsequent interviews elaborated, clarified, and rounded out descriptive data. Where the purpose of interview was not therapeutic, mothers shared that opportunity to retell their stories had beneficial consequences.

Data Collection, Storage, and Analysis. Interviews were audiotaped, transcribed, and printed, preserved on a floppy and hard disc and used for analysis of data. Transcriptions were done, in most cases, by a contract transcriber. Interviews were listened to initially by the researcher, and along with a hard copy of the transcript, corrections were made when errors were found. Analysis of meaning was begun with each first interview and continued throughout data collection and writing. The articulation, writing and rewriting, gleaning phenomenological understanding was concurrent throughout the research process and continues in presentation of findings. Presentations continue to validate both findings and the reflective research process used.

Human Subject Considerations. This researcher acknowledged that the sensitivity of the inquiry required that care be taken to provide participants with protection of human rights. This concern about protection and human rights was implemented by development of an advocacy role during recruiting participants, informed consent, ongoing assessment of effects of inquiry on participants, and establishment of referral in case of need.

Time Frame of Study. Data collection took place over an eight-month period. Validation of findings was begun before data collection was completed. Theme analysis began following the first interviews and was confirmed during interviews with individual mothers.

PHENOMENOLOGICAL REFLECTION

The third procedural activity in Van Manen's (1984) method, phenomenological reflection, includes two major steps: conducting thematic analysis and determining essential themes. A theme is defined by Van Manen as a description of the structure of the lived experience,

> *themes are more like knots in the webs of our experiences, around which certain lived experiences are spun and thus experienced as meaningful wholes. (p. 20)*

Uncovering thematic aspects in the descriptions was accomplished by reviewing the data carefully and repeatedly. The researcher brought into reflection other data from creative sources and scholarly literature. As themes were identified, notes and paragraphs were written to capture in more phenomenologically sensitive terms ideas from the research process. The writing and rewriting phase described below was concurrent with phenomenological reflection.

PHENOMENOLOGICAL WRITING

The fourth and final procedural activity in Van Manen's (1984) method was ongoing throughout investigation, from proposal to final writing. Written and rewritten descriptions of the phenomenon have provided the researcher with a linguistic understanding of meaning of mothers' lived experience. Reflection on data of existential investigation assisted in articulation and rearticulation of meaning. The final draft of findings took place over an approximate four-month period.

RELIABILITY AND VALIDITY

According to Guba and Lincoln (1981), four issues are considered to determine methodological rigor of qualitative scientific inquiry: truth value, applicability, consistency, and neutrality. Whether a description of experience is credible to the person with experience is a primary consideration. For the present study, participant mothers have concurred with credibility of findings. The second test of validity is the applicability of qualitative research which is evaluated by "fit" of data into contexts outside the study situation. The consistency of results generated by multiple methods of data collection and existential investigation of artistic sources contribute to validity. Findings were consistent throughout data collection during interviews and were confirmed with participants as the study was completed. Preliminary findings were shared and tested with mothers during third and final interviews.

Reliability in qualitative research relates to how well methods focus on

> *identifying and documenting recurrent, accurate, and consistent (homogenous) or inconsistent (heterogenous) features, as patterns themes, values, world views, experiences, and other phenomena confirmed in similar or different contexts. (Leininger, 1985, p. 69)*

The use of multiple methods further helped to elaborate, clarify, and support findings. The real tests of reliability and validity are in the hands of readers who have experience of the phenomenon either through personal or professional experience.

FINDINGS OF STUDY:
BEING-A-MOTHER IN ANOTHER WORLD

Merleau-Ponty stated that language as it is used by,

> *the operative language of literature, poetry, of conversation, and of philosophy, which possesses meaning less than it is possessed by it; does not speak of it, but speaks it, or speaks according to it, or lets it speak and be spoken within us, breaks through our present. This language "is open upon the things, called forth by the voices of silence, and continues an effort of articulation. (p. iii)*

Using mothers' voices and stories, the phenomenon as depicted in data from the artistic and creative investigation were used to bring from, the depths of silence, an understanding of meaning of mothers' experience of death of a wished-for baby. It was discovered that experiencing perinatal death of a baby, leaves a mother abandoned in another world, constituting an existential experience of being-a-mother in another world.

Meanings in mothers' experience were found to be experiences in temporality, lived within mothers' intimate connections within multiple changing contexts of mothers' lives. Figure 5-5 depicts "essences" discovered in meaning of mothers' experiences.

Being-a-Mother in Another World

A central theme related to Being in the data from this study was that mothers experience an existential abandonment by their baby following its death. Heidegger's (1962) discussion of Being-towards-death was found helpful in analysis and interpreting the data of mothers' experience. He stated that,

> *in Being-with the dead [dem Toten], the deceased himself is no longer factically "there". However, when we speak of*

IN ANOTHER WORLD:
Discovery of Meaning in Mothers' Experience
of Perinatal Death of a Baby

Temporality • Connection • Context

ESSENTIAL THEMES:

- The Essence of Perinatal Loss

- Reflective Pulling Back, Recovering, Reentering

- Embodiment of Mourning Loss

- The Narcissistic Injury

- The Finality of Death of the Baby

- Living through and "with" Death

- Altering World Views

- Death Overlaid with Life

- Failing and Trying again

Figure 5–5.   Findings of study.

"Being-with," we always have in view Being with one an-
other in the same world. The deceased has abandoned our
"world" and left it behind. (p. 282)

Listening carefully to mothers' descriptions and stories, many examples of mothers experience of being abandoned were found.
Mothers experienced a profound feeling of isolation, of Being-a-
mother in another world, and loss of the world of mothering that
follows death of a particular, wished-for baby.

Mothers in this study found that mourning provided them with an experience of "Being-with" the dead baby and allowed them the necessary time to mourn and experience the reality of loss gradually. This often presents a dilemma to the mother as acute grief unfolds and passes. Mourning that follows death of a baby involves a separation of mother from the baby and from the lost world of opportunities involved in mothering the particular baby.

Mothers in this study experienced a devastating period of grief and loss, isolated from the world of mothering and from people who would have been available had their babies been born healthy. The experience of existential abandonment by their dead infants left them suspended in another world, a world of isolation and silence. The transition from the world of Being-a-mother, the prospective Being-a-mother of a newborn to Being-a-mother of a dead infant, left them without a baby to nurture, as well as with few connections. Mothers were unanimous in their opinions that personal support systems and the working world surrounding them invalidated the significance of experience by inattention, oversight, and by just not "being there."

In addition, participant mothers' experience reflected a dilemma in Being, that of Being-a-mother of a dead baby. The baby's death left them suspended in a transition world between Being in a mother's world and Being in a nonmother's world. One mother stated that the memorial service was an important event, that she experienced it as Being-a-mother in public. The isolation that accompanies the state of Being-a-mother in another world, the world of Being-a-mother without a baby, and resultant invalidation of mothers' experience by the social world hinders a mother's mourning and bereavement.

Mothers found themselves after subsequent babies continuing to grieve the dead baby, often with little time and opportunity to do so. Those with babies and toddlers at the time of the research interviews were concerned about how to meet their own needs for remembering and mourning and protect their young children from their possible preoccupation with the dead child. Mothers sought out the grieving support network because they found that other mothers with experiences of perinatal death could relate to issues of continuing concern for their dead babies. As one mother nursed her baby girl during the interview, she said,

I am really the mother of three girls, not just one baby girl. And I find myself saying, "Alright, girls, we're going to do so and so."

Another mother described the months that followed her still-birth to be "a time of loss," a time when she needed pictures of her pregnancy and her dead baby within arm's reach. This same mother described the nine months that followed her baby's death as like a "cocoon:"

It was very protective. The things that had always bothered me didn't bother me. It had a niceness to it. . . . That's where you go. There's nowhere else to go.

On reflection, the "other world" is perhaps the period of time during which the mother is continuing to experience palliative effects of denial that accompany crisis events and death. This mother, and other mothers, spoke in detail about one of the most difficult periods, of confronting the public, of Being "without" their babies, and the poignant pain of Being in that reality.

I remember standing outside a baby store, on the second level of the mall. My tears were falling down to the first level. It was so hard trying to find something. I mean, just the idea of going and looking for something to bury your child in. But, we did . . . We found a very pretty dress.
I don't know how I did it, but I went out to dinner with friends, on two different occasions . . . two, three, days after I buried my child. Here I am sitting in a waiting room, a bar on one side, and a restaurant on the other, waiting for a table. And I think back later . . . I know I was in shock. I mean . . . this was just impossible to believe that I was doing it. But, I did it two nights in a row . . . One, with one girlfriend and one, with another. It's almost ridiculous now. I think my friends didn't know what to do or what to say. They thought that being company for me was helpful, but at the same time they weren't helpful. Whenever I mentioned anything, I would be quieted and not allowed to talk about it.

After having a first baby die of a genetic problem shortly after delivery, this mother learned early in pregnancy that her second baby probably had the same defect. She had to be ready to resort to the legal system in order to be assured of maternity leave. Her employer argued that she was not entitled to leave because she was not carrying a viable baby. Her co-workers were significantly bothered that, since she knew the baby was defective, she did not elect therapeutic abortion.

Even before this mother experienced her baby's death, the mother was placed in another world, abandoned by her social world at work because of her knowledge that the fetus was probably going to die and her refusal to terminate the pregnancy prematurely because of the slim possibility that the baby would be all right. This mother thought her experience with perinatal death had prepared her to face issues the second time around that would have been devastating had she not had that first experience. She was somewhat comfortable with Being-a-mother to a possibly defective baby and committed to mothering her baby until its natural death. She carried her baby to term, nurturing and experiencing the only reality available, of Being-a-mother to her baby during the completion of her pregnancy. During delivery, the baby died, evidenced by the monitored heart rate. The mother, her husband and father of the baby, and the attending staff took a moment of silence during which they acknowledged the death. A stillborn baby girl was delivered a short time later.

Temporality of Being-a-Mother in Another World

The researcher found in analysis that the mothers had an existential experience of being abandoned by the baby in another world. The experience of abandonment of the mother was further complicated by subsequent abandonment by the larger social world. This experience is an experience in temporality, bound in time by the nature of the loss, meanings of loss for the mother, the mourning process, and the sense she made of it over time.

The experience of motherhood and mourning death of a child is an experience in temporality. It is constantly evolving and changing with exacerbations in connections of Being with others and with events of life.

The concept of temporality is immersed within writings of T. S. Eliot (1936, 1955). In "Burnt Norton," from *Four Quartets,* temporality of meaning in past, present, and future is captured and further illuminates and validates the discovery of temporality in mothers' experiences. One mother expressed that, "No one understood that when Mary died, part of my future was gone forever." Another mother stated,

Sometimes it's a way of making your baby real, a kind of peeling away the denial. You had lost something that was going to be with you, not just for the moment, but over the years. You've lost that.

Connection of Being-a-Mother in Another World

Merleau-Ponty (1968) stated in his last work,

But at the very moment that I think I share the life of another, I am rejoining it only in its ends, its exterior poles. It is in the world that we communicate, through what, in our life, is articulate. It is from this lawn before me that I think I catch sight of the impact of the green on the vision of another, it through the music that I enter into his musical emotion, it is the thing itself that opens unto me the access to the private world of another. But the thing itself, we have seen, is always for the thing that I see. . . . It is therefore indeed true that the "private worlds" communicate, that each of them is given to its incumbent as a variant of one common world. The communication makes us the witnesses of one sole world, as the synergy of our eyes suspends them on one unique thing. (p. 11)

The researcher found that mothers' experience of being abandoned in another world without the baby is a connected experience, one that is shared relationally with very few others who dare to "be there" with concern. Having had a personal experience with perinatal loss, the researcher discovered that this experience provided a connection with mothers that facilitated sharing.

Shared understanding facilitated investigating and interpreting mothers' experiences.

Mothers described sharing the world of mourning of their babies in relationships with their husbands or partners, families, friends, and with other mothers and fathers in support processes offered in groups. They wondered about and missed the presence of nurses, of nurses "being there" to assist with postpartum care, of their not "being there" to discuss issues related to their mothering, performing mothering activities with ill or dead babies, decisions regarding seeing and holding the babies again, and planning ritual, memorial funerals. They missed opportunities to share their brief mothering of dead babies with relationships in the larger social world at the time of the experience, and they subsequently sought withdrawal from that more public social world around them. Memorial services were found to be very important events, symbolic of the brief public role as mothers, a transition that was incomplete with the death of the baby.

Mothers were able to find those who were "there" with concern and understanding and used opportunities to share and connect and reflect on their feelings and experiences. In this regard, relational reality and possibility, though limited, were integral to meaning of mothers' experience.

Through the support group we met a lot of couples who had lost children and they were very helpful, both before the baby died and afterwards. They rallied around us when we were back home. They phoned, they visited if we wanted them to visit. Most of the time we didn't want anybody to visit, but they phoned. Sometimes I answered the phone, sometimes I didn't. Sometimes I unplugged it so I wouldn't even hear it ringing. And that was all helpful. We continued to go to the support group and that's how we got through it.

This mother stated also,

There's only one person at work who came up to me and put her arms around me and said, "I'm so sorry about what happened." I had gotten cards from people here and there

. . . sympathy cards, but one would think that in addition to sending a sympathy card, the first time you saw that person, you would make a comment about the death. But only one person did. It was more than the fact that I was away from the office, it was the fact that I had a daughter, and I didn't want that daughter to be forgotten. It was a rare person who asked me how I was doing, and really wanted to know how I was doing.

Another mother reflected that in the weeks after her baby was stillborn,

I started to work gradually. It was very hard to go back to work. Everyone had seen me come along in my pregnancy . . . and nobody called. One clinician said to me that he was very concerned. It was like living in a twilight zone. It was horrible. I literally snuck in and out, trying to avoid everybody for weeks.

Context of Being-a-Mother in Another World

The meaning of the experience of Being-a-mother in another world was found to be related to the context of mothers' lives. This included the contexts of connection in life and work of mothers' lives, relationships in the mothers' private as well as social world, and temporality of mourning. The contexts of circumstances, relationships, work, and temporality surrounding the pregnancy were found to be related to a multiple, complex meaning of mothers' experience.

The context of relationships in mothers' lives greatly affected mothers' attribution of meaning to the experience of perinatal loss and eased exacerbations of acute grief and subsequent mourning. Intimate relationships with partners and husbands were supportive and enabled mothers to carve out their particular private cognitive and behavioral experience of grief. Relationships with family and friends were described to vary, were important, but were less integral to their experiences. Relationships with the larger social world, including the working world of the mother, with the exception of a grief support network, were described and characterized by a conspiratorially silencing of the mother and, in most cases, required her withdrawal.

Of particular interest was the context of mothers' work, an area of life that was particularly affected by the death. One mother stated,

> *I think what I'm doing and how I'm doing it is very differ-*
> *ent. This is one of the points in which my friends differed*
> *from me because I started changing my philosophy after the*
> *baby died. I think they thought I was going bananas. I*
> *wasn't doing anything extreme, but before, I never revealed*
> *anything about myself. I guess I got more directive with*
> *clients. When somebody comes in with a problem I probably*
> *work harder. I also found out I was much more confronting.*
> *In fact, I had nothing to lose. I had been through the worst*
> *possible thing, so I was going to sit there and work with*
> *these people in the best way I thought. I came out of the ex-*
> *perience that way about everything. From that came more*
> *interest in my work.*

Three of five participant mothers described particularly important changes in the conduct and meaning of work following death of their babies. These mothers work within the support network for families experiencing pregnancy loss. Two mothers have written professionally on topics of loss using personal experiences and experiences with mothers to articulate issues in need of attention. These writings were consulted during data analysis and used to validate interview data.

Another area of particular interest is in the context of Being-a-mother that changed in mothers' subsequent planning and/or becoming pregnant again.

> *I started trying to get pregnant in February after the still-*
> *birth at Thanksgiving. I remember I got my period at the end*
> *of January. It was like the beginning. I remember feeling*
> *very good, that I could start looking ahead again. The*
> *third time, I got pregnant. All during that period from*

Thanksgiving until I got pregnant, I was operating on about fifty percent. I was really intent on getting pregnant again.

Four of the mothers in the study did have subsequent mothering experiences with another baby. Again, very related to findings regarding altered world views, mothers experienced a heightened and enhanced valuing of opportunities and risks of motherhood, and a greater awareness of what had been forever lost to them in the death of the particular wished-for baby. Mothers found it difficult to continue grieving while caring for a child, though many found themselves confronting grief in daily routine activities of nurturing the subsequent baby. "I have her, but I still cry."

Mothers also found it difficult to know what is the "right" way to go about making their grief known either to other children in the family or to subsequent children. The research interview provided opportunity to explicate this mothering and nurturing issue, to bring up the issue from the private world of silence to the consideration of Being-a-mother to another child. Two mothers had other children at the time of perinatal death: one mother had two young children, one had a young adolescent child. The deliberations and decisions of a mother and father about informing and Being-with their two-year-old child in regard to death of their first baby, was a concern expressed by all of the mothers who had other babies. At the time of the completion of the study, this couple, pregnant with another child, were continuing to deal with the death along with the new birth with their two-and-a-half-year-old daughter.

ESSENTIAL THEMES IN MOTHERS' EXPERIENCES: "ESSENCES" OF MEANING

The "Essence" of Loss

The theme of loss was ever present in mothers' descriptions of their lived experiences with perinatal death. Losses took many forms: loss of a dream, loss of unfulfilled dreams, loss of many missed opportunities. The particular perinatal loss was further colored by multiple and recurrent losses. As shared earlier, one mother described the nine months following her stillborn baby's birth as a "time of loss" of the lived experience of being in a "cocoon," "a place where no one goes," of needing to be within arm's reach of the pictures of her stillborn baby for weeks on end. "There was no way out, but through it."

The theme of loss was persistent, consistent, and recurrent in mothers' lives following perinatal death of a wished-for baby. Each mother described experiences of living through loss with poignant examples depicting how loss had colored and had been colored in their lives.

One mother describes the period of time following her still-birth,

> *I think that's why I didn't get depressed. It took me a long time to get depressed. I was in a cocoon that lasted a good nine, ten, eleven months. It was during that period that I was grief stricken and angry, but I was not depressed. It was as if I were in this holding place, that was very vital. There was nothing dead about it, and the work I did during that period was really in the journal. It was very vivid, but I was not depressed. It was a "loss time." When that period ended, I really missed that cocoon. The reentering is really the critical part that nobody looks at and I think that that's the point where the trouble comes.*

Reflective Pulling Back, Recovering, Re-Entering

Mothers unanimously described their withdrawal from the larger social world following the first indication that "something was wrong." Only those most intimately connected were allowed in the "other" world. The mothers were assisted by husbands, partners, and families to pull back from the larger social world. The subsequent abandonment of the mother by the larger social world actually assisted the mother to create a boundary for herself within which she privately grieved in the manner she chose. The mourning experience was a narcissistic personal commitment of the mother to herself, which validated her mourning, her loss, her separating herself from her baby by "being with" her baby in death. Mothers were adamant about how, in the immediate period following the baby's death, they behaved in grieving, "any damn way I chose."

In addition to the withdrawal from the larger social world, mothers were selective in withdrawal from intimate relationships following the babies' deaths. The withdrawal from connections and relationships was both preceded and followed by a period of feeling isolation and fear that no one would know the extent of the suffering and disappointment. It was during the acute phase that many mothers made new connections with other people who had experienced perinatal loss. The "old" social and intimate world of the mother often invalidated the loss and became impatient for the mother to move "on" or "away" from the particular death and her experience of mourning. The isolation and experience of loss is interpreted to have propelled the mother into initiating and forming new connections, reflecting her altering views of the world based on her new experience of Being-a-mother in another world.

Eventually, all of the mothers became reinvolved with their "old" social world and the larger world, but with changes in world views that dictated changes in personal behavior. One mother described her withdrawal from her social world in the months that followed and her gradual re-entry to that world following the death.

> *I couldn't open my front door. I just sat here looking out the window at what I would never have. . . . a little girl across the street, who was just learning to walk. I couldn't get the mail. I didn't have the strength to open the door, to face anybody, or see anybody. I called a person the support group had recommended, and she made me promise to go out. And for a while if I saw anybody, I would automatically move to the other side of the street.*

This mother described mourning behavior, which included audible, verbal, and behavioral expressions of feelings. She described throwing pillows, taking care to miss her prized collection of ceramic angels. She gradually ventured down the street, crossing to avoid children and people; timing her daily outing to avoid children coming home from school and trolley stops delivering people to the neighborhood.

Embodiment of Mourning and Loss

Each mother described similar experiences, of the emotional and physiological, cognitive and behavioral symptoms characteristic of acute grief. The data of the immediate period following the death is interpreted phenomenologically as being the embodiment of loss. Mothers described in exquisite detail the lived experience: agony of the physical experience of acute grief; ache of empty arms; vivid memories and images of the time surrounding the first awareness that something was wrong; thoughts and feelings relating to the idealized baby; emotional and mental pain; gradual realization and consequences of experience of loss of the particular baby; months that followed and gradual return of interest in daily life.

> *So, some days I didn't get out of bed at all. I tried to. It was winter, and days were very short, and nights were very long. There were times that I wouldn't get out of bed until it was dark. I tried to get out of my nightgown by the time my husband walked in the door. Sometimes I succeeded, sometimes I didn't. It took me a long time before I felt like there was something to do in the day. I'd try to do a load of dishes, and it would take me all day to do the glasses. I'd start the water, start things soaking, and get back to it about three hours later.*
>
> *I cried, I screamed, and cried. I had a white bear that my sister had given to me as a birthday present a number of years ago. Well, that was my child, after she died. I had aching arms, empty arms. They were like weights. They hurt so much. At the time no one lived next door. It made it easier.*

As time passed, mothers described realization of impact of the experience on their subsequent life and its value, of their gradual move to another level of mourning. They described their subsequent preoccupation at times, of their suddenly being pulled back into feelings of acute loss resulting from reminders in the world about them, the reactions to anniversaries and opportunity for remembrances. They described the process of gradually incorporating the experience as part of their changed world view and family history.

For all of the mothers, unfulfilled and lost dreams, missed and lost opportunities, essence of loss was felt and experienced as losing the child forever. It was described as losing a part of the future, of losing a relationship with the child in the future, of losing the personal and social role of mother to the baby, of the forever lost context of Being-a-mother to the child. The experience of the brief, but intense, experience of Being-a-mother to the dead child was captured in thoughts, memories, and life experiences since the death.

Losses experienced by mothers included loss of feeling invulnerable, loss connected with realization that bad things can happen during pregnancy, loss of protective denial pregnant experienced by mothers as they live through pregnancy, loss of denial that helps them deal with anxiety connected to Being-a-mother. As one mother put it,

> *Part of the shock of his death was that anything so consciously planned and worked on could not have not worked, and something that was so . . . that had a technical aspect right from the beginning . . . there was nothing at the end to do, clinically, that would have saved him.*

This mother whose baby was stillborn experienced a second loss, an early pregnancy loss following artificial insemination. She found herself very angry following the second loss. It was just "too much."

Another mother, following the birth of another baby, a girl a year and a half after the death of her baby son, said, "I still cry. I have her but I still cry." Having experienced the worst possible thing imaginable, another mother was able to withstand tremendous social pressure to make a decision to carry her second baby to term even though she was almost certain that the baby suffered from the same genetic defect as her first stillborn baby. This mother thought that the first loss had prepared her for the second experience.

The Narcissistic Injury

Perinatal loss is experienced by the mother as personal loss, constituting a narcissistic injury to self-esteem, her identity as a mother, and her ability to provide protection for her child. As one mother stated, "I felt as if part of me died, too."

Another mother stated,

> *I don't remember how I functioned during the day. I don't remember it at all. I do remember going to bed at 5:00 P.M. My best friend had given me a stuffed animal when I was in the hospital, so that was my security blanket. So, I'd get into bed with my stuffed animal and my nightgown, and the kids would come in and I would read to them in bed. I didn't want to read to them in their rooms. I don't have much memory about it.*

As one mother said, "I couldn't understand what was wrong with me." This mother articulated how she found herself seriously depressed, not because of loss, but because of narcissistic damage of the experience she confronted long after the agony of the acute grieving period was over.

The death of the child also represented death of the world of Being-a-mother to the lost baby, at that time, even though mothers were described to acquire an almost reflexive thought about having another baby immediately. Four of the mothers, plus the pilot mother began actively planning for another baby within the first few months. Another mother, finding herself pregnant again, began the long anticipated prospect of Being-a-mother to another baby. All of the mothers describe the anticipation, of another baby within a few months of the death. All of the mothers had subsequent pregnancies following perinatal death. Only one mother, unsuccessful in attempting to have another baby, is gradually accepting the reality that she will probably not become a mother again.

The Finality of the Death of the Baby

The ultimate loss for mothers who experience the death of a wished-for baby is the loss of the particular child, the loss of Being-a-mother to the child, of a future relationship with the child. The finality of the death is only gradually experienced and accepted. Even though the realization is gradual, each mother described living through the process and her poignant acceptance of the finality of the death. Even though mothers, in some cases, were unable to come up with answers to why it happened and what was wrong, in this sample at the time of interviews, all five mothers and the pilot mother had learned to live "with" the idea of death and the finality with which it strikes.

It happened like a blow. He was dead. There was no way to deny it. My baby was dead. He would always be dead. There was nothing I could do but live with it.

Another mother stated,

It was incredible, really. In the midst of the most horrible thing that had ever happened to me, I was thinking, planning, doing it by the book. I was devastated, really.

Living with and Through Death

In the preceding discussion regarding the mother being abandoned by the dead baby and her social world, and the necessity of living through death, it was discovered that mothers use isolation as a protective world that provided space and time for personal expressions of mourning. The experience of Being in another world, enabled mothers to live "through" experience and be "with" the dead baby. In this other world, mothers were able to prepare for Being-a-mother without a baby. The experience was accompanied by a changed relation with the world, a changed and altering view of the world, and a choice of continuing to live within the world and Being-a-mother to another child.

> *There was nothing I could do about it. I had no choice. I just moved through it day by day. Time seemed suspended. I had my pictures, my privacy, and my memories. I could close my eyes and see the experience all over again. I could be pregnant . . . before it all came crashing down. I was afraid I'd forget what he looked like. And in time it became more and more OK.*

The description of one mother's experience was that for nine or so months that it was like being in a "cocoon." She stated that she had not read about this perception or had not heard other mothers talk about mourning in this way.

Altering World Views

The experience of having a baby die was discovered to have greatly affected views mothers had of the world before, during the crisis, and after death. The changing and altering world view is related to personal meaning of the experience, meaning which, as stated before is temporal, connected to people, and bound in the context of experience in the mothers' world.

Where mothers varied in their mourning experiences, some common features were shared. The degree to which mothers had integrated the experience into other aspects of their lives, the degree mothers had incorporated the experience into life stories and histories, the degree to which experience had changed the mother's world and the relationship of the mother to world, varied from mother to mother. However, each mother voiced change in the following areas: change in *what, how, why,* and change with *whom* mothers connected. In addition, the sense mothers make of experience, though different from each other, reflected a greater, heightened awareness of value of life and death and value of the wished-for baby. The mother of the baby who was stillborn following conception by artificial insemination stated,

I know that no matter what's going on now, whether it's good or bad, that it's going to change. Something else is going to happen. That's really comforting, because I don't think that I had that longer range vision before.

This was so bad that it put everything else in perspective. It was one of my worst fears. Now that it's happened, I feel freed up. I had always wanted to write. I can be comfortable alone. Relationships are more important to me, but I'm less desperate.

I'm not as easy as I used to be. I think I was much more obliging before. I don't feel as much like a cheerleader. I've incorporated the idea of evil and disaster into my view of life and through that have gotten more interested in my spiritual life. My perspective has altered violently. The whole idea of good and bad are both part of the same swing. I'm much more confrontive than I was before. I've gotten interested in death and loss.

Death Overlaid with Life

The theme that death is overlaid with new life and rebirth was discovered to be very present, very strong, and unanimous in mothers' experience of perinatal loss. This, along with the theme of loss was a persistent, consistent, and recurrent theme running throughout the data and was present from the first piloted interview throughout inquiry into the final interviews. The existential descriptions found in artistic, literary, and creative findings support this finding, especially excerpts from Lindbergh (1971), T.S. Eliot's work (1936), and an anthology of literature (Enright, 1987). This theme is present in poetry by T.S. Eliot, in *The Waste Land,* "The Burial of the Dead."

The theme of death overlaid with life, renewal, and rebirth took varying forms. The pregnancy and birth of the baby who died was connected in mothers' minds with another personal loss. Each mother spoke of renewed respect for value of qualitative aspects of their lives.

Several stories of mothers' experiences, their baby's lives and deaths were connected with lives and deaths of significant others.

*My cousin was killed in a car accident that May, before.
She had been named for my father. So when I got pregnant, we named this child for her. We called our baby by
name throughout the pregnancy.*

Another mother described how the pregnancy was like a breath
of fresh air during a period when her husband's father was terminally ill, that the pregnancy and wished-for new baby, helped them
cope during a period of stress.

*My husband's father died that January and we went to
the viewing. A pretty awful time in terms of illness and
death. But, the pregnancy kind of kept me going. There was
a memorial service and people were commenting that at
least there was one bright spot. We had told him we were
expecting a baby before he died. We were so glad he knew
about the baby.*

A mother whose brother had died in an accident stated that her
baby was buried with her brother.

*My brother and baby are buried together in the same ceme-
tery plot my father bought when my brother died. My dad
visits the cemetery daily. He plants spring pots and a little
window box in front of the tombstone each year. . . . We
bought a tree and planted a tree on the side of the tombstone.*

Each mother discussed importance of ritual memorial service, funerals, and/or burials of their babies.

Failing and Trying Again

This theme pervades data of mothers' lived experience of loss.
Each mother described a reflexive focusing on beginning another
pregnancy whether by choice or indecision. The transition into the
world of Being-a-mother was incomplete with death of the baby.
The mothers' view, her identity as a mother, necessitated another
attempt at Being-a-mother.

DISCUSSION, SIGNIFICANCE AND LIMITATIONS OF STUDY

The data of mother's lived experience of loss is messy, indeterminant, and required one's descent, as Schon (1990) describes, to the swamp, the low lying land of human experience of living through death. It promised a discovery of meaning in mothers' experience and a greater depth of understanding. The use of mothers' stories of loss and mothers' voices in inquiry was perhaps the reason that mother's existential experience of Being-a-mother in another world was articulated and amplified so loudly.

The study discovered that connections and relationships with people were integral to personal meaning of mothers' experiences. Mothers in this inquiry carefully selected connections they needed and desired, and initiated new connections when old ones did not serve their needs in mourning. In addition, the current study discovered that interrelatedness of experience, mothers' world views, temporality, experience over time, and the nature and quality of contextual aspects of mothers' lives were intimately related to meaning.

Where a credible discovery of meaning has been described, the reader is cautioned regarding making far-reaching generalizations. Mothers in this study may not represent the larger world of mothers and meaning identified may not be generalizable to represent all mothers with experience of the phenomenon.

The phenomenological perspective and research process resulted in discovering meaning of mothers' experience while meeting mothers' needs of increased self-understanding. Feedback from mothers and others with whom these study results have been shared point to the need for continuing further study.

Even though knowledge reflected in literature and research in the area of perinatal loss has been substantial in recent years, qualitative aspects of the meaning of mothers' experience has been poorly understood. This study used an inquiry which served to bridge the discrepancy of understanding. By using mothers' memories and stories, meaning or "essences" of mothers' experience was uncovered, articulated, and further amplified by voices of mothers themselves. Significance of the study exceeds nursing care reform with mothers experiencing perinatal loss. It provides opportunity to reflect more deeply with greater understanding on a phenomenon of human experience and facilitates the process of becoming more fully human and allows action on meaning illuminated.

IMPLICATIONS FOR RESEARCH, EDUCATION AND PRACTICE

As a result of inquiry, an evolution of a preliminary graphic depiction of a conceptual model of meaning of mothers' experience of perinatal loss is shown in Figure 5-6. The model has three integrally related dimensions: temporality, connection, and context. Essential themes run throughout the dimensions to produce the "essences" of meaning of mothers' experience with perinatal death of a wished-for baby.

The study is especially timely in light of current interest within the nursing profession in qualitative research. The particular phenomenological research methodology selected for investigating the phenomenon facilitated an emergence of a wealth of quality phenomena of loss. The rich sources of data identified and quality of data, coupled with the process of phenomenological reflection, promoted understanding of the meaning of experience "for" mothers and their families as well as "with" mothers themselves.

It is especially important to acknowledge that the meanings and "essences" revealed in the study illuminate the research and discovery process facilitated by phenomenology, as well as highlighting meanings found. The phenomenological method provided by Van Manen (1984) and Munhall (1992) allowed the researcher to address multiple and complex meanings surrounding the phenomenon. It uncovered meanings hidden and concealed from immediate view in the public world, and directed the researcher to go beneath the "silence," that is, beneath the surface, to uncover and generate data surrounding the phenomenon. It also directed the researcher to identify meanings readily revealed and described through analyzing mothers' experiences in light of this larger world of data surrounding the phenomenon.

An important outcome from this study is that phenomenology offers an approach to nursing research that has direct impact on

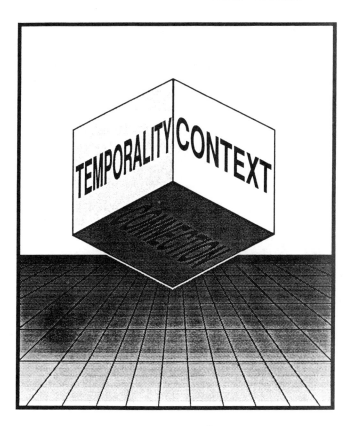

Figure 5–6. Conceptual model of meaning in mothers' experience with perinatal death of a wished-for baby.

practice and education. As a research methodology, phenomenology offers an opportunity for investigating a particular phenomenon of human experience, while at the same time gleaning a depth of human understanding from the bigger, more farsighted picture. It involves a process of reflection on personal and professional experience, as well as human experience, which is crucial to changing and articulating more informed human care. The direct practice applications from this research are many, and stem from the enhanced understanding of experience.

Implications from this research also speak to a need for nurse researchers to commit themselves to inquiry into phenomena for which there is great professional and/or personal knowledge and interest. Reflection on personal and professional experience facilitates understanding and assists in critical analysis of experience. As a process in this investigation, reflection on personal experience facilitated bracketing of personal biases and at the same time provided a connection between the researcher, support network, and mothers. In the view of the researcher, the discovery in this study is related to a relative goodness of "fit" among the phenomenon, research methodology process, human experience and potential for understanding.

REFERENCES

Becker, E. (1973). *The Denial of Death.* New York: The Free Press.

Burns, S. (1990). *Sleeping Beauty: Memorial Photography in America.* New York: Twelve-Trees Press.

Campbell, J. (1988). *The Power of Myth.* New York: Doubleday Dell Publishing Co.

Chute, M. (1962). *Shakespeare of London.* London: The New English Library, Ltd.

Eliot, T. (1936). *Collected Poems 1909-1962.* New York: Harcourt, Brace & World.

Enright, D. (Ed.). (1987). *The Oxford Book of Death.* Oxford: Oxford University Press.

Flowers, B. (1988). *The Power of Myth / Joseph Campbell with Bill Moyers.* New York: Anchor Books Doubleday.

Freud, S. (1915). "Thoughts for the times on war and death, *Collected Papers, Vol. IV.* 316–317. New York: Basic Books.

Greene, D. (1985). *Greene's Biographical Encyclopedia of Composers.* New York: Doubleday & Co.

Guba, E. & Lincoln, Y. (1981). *Effective Evaluation.* San Francisco: Jossey-Bass.

Heidegger, M. (1962). *Being and Time.* (J. Macquarrie & E. Robinson, Trans.). New York: Harper & Row, Publishers, Inc. (Original work published 1927.)

Husserl, E. (1952). *Ideas: General Introduction to Pure Phenomenology.* (W. Gibson, Trans.). New York: Macmillan.

Knapp, R. (1986). *Beyond Endurance: When a Child Dies.* New York: Shocken Books.

Leininger, M. (1985). *Qualitative Research Methods in Nursing.* Orlando: Grune and Stratton, Inc.

Lewis, C. (1961). *A Grief Observed.* New York: Harper Collins Publishers.

Lindbergh, A. (1973). *Hour of Gold, Hour of Lead.* Orlando: Harcourt, Brace, Jovanovich.

Linscott, R. (1932). (Ed.). *The Stories of Anton Tchekhov.* New York: The Modern Library.

Lloyd, P. (1980). Post humous mourning portraiture. In M. V. Pike & J. G. Armstrong (Eds.). *A Time to Mourn.* New York: The Museums at Stony Brook.

Mason, J. (1970). *Gilgamesh.* Boston: Houghton Mifflin Company, Inc.

Merleau-Ponty, M. (1973). *Adventures of the Dialectic.* (J. Bien, Trans.). Evanston: Northwestern University Press.

Merleau-Ponty, M. (1962). *Phenomenology of Perception.* London: Routledge & Kegan Paul.

Merleau-Ponty, M. (1974). *Phenomenology, Language & Sociology.* London: Heinemann Educational Books Ltd.

Merleau-Ponty, M. (1973). *The Prose of the World.* (C. Lefort, Trans.). Evanston: Northwestern University Press.

Merleau-Ponty, M. (1964). *Sense and Nonsense.* (H. Dreyfus & P. Dreyfus, Trans.). Evanston: Northwestern University Press.

Merleau-Ponty, M. (1968). *The Visible and the Invisible.* (C. Lefort, Ed., A. Lingus Trans.). Evanston: Northwestern University Press.

Meryman, R. (1991). The Wyeth family: American visions. *National Geographic. 180*(1) 78–109.

Munhall, P. (1992). Unpublished manuscript.

Pike, M., & Armstrong, J. (1980). *A Time to Mourn.* New York: The Museums at Stony Brook.

Sartre, J. (1965). *What Is Literature?* (B. Frechtman, Trans.). New York: Harper & Row. (Original work published 1949.)

Schutz, A. (1967). *The Phenomenology of the Social World.* (G. Walsh & F. Lehnert, Trans.). Evanston: Northwestern University Press. (Original work published 1932.)

Schon, D. (1990). *Educating the Reflective Practitioner.* San Francisco: Josey-Bass.

Schorsch, A. (1976). *Mourning Becomes America.* Philadelphia: Pearl Pressman Liberty.

Spiegelberg, H. (1965). *The Phenomenological Movement/Volumes I. & II.* The Hague: Nartinus Nijhoff.

United States Department of Health and Human Services. (1990). *Monthly Vital Statistics Report. 39*(3).

Van Manen, M. (1984). *"Doing" Phenomenological Research and Writing.* Alberta: The University of Alberta Press.

Wilcox, L. (1911). Facing death. *Harper's Bazaar.* January, 21.

6

Grounded Theory:
The Method

Sally A. Hutchinson

Those, however, who aspire not to guess and divine but to discover and know; who propose not to devise mimic and fabulous worlds of their own, but to examine and dissect the nature of this world itself; must go to the facts themselves for everything. Sir Francis Bacon

The writings of Sir Francis Bacon, an initiator of the scientific revolution, prefigure the underlying philosophy of grounded theorists. Bacon worked diligently toward "the regeneration and restoration of the sciences" (Warshaft, 1965, p. 35). Although the facts to which he referred differed radically from the facts examined by grounded theorists today, Bacon's aim, like ours, was to shed dogmatic beliefs in order to perceive reality more clearly. (In Bacon's time, scientists were interested in facts related to the earth and the universe. Grounded theorists search for social processes present in human interaction.) Such intellectual revolutions guard against the eternal danger that scientists lean too heavily on inherited dogma or theories. Grounded theory contains an inherent safeguard against this danger in that its explanation of key social structures or processes is derived from or grounded in the empirical data themselves. Speculative theory, in contrast, originates and develops in the researcher's mind, with varying regard for these empirical phenomena.

Grounded theories may be formal or substantive. Formal theories address a conceptual level of inquiry, such as status passage, socialization, stigma, or illness (Morse & Johnson, 1992). Substantive theories are generated for a specific, circumscribed, and empirical area of inquiry, such as family caregiving for relatives with Alzheimer's dementia (Wilson, 1989), people with bipolar disorder (see Chapter 7), or dying patients (Glaser & Strauss, 1968). Substantive theories can be used to build formal theories.

Barney Glaser and Anselm Strauss, two sociologists at the University of California, San Francisco, developed the grounded theory method in the 1960s. Trained at Columbia University and the University of Chicago, respectively, Glaser and Strauss embarked on a study of dying. Their research resulted in two classic books, *Awareness of Dying* (1965) and *Time for Dying* (1968), and a book on method, *Discovery of Grounded Theory* (1967). Their student, Jeanne Quint Benoliel, a nurse sociologist, became the first nurse to do both collaborative and individual work in grounded theory. Her excellent book, *The Nurse and the Dying Patient* (1967), and her many articles on research and cancer nursing reflect her years with Glaser and Strauss.

Research methodology is not a haphazard bag of tricks. Rather, each research method is linked to a perspective on a philosophy of science. Symbolic interactionism, described by sociologists George Herbert Mead (1934) and Herbert Blumer (1969), provides the philosophical foundations for grounded theory and guides the research questions, interview questions, data collection strategies, and methods of data analysis (Bowers, 1988; Hutchinson & Wilson, in press). Nurse sociologist Bowers (1988) and Stern, Allen, and Moxley (1982) presented a history of grounded theory methods and articulated the symbolic interactionist perspective. "Symbolic interactionism is a social-psychological theory of social action" that is organized around the self, the world, and social action (Bowers, 1988, p. 36). The self and the world are socially constructed, and, as such, they are ever changing through processes of social interaction. Thus, individuals and their actions cannot be understood out of social context. Stern et al. (1982) noted:

> *Symbolic interactionism posits that humans act and interact on the basis of symbols which have meaning and value for the actors. Examples of symbols include words for an object rather than the object itself, body language which communicates messages to others with or without words.* (p. 203)

How people dress, how they speak, and the artifacts they use all contribute to their presentation of self to the world. Both the behavioral or interactional level and the symbolic level of behavior are important to symbolic interactionists (Chenitz & Swanson, 1986). Grounded theory research is aimed at understanding how a group of people define, via social interactions, their reality (Stern et al., 1982). The purpose of this chapter is to present the method of grounded theory that aims toward this goal of accurately perceiving and presenting another's world.

The generation of grounded theory relies on the inquiring, analytical minds of its researchers/theorists. Their task is to discover and conceptualize the essence of complex interactional processes. The resulting theory emerges as an entirely new way of understanding the observations from which it is generated. It is this understanding that permits the development of relevant interventions in the social environment under consideration.

Denzin (1970) makes the point that all data, qualitative or quantitative, serve four basic functions for theory: to initiate new theory and to reformulate, refocus, and clarify existing theory (p. 120). The grounded theory method serves each of these functions well. If little is known about a topic and few adequate theories exist to explain or predict a group's behavior, the grounded theory method is especially useful. The grounded theory method can also offer an existing new approach to an old problem (Stern, 1980). Interventions resulting from grounded theory may result in the improvement of patient care (Glaser & Strauss, 1965, 1968; Morse & Johnson, 1992; Wilson, 1989) or curriculum enrichment (Glaser & Strauss, 1965, 1968; Hutchinson, 1992). Because of its practical implications, grounded theory research can be classified as applied research.

VERIFICATIONAL RESEARCH

It is useful for the reader to understand some differences between verificational research and grounded theory generation. In verificational research, the researcher chooses an existing theory or conceptual framework and formulates hypotheses, which are then tested in a specific population. Verificational research is linear; the researcher delineates a problem, selects a theoretical framework, develops hypotheses, collects data, tests the hypotheses, and interprets the results. On a continuum, verificational research is more deductive whereas grounded theory research is more inductive. Verificational research moves from a general theory to a specific situation, whereas grounded theorists aim for the development of a more inclusive, general theory through the analysis of specific social phenomena.

It is not unusual for nurses to apply research instruments or theories indiscriminately in a variety of settings. Uncritical reliance on preexisting research instruments precludes even a preliminary exploration of the research problem and results in limited conceptualization, premature closure, and doubtful utility. The misapplication or untimely use of theories from other disciplines produces only a superficial fit between theory and reality and does not adequately explain observed variations in behavior.

A researcher using an existing theory approaches the problem from the top down (from theory to practice) rather than from the ground up (from practice to theory). Grounded theory employs an inductive, from-the-ground-up approach using everyday behaviors or organizational patterns to generate theory. Such a theory is inherently relevant to the world from which it emerges, whereas the relevance of verificational research varies widely.

NURSING RESEARCH, A HISTORICAL PERSPECTIVE

From its inception, the focus of nursing research has been on theory testing—that is, verificational research. This bias is evidenced in nursing research journals, funded research, research presented at conferences, and the curriculum content in colleges of nursing. The excessive respect accorded to quantitative methods indicates a premature rigor and misplaced emphasis in nursing research. The exclusive focus on verificational research also creates a false dichotomy between theory building and theory testing.

The past ten years in nursing research have evidenced a trend toward some appreciation of the contributions of qualitative research, yet the majority of critics still bring the canons of empirical science to bear on qualitative proposals. An increasing number of grounded theory studies, and studies using other qualitative methods, have been published in leading nursing research journals such as *Nursing Research, Image, Advances in Nursing Science, Research in Nursing and Health,* and *Western Journal of Nursing Research.* Nurse researchers who have expertise in qualitative methods review grant proposals at the National Center for Nursing Research and other National Institutes of Health, and they review manuscripts for research and clinical journals. These outspoken nurse researchers are responsible for altering the research climate so that grounded theory studies, and studies using other qualitative methods, are funded and published. The caliber of qualitative studies is rapidly improving, giving credibility to the method and the product.

ASSUMPTIONS OF GROUNDED THEORY

Grounded theories are guided by the assumption that people do, in fact, order and make sense of their environment, although their world may appear disordered or nonsensical to observers. Reality is a social construct, or, as Berger and Luckmann (1967) described it:

> *The world of everyday life is not only taken for granted as reality by the ordinary members of society in the subjectively meaningful conduct of their lives. It is a world that originates in their thoughts and actions, and is maintained as real by these. (pp. 19–20)*

People sharing common circumstances, such as neonatal intensive care unit (NICU) nurses or people with bipolar disorders, experience shared meanings and behaviors that constitute the substance of grounded theory. Grounded theorists base their research on the assumption that each such group shares a specific social psychological problem that is not necessarily articulated. This fundamental problem is resolved by means of social psychological processes. After spending a few months in a level III NICU* (Hutchinson, 1984), I discovered that the nurses' unarticulated problem was one of horror resulting from dealing with the repetitive death and deformation of newborns. This problem of horror initiated the basic social psychological process of "creating meaning." Nurses in an NICU create a variety of meanings for themselves, and these meanings permit them to derive satisfaction from their work with critically ill newborns. If a nurse is unable to create meaning, he or she evidences signs of burnout, such as depression, low morale, and irritability.

In research on family caregivers for relatives with Alzheimer's dementia, Wilson (1989) discovered that the unarticulated problem for the caregivers was "coping with negative choices" because all the possible alternatives were undesirable. The resulting process, "surviving on the brink," describes a "consciously examined, self-reflective, strategic, and difficult means of surviving on a day-to-day, if not moment-to-moment basis under conditions of initial uncertainty and unpredictability, pressing demands with a paucity of support, and a dreaded future" (p. 95).

---

* Level III units provide a range of complex newborn intensive care services, including long-term ventilating management.

When a previously unarticulated problem and its resultant basic social psychological process are uncovered and conceptualized, one can explain and predict behavioral variation in a group. Glaser and Strauss advocated the search for social psychological problems and processes, viewing them as central to the understanding of people's behavior. Thus, research questions for grounded theory studies focus on discovering social processes. The research question for the NICU research was: "What are the social processes involved in being an NICU nurse?" The research question for Wilson's (1989) study was: "What is the process of family caregiving for elderly relatives with Alzheimer's dementia as experienced from the perspective of the caregiver?"

DATA GATHERING

In grounded theory research, data gathering generally follows the pattern of field research. The field research method has been traditionally practiced by anthropologists and sociologists, who, in fact, lived in the field. Once the researcher/theorist chooses a group or a setting to study, he or she becomes immersed in that social environment. Initial observations are used to understand and describe the typical social structure and observed patterns of behavior in this environment. Chenitz and Swanson (1986) noted:

> *The focus of observation is on the interaction since it is in both verbal and nonverbal behavior that the symbolic meaning of the event is transmitted. The analysis of interaction includes participants' self-definitions and shared meaning. Observation focuses on the interaction in a situation and analysis focuses on the symbolic meaning that is transmitted via action. Analysis focuses on interaction, patterns of interaction, and their consequences. (p. 6)*

Observations form the matrix from which the basic social psychological problem and process are derived. Initially, the researcher's observations are tentative and become focused only after a problem and basic social psychological process emerge.

Because grounded theory research requires interpersonal interaction, the researcher is inevitably part of his or her daily observations. Therefore, one must become aware of personal preconceptions, values, and beliefs. Only through self-awareness of mind-set can the researcher begin to search out and understand another's world. Such understanding is vital to field research, as Berger and Kellner (1981) reminded us:

> *If such bracketing (of values) is not done, the scientific enterprise collapses, and what the [researcher] then believes to perceive is nothing but a mirror image of his own hopes and fears, wishes, resentments or other psychic needs; what he will then not perceive is anything that can reasonably be called social reality. (p. 52)*

A daily journal or diary in which the researcher can express personal feelings and reflections is often helpful in sustaining this heightened level of awareness.

As a participant in the social scene, the researcher begins to make observations. Interviews, generally informal in nature, augment these observations and serve to clarify the meanings the participants themselves attribute to a given situation. For example, in the NICU, I noticed numerous babies shaking and quivering. I assumed they were cold and asked a nurse to check them. She informed me that they were not shivering but were having seizures. Had I not asked her (informal interview), I would have misunderstood what I saw. Interviews help the researcher understand a problem through the eyes of the participants. The observer searches for their concepts of meaningfulness rather than viewing a situation from his or her own perspective or that of any other group. The human touch—the capacity to empathize with these participants—is essential for this type of research.

Formal, semistructured interviews are also foundational for grounded theory research and, in certain studies, may be the only source of data. For example, in studies of past experiences such as incest, rape, or giving birth to a deformed child, interviews may be the only way to capture the participants' feelings and experiences. Issues of time and access may preclude fieldwork with people or groups currently experiencing similar situations.

Formal interviews occur at a time and a place acceptable to the participant, generally last from one to two hours, and may occur over time, depending on the research. The researcher aims to generate a theory that accounts for all behavioral variation within a group. To accomplish this, a diversity of perspectives is necessary. In the same setting, people who are of varying ages, socioeconomic groups, educational status, and cultures will be interviewed. Participants are chosen purposefully because they are knowledgeable about the area of study.

Interview questions move from the general to the particular; ultimately, they elicit information fundamental to grounded theory studies, such as dimensions, phases, properties, strategies, consequences, and contexts of behavior. For example, a beginning general question in the NICU study was: "Tell me what it is like to be an NICU nurse." A specific question much later in the research process was: "What do you do [a strategy question] when you disagree with the physician's care of a baby?" The researcher asks different participants different questions as the theory evolves; interview questions are guided by the emerging theory.

Additional data might include organizational charts, patient records, hospital policies, newspaper and television coverage, and fictional and anecdotal descriptions that expand and further substantiate the data base from which the theory emerges. NICU nurses shared diaries and termination letters. People with bipolar disorders offered poetry and photographs. One woman shared editorials she had written to the newspaper. Such diverse "slices of data" (Glaser & Strauss, 1967, p. 66) ensure density and provide multiple perspectives for illuminating social phenomena. Dense data contain numerous examples of specific incidents and behaviors. Too few examples yield an inadequate, incomplete theory. A dense theory has numerous propositions that are indicative of complexity, and such a theory cannot be easily summarized.

RELIABILITY AND VALIDITY

Researchers should and do ask the question: "Does such an eclectic array of data accurately reflect the milieu under study?" Quantitative researchers frequently describe qualitative research as "too subjective" and inherently unreliable and invalid. They regard the presence of the field researcher as an intrusive factor that inevitably influences the behavior of the participants. They also maintain that, in both informal and formal interviews, these participants may lie, distort the truth, or withhold vital information, in which case the researcher is misled by incomplete, inaccurate, or biased data.

A rebuttal to such assertions would propose that, although a participant observer may initially influence the setting, social and organizational constraints will invariably neutralize this effect. Participants will become more concerned with meeting the demands of their own situation than with paying attention to, pleasing, or playing games with the researcher (Becker, 1970, p. 43). In an NICU, for example, babies must be taken care of in spite of the researcher's presence.

The temporal reality of fieldwork provides an additional check on the data. Grounded research is conducted in the field, through interviews over a protracted period of time. The researcher continually formulates hypotheses and rejects them if they do not seem accurate. A grounded theorist looks for contradictory data by searching out and investigating unusual circumstances or occurrences. If such data do not fit what has already been found, they will not be discarded but will contribute to the richness of the theory in process. Data are compared and contrasted again and again, thus providing a check on their validity. Distortions or lies generated by the participants will gradually be revealed. The multiple methods of data collection used in grounded theory research—direct observation, interviews, and documents—prevent undue bias by increasing the wealth of information available to the researcher.

Can a theory generated in a specific context be generalized to a larger group? Can a theory of NICU nurses in one setting be expected to be relevant to NICU nurses in another? A substantive theory can be said to be valid only for the studied population. A quality theory, however, will inevitably identify a basic process that is also relevant to people in general.

One of the criticisms of grounded theory is that the purposeful sampling strategy does not meet the requirements for statistical generalizability. However, the concern in qualitative research is with analytic generalizability, not statistical generalizability. Analytic generalizability refers to the utility of the concepts/ constructs to explain a given situation. To assess analytic generalizability, one might ask: "Is the theory with its concepts/ constructs useful in understanding particular social phenomena? In the area under study and/or in other related areas?" For example, the basic social psychological process of creating meaning was generated in a specific NICU, yet nurses from many other NICUs acknowledged that it was relevant to them. Many people may use the process of creating meaning at difficult times in their lives (e.g., divorce, death of a loved one), but it may not be one of their basic processes. Further research into key processes should establish their validity in other areas.

Another question might be: "Is grounded theory research replicable?" The answer is: "Probably not." Grounded theory process depends on the interaction between the data and the creative processes of the researcher. It is highly unlikely that two people would generate the same theory. Berger and Kellner (1981) noted:

The social location, the psychological constitution and the cognitive peculiarities of an interpreter are inevitably involved in the act of interpretation, and all of them will affect the interpretation. (p. 48)

The question of replicability is not especially relevant, because the point of theory generation is to offer a new perspective on a given situation and good and useful ways of looking at a certain world. Honigman (1976) pointed out:

[Data are] not reflections of facts or relationships, existing independently of the observer. In the process of knowing, external facts are sensorially perceived and immediately transformed into conceptualized experience, the observer being an active factor in the creation of knowledge, not a passive recipient or register. (p. 245)

The question of reliability, or the consistency of data over time, is taken care of in part by the duration of field research. Because a theory is modifiable, changes in relevant variables can be accounted for by way of modifications.

Lincoln and Guba (1985) suggested terms, other than validity and reliability, that are more in keeping with the nature of qualitative research. These terms include credibility, transferability, dependability, and confirmability. In their book, *Naturalistic Inquiry,* Lincoln and Guba provided detailed strategies that enhance these qualities.

DATA RECORDING

The immediate recording of data is vital to the success of grounded theory generation. Researchers rely on taped interviews and/or written notes prior to using a word-processing program to expand their data with memory. Field notes are typed double-spaced, with page numbers and appropriate headings (place, date, and time). (See Figure 6–1.) Wide left and right margins facilitate working with the text. Word-processing programs provide specific instructions about formatting the files (ASCII or DOS text files) so that they are retrievable for data analysis.

The type of research setting and the skills of the researcher are variables that influence the choice of the data recording method. The researcher must be sensitive to the social environment before making this choice. The use of a tape recorder in a hospital that had recently experienced a grand jury investigation inspired an understandable fear on the part of the interviewees. Even the unobtrusive use of pen and paper can be offensive to participants in highly stressful settings, such as disciplinary hearings for hospital employees or an NICU where parents are in the process of making decisions about the treatment of their critically ill child. In such cases, dictating notes after the proceedings/interactions is the most reliable method possible.

THE METHOD OF THEORY GENERATION

The Discovery of a Core Variable or Basic Social Psychological Process

The discovery of a core variable is an essential requirement for a quality grounded theory. Continuous reference to the data,

Place: Neonatal ICU   Time: 9–11:30 AM   Date: May 27, 1981

It's May 27th, the first day of the research. I called the Director of Nursing last week and she said, yes, I could start the research but to please start in the neonatal unit because she said she had never seen so much anger in her whole life. Nurses were quitting and there was a lot of stress over there. Doctors were blaming the nurses for infant deaths. I talked with Dr. 1 and he said, "Yes, the unit had always been quite stressed." So, I'll start the research there.

Problems that were suggested to me by different people were that the physical space in the unit was small, that it was very crowded, that there were no windows, that the nurses were suffering from depression. A doctor suggested that they switch off with other nurses in Pediatrics, but that idea was met with disapproval by all the nurses.

Met with Mrs. X and Mrs. Y. Both of them seemed very responsive to the research. Some humorous comments were made. Mrs. X said that because I was a "psych" nurse, I was in the right place; that some of the staff on the unit had psychiatric problems, although they didn't realize it. She told me that they had had 19 deaths the first 19 days of May—4 deaths in 1 day. That had really stressed everybody. Mrs. X then took me to the unit.

Figure 6–1.   Field notes.

combined with rigorous analytical thinking, will eventually yield such a variable. The researcher undertakes the quest for this essential element of the theory, which illuminates the "main theme" of the actors in the setting and explicates "what is going on in the data" (Glaser, 1978, p. 94). The core variable has six essential characteristics:

1. It recurs frequently in the data;
2. It links the various data together;
3. Because it is central, it explains much of the variation in the data;
4. It has implications for a more general or formal theory;
5. As it becomes more detailed, the theory moves forward;
6. It permits maximum variation in analysis (Strauss, 1987, p. 36).

The core variable becomes the basis for the generation of the theory. The categories, properties, phases, and dimensions of the theory are inextricably related to the core variable. The integration and density of the theory are dependent on the discovery of a significant core variable.

Basic social psychological processes (BSPs) are core variables that illustrate social processes as they continue over time, regardless of varying conditions (Glaser, 1978, p. 100). Another kind of core variable is called a basic social structural process (BSSP) (Glaser, 1978; Glaser & Strauss, 1967). Strauss (1987) advocated searching for both interactional/processural and structural conditions and linking the two together. Most commonly, grounded theory studies are either one or the other. Most of the grounded theory studies in nursing focus on the microanalysis of social processes (see Chapter 7 and Wilson, 1989) and do not address the relevant macroanalysis of structural processes. However, with further data collection and analysis, relevant structural processes can be discovered and woven in with the theory. Fagerhaugh and Strauss (1977), in *The Politics of Pain Management,* provided a good example of the interrelationship of social structural and social psychological processes. They analyzed the organizational settings in which pain occurs, along with staff–patient interaction around the issues of pain.

In her caregiving study, Wilson (1989) discovered surviving on the brink as a BSP that was a response to the problem of coping with negative choices. Creating meaning is a BSP that emerged in the NICU research as a response to the problem of horror. This process unfolds in stages, including creating meaning emotionally, technically, and rationally. These stages, with the individual properties and conditions, form the structure of the theory. Creating meaning may not be the only BSP of theoretical importance in NICU work, but it explains much of the behavioral variation in the data.

Once a BSP or BSSP emerges, the researcher selectively codes only those data that relate to it. (Coding is elaborated on in the next section.) Thus, the BSP becomes a guide for further data collection and analysis. With selective coding, many codes emerge either as separate categories or as conditions, strategies, or phases of categories. For example, creating meaning technically was initially a substantive code; on further analysis, it became a stage in creating meaning.

BSPs evidenced in the social organization of a particular group may be found in other groups and settings. Creating meaning as a survival strategy for NICU nurses is not specific to the NICU but may emerge in many different situations. As a process, it is independent of the structural unit in which it was discovered.

Several steps precede the selection of the BSP. These steps include different levels of coding, memoing, theoretical sampling, and sorting. Table 6–1 and Figure 6–2 help set the theory generation process into linear and temporal patterns.

Coding

The process of doing grounded theory is both systematic and intense (Strauss, 1987) because it requires that the researcher simultaneously collect, code, and analyze the data beginning with the first interview and/or the first day in the field. The method is circular, allowing the researcher to change focus and pursue leads revealed by the ongoing data analysis. A month of observations

Table 6–1
Grounded Theory

Process	Product
Primary literature review	Discovery of sensitizing concepts, gaps in knowledge
Data collection: interviews, observations, documents	Masses of narrative data
Coding: coding paradigm, axial coding, constant comparative method	Level 1 codes—called in vivo or substantive
	Level II codes—called categories
	Level III codes—called theoretical constructs
Memoing	Theoretical ideas
Theoretical sampling	Dense data that lead to the illumination and expansion of theoretical constructs
Sorting	Basic social psychological process (BSP)—a central theme and/or Basic social structural process (BSSP)—a central theme
Selective coding based on BSP	Theory delimited to a few theoretical constructs, their categories, and properties
Saturation of codes, categories, and constructs	A dense, parsimonious theory covering behavioral variation; a sense of closure
Secondary literature review	Discovery of literature that supports, illuminates, or extends proposed theory
Writing the theory	A piece of publishable research

and informal interviews in a medical intensive care unit (MICU) yielded little relevant information on nonprofessional behavior, the focus of the research. If I had not been reading and rereading and questioning my data daily, I would have lost my focus entirely by not recognizing the paucity of relevant information in my field notes. I concluded that the absence of a frame of reference by which to identify such behavior made it difficult to see what was

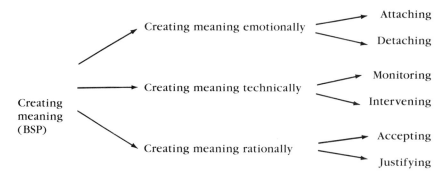

Figure 6–2. Theoretical codes for NICU research.

going on. Consequently, I decided to move to a psychiatric unit, where I shared common meanings and was known to some of the nurses. In this setting, it was easier for me to ask direct questions about nonprofessional behavior and to perceive such behavior when it took place. I began to identify categories of nonprofessional behavior and planned to explore their relevance in the MICU. For example, if rough and insensitive treatment of a patient on a psychiatric floor is nonprofessional, are there similar (or different) kinds of nonprofessional behaviors in an MICU? Preliminary experiences from the psychiatric unit guided my focus into other, less familiar areas.

Level I coding begins with words that describe the action in the setting. Such codes are the in vivo or substantive codes and may be the exact words that the actors use. As such, they tend to be catchy and meaningful. Examples of early substantive coding on nurse behaviors in the NICU research were "feeling personally depleted," "losing it," "crying," "monitoring," "changing a catheter," and so on. Wilson (1989) used such codes as "giving my all" and "feeling burnt out." Substantive coding based only on the data prevents the researcher from imposing preconceived impressions.

Open coding refers to the coding of each sentence and each incident into as many codes as possible, to ensure full theoretical coverage. For example, an incident may be coded as both "monitoring" and "being vigilant." All data must be coded or the emerging theory will not fit the data and explain behavioral variations. For example, if the NICU nurses spend much time complaining about their problems with respiratory therapists, these data must be coded as well as the data that indicate how they care for the babies.

Level I codes break the data into small pieces; later, level II and level III codes elevate the data to more abstract levels. Level II codes can also be called "categories" and may result from the condensing of level I codes; that is, some level I codes may be subsumed in a larger category. In the process, some data may be discarded if they seem irrelevant. Decisions about categories are made by asking the following questions of the data: "What does this incident indicate?" Each incident is then compared with other incidents. "What category would include these similar incidents?" Finally, the emerging categories are compared with each other to ensure that they are mutually exclusive and cover the behavioral variations.

Level III codes, or theoretical constructs, are derived from a combination of academic and clinical knowledge. The constructs contribute theoretical meaning and scope to the theory (Glaser, 1978, p. 70). Creating meaning is a theoretical construct from the NICU study, whereas privatized discovery is the main theoretical construct from Swanson's (1988) study, and surviving on the brink is the main theoretical construct from Wilson's (1989) study. These theoretical codes may or may not be BSPs, depending on the amount of behavioral variation for which they account. Theoretical constructs conceptualize the relationship among the three levels of codes, "weaving the fractured data back together again" (Glaser, 1978, p. 116). This comprehensive pattern is, in fact, the theory. The theoretical constructs are grounded in substantive or categorical codes, precluding the possibility of unfounded, abstract theorizing.

Families of Theoretical Codes

Grounded theorists use a repertoire of theoretical coding families that suggest the posing of certain questions during coding. The questions enable the researcher to grasp the data more easily and to establish theoretical codes for the empirical indicators. The aim is to saturate the properties of the concept/construct. Some questions I asked about my data involved "The Six Cs" coding family: causes, contexts, contingencies, consequences, covariances, and conditions. For example, what is the cause of nurse crying behavior in the NICU? I learned that new nurses, confronted with the horror of deformity, cried. Nurses who had cared for a baby over a long period of time, who had been involved with the family, and who had experienced the baby's death, cried. Some nurses who felt abused by physicians cried. The context refers to the environment or setting where the behavior occurs. Some nurses left the unit to cry in private. However, if a baby died and several nurses and/or physicians were expressing grief, a nurse might feel free to cry in the presence of others.

I might also ask: "What is this behavior contingent on?" For example, being able to create meaning technically was contingent on nurses' having enough experience to make them skilled with the technology and with special procedures. What are the consequences (for patients, families, nurses, physicians) of crying? Nurses who cry "too much" are unable to create meaning and eventually leave the unit. Nurses who cannot cry are often viewed as "hard." Families often appreciate a nurse who demonstrates feelings for their child, and physicians at times are envious of a nurse who expresses feelings of grief.

Covariances were not relevant to this research. Conditions or qualifiers (Glaser, 1978, p. 74) refer to those factors essential for the actualization of the social psychological processes under study. For example, nurses who bend the rules for the sake of their patients (Hutchinson, 1989) have knowledge, an ideology, and experience. They have knowledge about the patient's disease process, about the rules that the nurse bends, and about how the patient will respond to the rule bending. They share an ideology about patient care that involves patient advocacy; their experience helps them to assess the patient adequately and to anticipate the consequences for the patient when the rules are bent. All these conditions are prerequisite for their knowing how and when to bend the rules to benefit the patient.

Other coding families include the degree family, the dimension family (for an example of dimensional analysis, see Bowers, 1987), the type family, the strategy family, the cutting point family, and so on (Glaser, 1978). The use of these families of codes enhances theoretical sensitivity. Glaser (1978) pointed out that every study is "of" one of these codes; the researcher must recognize which one "infuses the study theoretically while broadening its perspective" (p. 77).

In recent work, Strauss (1987) and Strauss and Corbin (1990) advocated the use of a coding paradigm (specific families of codes) that encourages the development not only of categories but also of subcategories that are present in the context. The coding paradigm involves asking pertinent questions about each category in order to assess conditions, interactions, strategies/tactics, and consequences. Such questions provide a structured way to analyze the data. Strauss (1987) reminded us that, "without inclusion of the paradigm items, coding is not coding" (p. 28).

It is important to think of the codes as provisional and not to censor ideas during the initial open-coding phase. Further analysis and delineation of codes will yield codes that fit the data. Remaining open to theoretical ideas is essential to generating theory that is interpretive rather than merely descriptive.

Axial coding refers to the use of paradigm coding around one category at a time. The analysis revolves around the axis of the category and is necessary to ensure dense data. For example, monitoring was a category in the study on NICU nurses. When looking at monitoring as a code, I asked: "What are the conditions for monitoring? What are the interactions that surround monitoring behaviors? What are the strategies/tactics of monitoring? What are the consequences of monitoring?" This intense focus on each category helps to show the relationship among data, such as what specific conditions fit with what specific interactions, strategies, and consequences (Strauss, 1987, p. 78). Strauss (1987) also emphasized the need to "analyze the data minutely" (p. 31). Line-by-line coding with the coding paradigm and the use of axial coding with each category facilitate the generation of a dense theory that covers all behavioral variation.

Questions asked during coding should emphasize both interaction and structure, in an effort to link one with the other. For example, when examining the interactions/behaviors of NICU nurses, I should ask what effect the unit and/or hospital structure has on their interactions. If I have discovered a social structural process in a hospital, I might question how nurse/physician/administrator/patient interactions affect the structural process.

As mentioned earlier, the fundamental aim of coding is to discover a BSP and its related properties. Selective coding refers to coding that aims to generate the BSP and all the codes that relate to it. The researcher searches for the BSP, the conditions of the BSP, the phases of the BSP, the consequences of the BSP, and so on. Certain questions asked of the data, while coding, aid the generation process:

1. What is going on in the data?
2. What are these data a study of?
3. What is the basic social psychological problem with which these people must deal?
4. What basic social psychological process helps them cope with the problem?

These questions force the researcher to transcend the empirical nature of the data and to think in theoretical terms.

Good theories are both dense and parsimonious. A parsimonious theory—one that is comprehensive without being unwieldy—consists of a few theoretical codes, a greater number of categorical codes, and a majority of in vivo or substantive codes. The researcher returns to the field and interviews repeatedly throughout the research process; coding takes place until the final draft of the paper is begun.

Constant Comparative Method

The constant comparative method is the fundamental method of data analysis in grounded theory generation. The aim of this method is the generation of theoretical constructs that, along with substantive codes and categories and their properties, form a theory that encompasses as much behavioral variation as possible. The proposed theory is molecular in structure rather than causal or linear.

While coding and analyzing the data, the researcher looks for patterns. He or she compares incident with incident, incident with category, and, finally, category with category or construct with construct. By this method, the analyst distinguishes similarities and differences of incidents. By comparing similar incidents, the basic properties of a category or construct are defined; certain differences between incidents establish boundaries; relationships among categories are gradually clarified. Comparative analysis forces the researcher to expand or "tease out" the emerging category/construct by searching for its structure, temporality, cause, context, dimensions, consequences, and relationship to other categories. An in-depth examination of these properties is likely to yield a dense theory that also accounts for behavioral variation.

In addition to incidents, the researcher compares the behavior patterns of different groups within the substantive area. Eventually, categories and their related properties emerge. This process of categorization yields groups of categories/constructs that encompass smaller categories. Thus, major processes or clusters are revealed. Subgroup comparisons maximize differences and variation and, thus, yield a more dense theory (Wilson, 1974, p. 43). In the NICU research, I compared behaviors of new nurses versus those of the "old guard," black nurses versus white nurses, nurses with associate degrees versus those with baccalaureate and master's degrees. I found, for example, that new nurses had a difficult time with the horror and with finding ways to create meaning. The seasoned nurses had, for the most part, made their own peace. Those comparisons contributed substantially to the richness of the theory.

Memoing

In order to generate a quality theory, the descriptions of empirical events must be elevated to a theoretical level. Memoing is a vital part of this process. On index cards, in a journal, or on a computer, the researcher quickly and spontaneously records his or her ideas in order to capture the initially elusive and shifting connections between the data. Memos on memos accumulate. Memos may be long or short and can be written without concern for style or formal punctuation. The emphasis is on conceptualization of ideas. One ends up with hundreds of memos documenting the thinking process. The ideas are retrievable because each memo is headed by the code or codes it describes. Even in the computer, memos can be shifted around to check the relationship with other codes. Irrelevant codes can be discarded and core codes retained. The emerging theory is, therefore, always modifiable.

While memoing, the researcher asks what relationship one code has to another. Are they separate codes? Is one code a property or a phase in another? Is one event the cause of another or the consequence? What are the conditions that influence the codes? The intent of the questioning is to develop freely codes that can be sorted and compared again and again. Through repetitive questioning, the theory evolves. The basic social psychological process emerges, and its properties become integrated. The rapid generation of linkages occurs throughout the research process. Even during the writing phase, new insights may occur.

During the memoing phase, the thinking process is both inductive and deductive. One conceptualizes (inductive) when coding and memoing and then assesses (deductive) how the concepts fit together. Repetitive examination of the data, combined with theoretical sensitivity, aids both processes.

Memoing is a regular and critical part of the grounded theory process, beginning with data analysis after the first interview or observation. Strauss (1987) described changes in memoing during the analytic process that yield different types of memos. Among them are: initial, orienting memos; preliminary memos; memo sparks; memos that open attacks on new phenomena; memos on new categories; initial discovery memos; memos distinguishing between two or more categories; memos extending the implications of a borrowed concept (pp. 138, 139). Other memos or notes (Schatzman & Strauss, 1973) may include methodological memos that focus on strategies for data collecting, and personal memos that illuminate the researcher's introspective process. In a methodological memo I wrote for the NICU study, I reminded myself to observe and do informal interviews with the night shift to determine whether those nurses' interactions with physicians were different from those of the nurses who worked days and evenings. In a personal memo in the same study, I documented my varied and changing feelings about specific babies/situations and compared and contrasted them with feelings of both new and experienced NICU nurses. Memos of all types leave an audit trail for the research and may provide data for presentations, publications, and/or additional research.

Theoretical Sampling

Experimental research compares predetermined groups on specified variables. The groups are chosen to be similar on all points except one, the treatment variable. In grounded theory, sampling decisions are made theoretically during the entire research process. One gathers information from any group that may be a source of relevant data. Relevance is determined by the requirements for generating, delimiting, and saturating the theoretical codes. Saturation of codes refers to their completeness; a code is saturated if the researcher can answer, via the data, questions regarding the cause, context, consequences, and so on, of the particular code. One can see how the code fits in the theory. One engages in a constant dialogue with the data, in order to establish direction for further sampling. For example, studying monitoring behaviors and interactions of NICU nurses could lead me to study monitoring of air traffic controllers or mothers of adolescents. If I wanted to develop a formal theory of monitoring, it is these groups that I would study. The substantive theory about NICU nurses was generated, in contrast, by sampling the subgroups within those nurses.

Diversity in sampling ensures extensive data that cover the wide ranges of behavior in varied situations. My study on bipolar patients (see Chapter 7) revealed that they required different amounts of time to accept (to "own") their diagnosis and illness. I began to collect more data from people with bipolar disorder, to assess the conditions that influenced the different acceptance rates. A patient's symptoms, the time of diagnosis, the method of treatment, and personal illness history all affect when and how the patient owns his or her diagnosis. Theoretical sampling causes the significant variables to become apparent through the expansion and elaboration of the developing codes.

Sorting

Creating meaning as a core variable (and BSP) in the NICU research was discovered during the memo-sorting phase. Once codes are plentiful and memos are accumulating rapidly, sorting begins. One first decides on a core variable that explains most of the behavioral variation in the data. This BSP offers focus and direction to the sorting process. One then attempts to discover the relationship of the different levels of codes to the BSP. Gradually, an outline emerges from the sorted memos that is the basis for writing the theory. While sorting to produce an outline, one may draw and redraw integrative diagrams (see Chapter 7), including logic diagrams that illuminate categories and their relationships. (See Strauss, 1987, and Strauss & Corbin, 1990, for more detail about diagrams.) These diagrams are very helpful in setting forth the developing theory. Figure 6-2 is a diagram of the major theoretical codes for the NICU research.

The object of the sorting is to put the fractured data (Glaser, 1978, p. 116) together into a coherent and workable whole. Sorting the memos facilitates the generation of a theoretical outline that integrates the main ideas.

The mechanics of sorting require the researcher to separate all memos by code, delineating the causes, conditions, contexts, strategies, and dimensions of one's theoretical constructs. As the codes become saturated, their boundaries are defined. The relationship among these individual codes and their collective relationship to the basic social psychological process become the framework of the theory. One strives for a "parsimonious set of integrated concepts" (Glaser, 1978, p. 120).

Saturation

Saturation refers to the completeness of all levels of codes when no new conceptual information is available to indicate new codes or the expansion of existing ones. Although new descriptive data may be added, the information will not be useful unless the theoretical codes need to be altered. When all the data fit into the established categories, interactional and organizational patterns are visible, behavioral variation is described, and behavior can be predicted. The researcher, by repeatedly checking and asking questions of the data, ultimately achieves a sense of closure.

Review of the Literature

In both verificational research—for example, hypotheses testing studies—and grounded theory studies, a literature review is written prior to data collection and analysis. Existing theoretical and methodological literature is used to build a case or rationale for the proposed research. Because the literature used in grounded theory studies can provide only sensitizing concepts and an awareness of the gaps in knowledge, grounded theorists turn to an entirely new body of literature after generating their theory. This second literature review links extant research and theory with the concepts, constructs, and properties of the new theory.

In the NICU research, I identified the problem of horror and the resulting BSP of creating meaning. Literature, novels, and research on the paradox of creating meaning from such horror became relevant. Stories about the lives of cancer patients (*Cancer Ward*) or concentration camp prisoners (*Man's Search for Meaning; Sophie's Choice*) offered insight. Literature that illuminates, supports, or extends the proposed theory is interwoven with the empirical data. Through its correspondence with the real world, literature establishes a vital connection between theory and reality.

WRITING THE THEORY

Smith and Pohland (1976, p. 269) wrote:

> *Really knowing not only means having it conceptualized, but also being able to describe its day-to-day working as well as, if not better than, the man who is actually living and working in the setting.*

After the theoretical sorting and saturation, the researcher begins writing the conceptualization of the substantive theory, with the BSP as its central focus. The phases of the BSP (or any other theoretical coding family) serve as subheadings for the elaboration of the categories. At this point, as Glaser (1978) explained, the theory "freezes the on-going for the moment" in a "fixed conceptual description" (p. 129).

Both during and after the initial writing, the researcher continues to memo and to reconceptualize parts of the theory. Through constant dialogue with the data, the theory emerges, complete with properties, conditions, strategies, and consequences. During the reworking of the draft, the relevant literature is incorporated into the theory.

TEMPORAL CONSIDERATIONS

The grounded theory method requires a time orientation that differs from that of traditional verificational research. Because the time frame of verificational research is linear, the researcher can generally estimate the time involved in each phase of the research process. The generation of grounded theory is inherently circular in nature, requiring an indeterminate amount of time for conceptualization to occur.

During the process of grounded theory generation, the researcher experiences alternating periods of confusion and enlightenment. Recognizing this fact enables the researcher to approach realistically this difficult but exciting method of research.

THE EVALUATION OF GROUNDED THEORIES

Because the methods and aims of grounded theory research are substantially different from those of verificational research, the criteria for evaluation differ accordingly. In *The Discovery of Grounded Theory* (1967), Glaser and Strauss listed the significant criteria for evaluation. A quality grounded theory has codes that fit the data and the practice area from which it is derived. Data fall into place naturally; the researcher does not force them into a code where there is only a marginal fit. Readers of quality theories can actually sense or feel this fit.

A quality theory must work; it will explain the major behavioral and interactional variations of the substantive area. Such a theory can predict what will happen under certain conditions or given certain variables. For example, my theory about NICU nurses predicts that if they cannot create meaning (emotionally, technically, and rationally), they will exhibit symptoms of burnout.

A quality theory must possess relevance related to the core variable and its ability to explain the ongoing social processes in the action scene. If the actors in the setting immediately recognize the researcher's constructs ("Wow, that's it!"), he or she can be confident that the theory possesses relevance. Relevance is dependent on the researcher's theoretical sensitivity in enabling the BSP to emerge from the data without imposing his or her own preconceived notions or ideas.

Social life is not static, and a quality theory must be able to capture its constantly fluctuating nature. A theory must be modifiable; for example, if values or related variables differ, a theory can be modified to fit the setting. As new data surface, new categories must be constructed or current categories modified to incorporate them. Flexibility is required for theoretical relevance.

Density and integration are additional criteria for assessing the quality of a theory. A quality theory is dense: it possesses a few key theoretical constructs and a substantial number of properties and categories. Good integration ensures that the propositions are systematically related to one another into a tight theoretical framework (Glaser & Strauss, 1968, p. 243).

A quality theory meets all the above criteria, providing an explanation of relevant social processes that describe the social psychological interaction in a given setting or group. These processes cover, by virtue of their abstract nature, the major behavioral variations of the people involved.

In their recent work, Strauss and Corbin (1990, p. 253) proposed the following questions as guidelines for judging the adequacy of the grounded theory research process as reported in a research presentation or publication:

1. How was the original sample selected? On what grounds?
2. What major categories emerged?

3. What were some of the events, incidents, and actions that pointed to some of these major categories?

4. On the basis of what categories did theoretical sampling proceed? How did theoretical sampling guide the data collection? How representative are the categories?

5. What were some of the hypotheses pertaining to conceptual relations among categories, and on what grounds were they formulated and tested?

6. Were there instances when hypotheses did not hold up against what was actually seen? How were these discrepancies accounted for? How did they affect the hypotheses?

7. How and why was the core category selected? Was it sudden or gradual, difficult or easy?

The following questions (Strauss & Corbin, 1990, pp. 254-257) suggest criteria concerning the empirical grounding of the study:

1. Are concepts generated?
2. Are the concepts systematically related?
3. Are there many conceptual linkages and are the categories well developed? Do they have conceptual density?
4. Is much variation built into the theory?
5. Are the broader conditions that affect the phenomenon under study built into its explanation?
6. Has process been taken into account?
7. Do the theoretical findings seem significant? To what extent?

THE PITFALLS OF
GROUNDED THEORY RESEARCH

Certain pitfalls, all of which strongly influence the quality of the proposed theory, may confront a budding grounded theorist. Most pitfalls can be avoided with awareness.

Premature closure will cause the theory to be incomplete, to lack density, and to cover inadequately the behavioral variations. If a researcher is under time constraints, premature closure may be necessary. (I was forced to finish my NICU research after a few months. The core variable and major phases were clear, but some of the theoretical codes and categories, and the memoing and sorting, were incomplete.) The researcher then has the choice of completing the study at a later time or settling for a thin theory. Premature closure often occurs with theses and dissertations.

The failure of a BSP or core variable to surface is a significant pitfall. Because a BSP is the conceptual basis of a grounded theory, there simply is no theory without it. The question then becomes: "How can the study be salvaged?" However tempting the remedy, a core variable cannot be imposed on the data. Offering the research as a descriptive study may be a worthwhile endeavor. If key concepts have emerged, they can be used as headings for the write-up of the research. Although the study terminates at a descriptive rather than an interpretive level, it may offer potential for future research.

A third potential pitfall concerns the researcher personally. The choice of research question is a highly personal decision. The method one chooses to solve the problem also involves personal preferences. A researcher who thinks predominantly in the deductive mode has more difficulty generating a grounded theory than one who is skilled in abstract thinking. The abstract thinker may have less interest in and more difficulty doing verificational research. The choice of method should be made carefully. Good grounded theories have great appeal and may seduce the unaware into underestimating the difficulties involved. In order to generate a grounded theory, one must be a conceptual thinker. Deductive thinkers who get in over their heads may be able to salvage their research with a descriptive study, as suggested in the previous paragraph.

Recognition of the requirements for generating a quality theory should be of use to researchers considering the grounded theory method. The grounded theory process is always challenging and, at many stages, exciting. The lengthy time commitment and the necessity for rigorous thinking, however, are equally essential parts of the process. The generation of a quality theory makes this investment worthwhile.

RELEVANCE OF GROUNDED
THEORY FOR NURSING

Nursing, in its present stage of development, has few middle-range substantive theories that explain the everyday world of patients, families, nurses, and health care agencies. Nurses, because they are typically enmeshed in real-life dramas, need the freedom offered by grounded theory to explore intelligently and imaginatively issues and concerns that have social psychological consequences. Social psychological factors are perhaps the most relevant factors in human behavior. Grounded theory offers systematic, legitimate methods to study the richness and diversity of human experience and to generate relevant, plausible theory that can be used to understand the contextual reality of behavior. With this understanding, we can assess what is happening in the groups studied and plan interventions to improve the quality of patient care. Thus, grounded theory can help nurses better understand their own world—people in changing, complex social situations.

The nursing profession is, according to Meleis, Wilson, and Chater (1980), in a preparadigmatic state (Kuhn, 1970). As a neophyte discipline, the profession must encourage theory generation to develop a much needed theoretical base for nursing practice. The generation of grounded theory in our profession would provide substantive middle-range theories that are useful in their own right as bridges from theory to practice. Such theories would contribute to the building of formal theories, as Morse and Johnson (1992) demonstrated.

Grounded theory methods also can be used for evaluation of any aspect of our work. Instead of using only the traditional quantitative methods for evaluation, grounded theory offers us a qualitative approach to evaluation that takes into account people and their experience. We might use this approach to study patient evaluation, student evaluation, or program evaluation.

As nurses begin to generate grounded theories, new and relevant uses will emerge. For now, we need explorations into new areas with new methods, and grounded theory offers us this possibility. "It is up to us," as Goldman (1980) urged, "to accept the challenge of strange and difficult ideas and to abandon the complacency of converting all that is novel into clichés of the familiar" (p. 14).

REFERENCES

Becker, H. (1970). *Sociological work.* Chicago: Aldine.

Benoliel, J. Q. (1967). *The nurse and the dying patient.* New York: Macmillan.

Berger, P., & Kellner, H. (1981). *Sociology reinterpreted.* New York: Anchor Books.

Berger, P., & Luckmann, C. (1967). *The social construction of reality.* New York: Anchor Books.

Blumer, H. (1969). *Symbolic interactionism: Perspective and method.* Englewood Cliffs, NJ: Prentice-Hall.

Bowers, B. (1987). Intergenerational caregiving: Adult caregivers and their aging parents. *Advances in Nursing Science, 9*(2), 20-31.

Bowers, B. (1988). Grounded theory. In B. Sarter (Ed.), *Paths to knowledge* (pp. 35-59). New York: National League for Nursing.

Chenitz, C., & Swanson, J. (1986). *From practice to grounded theory.* Menlo Park, CA: Addison-Wesley.

Denzin, N. (1970). *The research act in sociology.* Chicago: Aldine.

Fagerhaugh, S., & Strauss, A. (1977). Politics of pain management: Staff-patient interaction. Menlo Park, CA: Addison-Wesley.

Glaser, B. (1978). *Theoretical sensitivity.* Mill Valley, CA: Sociology Press.

Glaser, B., & Strauss, A. (1965). *Awareness of dying.* Chicago: Aldine.

Glaser, B., & Strauss, A. (1967). *The discovery of grounded theory.* Chicago: Aldine.

Glaser, B., & Strauss, A. (1968). *Time for dying.* Chicago: Aldine.

Goldman, I. (1980). Boas on the Kwakiutl: The ethnographic tradition. *Sarah Lawrence College—Essays from the Faculty, 3*(4), 5-23.

Honigman, J. (1976). The personal approach in cultural anthropological research. *Current Anthropology, 17*, 243-261.

Hutchinson, S. (1984). Creating meaning out of horror. *Nursing Outlook, 32*(2), 86-90.

Hutchinson, S. (1990). Responsible subversion: A study of rule bending among nurses. *Scholarly Inquiry for Nursing Practice, 4*(1), 3-17.

Hutchinson, S. (1992). Nurses who violate the Nurse Practice Act: Transformation of professional identity. *Image: The Journal of Nursing Scholarship, 24*(2), 133-139.

Hutchinson, S., & Wilson, H. (in press). Research and therapeutic interviews. In J. Morse (Ed.), *A contemporary dialogue.* Newbury Park, CA: Sage.

Kuhn, T. (1970). *The structure of scientific revolutions.* Chicago: University of Chicago Press.

Lincoln, Y., & Guba, E. (1985). *Naturalistic inquiry.* Newbury Park, CA: Sage.

Mead, G. (1934). *Mind, self and society.* Chicago: University of Chicago Press.

Meleis, A., Wilson, H., & Chater, S. (1980). Toward scholarliness in doctoral dissertations: An analytical model. *Research in Nursing and Health, 3,* 115–124.

Morse, J., & Johnson, J. (1992). *The illness experience: Dimensions of suffering.* Newbury Park, CA: Sage.

Schatzman, L., & Strauss, A. (1973). *Field research. Strategies for a natural sociology.* Englewood Cliffs, NJ: Prentice-Hall.

Smith, L., & Pohland, P. (1976). Grounded theory and educational ethnography: Methodological analysis and critique. In J. Roberts & S. Akinsanya (Eds.), *Educational patterns and cultural configurations* (pp. 254–278). New York: David McKay.

Stern, P. (1980). Grounded theory methodology: Its uses and processes. *Image: The Journal of Nursing Scholarship, 12*(1), 20–23.

Stern, P., Allen, L., & Moxley, P. (1982). The nurse as grounded theorist: History, process and uses. *The Review Journal of Philosophy and Social Science, 7*(1,2), 200–215.

Strauss, A. (1987). *Qualitative analysis for social scientists.* New York: Cambridge University Press.

Strauss, A., & Corbin, J. (1990). *Basics of qualitative research.* Newbury Park, CA: Sage.

Swanson, J. (1988). The process of finding contraceptive options. *Western Journal of Nursing Research, 10*(4), 492–503.

Warshaft, S. (Ed.). (1965). *Francis Bacon: A selection of his works.* New York: Odyssey.

Wilson, H. (1976). Presencing: Social control of schizophrenics in an anti-psychiatry community. In C. R. Kneisl & H. Wilson (Eds.), *Current perspectives in psychiatric nursing.* St. Louis, MO: C. V. Mosby.

Wilson, H. (1989). Family caregiving for a relative with Alzheimer's dementia: Coping with negative choices. *Nursing Research, 38*(2), 94–98.

7

People with Bipolar Disorders Quest for Equanimity: Doing Grounded Theory

Sally A. Hutchinson

To behold is to look beyond the fact, to observe, to go be-
yond the observation.
Look at a world of men and women, and you are over-
whelmed by what you see;
Select from that mass of humanity a well-chosen few, and
these observe with insight,
And they will tell you more than all the multitudes
together.
This is the way we must learn: by sampling judiciously,

I thank the participants in this study for sharing their stories with me. This research would not have been possible without their willingness to talk, their candor, and their generosity of spirit.

213

> *By looking intently with the inward eye.*
> *Then, from these few you behold, tell us what you see to*
> *be the truth. P. L. Leedy (1989)*

*B*ipolar illness, also called manic depression, is a psychological condition that is primarily chemical and genetic (Egeland, 1988) in origin. It occurs in at least 3% to 4% and possibly as high as 8% to 10% of the general population (Fieve, 1989). The disorder is frequently misdiagnosed; only one in three manic depressives receives treatment, making the proportion of bipolar patients in treatment the lowest among all those with major psychiatric disorders (Goodwin & Jamison, 1990). Manic depression affects men and women equally.

A review of the nursing literature over the past few years, including such journals as *Archives of Psychiatric Nursing, Psychosocial Nursing,* and *Issues of Mental Health Nursing,* revealed one article (McEnany, 1990) on bipolar illness. The medical literature focuses on treatment issues such as medication management (Brown, 1989; Calabrese & Delucchi, 1989; Fawcett, 1989; Strober, Morrell, Lampert, & Burroughs, 1990); an integrated treatment approach that includes pharmacologic and nonpharmacologic methods such as group therapy (Schou, 1988; Van Gent, Vida, & Zwart, 1988; Wulsin, Bachot, & Hoffman, 1988); suicide prevention (Schou & Weeke, 1988); symptoms and relapse (Fox, 1988; Molnar, Feeney, & Fava, 1988; Silverstone & Romans-Clarkson, 1989). Goodwin and Jamison's (1990) excellent text, *Manic-Depressive Illness,* is the most comprehensive book available. Anecdotal works in the popular literature are especially interesting to read. They include radical feminist and writer Kate Millet's autobiography, *The Looney-bin Trip;* Patty Duke and G. Hochman's *A Brilliant Madness;* and the autobiography of Joshua Logan, *Josh, My Up and Down, In and Out Life.* Logan, a theatrical director, writer, and actor wrote such works as *South Pacific* and *Picnic.* Poets Robert Lowell and Ann Sexton were bipolar; both committed suicide. Their illness was clearly evident in their writings.

The present research contributes to the literature by providing an explanatory schema, a substantive grounded theory, about what it is like to live with a bipolar disorder. "The final goal—of which the nurse [researcher] should never lose sight—is to grasp the patient's point of view, his relation to life, to realize his vision of the phenomena of health and illness" (Ragucci, 1972, pp. 489–490). Grounded theory makes this possible.

Data collection methods appropriate to the purpose included in-depth semistructured interviews, participant observation, and document analysis. After meeting the "modulator" of the local support group for manic depressives, I used a snowball sampling technique: People referred me to friends or acquaintances who had volunteered to be interviewed. Interview questions included:

1. Please tell me what it is like to live with a bipolar disorder.
2. What are the difficulties you encounter? With family, friends, work, health care professionals?
3. Is there anything positive about being bipolar?
4. What would you tell a person who is newly diagnosed with a bipolar disorder?
5. What would you tell health care professionals?

The sample included 19 people (9 men, 10 women) whose ages ranged from 28 to 60. Some worked, some didn't. Some had been diagnosed in the past few years, others had been diagnosed up to 10 years earlier. One man had been diagnosed at age 17, others were not diagnosed until they were in their 40s.

Interviews lasted from one to two hours and took place at participants' homes and/or in my office, depending on their choice. Interviews were audiotaped and transcribed; data were anonymous and confidential.

Participant observation involved two parties—a New Year's party and a spring party—and a weekly 2½-hour support group that I attended for one year. I took notes after the parties and during the weekly meetings. All notes were dictated and transcribed.

Documents included volunteered poems, diaries, and letters that were placed with the field notes and analyzed as text. These modes of data collection yielded approximately 1,000 pages of typed field notes.

Theory generation transpired over a period of one year. Data collection and analysis occurred simultaneously and followed the

steps discussed in Chapter 6. Only after much coding and memoing did I discover the core variable and basic social psychological
process: the quest for equanimity. Subsequent to that discovery,
the core variable guided data analysis.

THE QUEST FOR EQUANIMITY

In accordance with the grounded theory method, the interpretive
analysis focused on the participants' basic social problem and the
process used to resolve the problem. The basic social problem for
these people with bipolar disorders was the "ceaseless undulations" of their moods. Although mood patterns or cycles have been
described by psychiatrists (3-month cycle, 6-month cycle, daily or
monthly cycle for those people called rapid cyclers), each person's
pattern was unique. The ceaseless undulations were always terror-
izing, keeping the people, as one person said, "living on the edge"
of depression or mania. Kate Millet (1990) eloquently described
depression:

> *Depression is death, the very tinge and certainty of decay.*
> *Paradoxically depression is when you finally contract the*
> *sickness they accused you of as manic. A delayed reaction if*
> *you will; the internalization of all the crimes of your high-*
> *and-mighty time in the suffering of your fallen, dying time.*
> *Depression is when you agree with them all and surrender.*
> *(p. 257)*

Participants described depression as "a neverending sadness," "a
black hole," having "no hope left to live for," feeling "alone and
scared," feeling "socially disapproved of," and being in "a dense
fog."

In contrast, being hypomanic was feeling on "top of the world,"
"superhuman," "invincible," and "elated"; "It's like a junkie fix."
However, for many, the escalation into the psychotic stage of mania was rapid. Elation was replaced by fear, paranoia, agitation, an
increase of the racing heartbeat, and an inability to eat and sleep
that heralded the manic phase. Feeling panicked and "having the
shakes" were common. The shift between mania and depression
was, as one man said, as if "alien force fields control my body."

With mania and depression, people feel off balance. Moods are powerful because, through moods, people discover and view their worlds. Moods condition understanding and guide actions. People with bipolar disorders are literally thrown by their moods.

The basic social process that helps people counteract these ceaseless undulations is "the quest for equanimity." The quest implies a search, a mission that is requisite to finding the elusive equanimity. Equanimity is hard won, never happening by chance or serendipity. Only equanimity permits these people to escape from being prisoners of their moods. Equanimity implies self-possession, levelheadedness, presence of mind, self-restraint, self-confidence, and equilibrium—all personal attributes that are missing in mania and depression. The quest for equanimity becomes a way of living for people with bipolar disorders. Certain phases are fundamental to the quest. Figure 7–1 presents a schematic diagram of the major constructs in the theory, each of which will be discussed in the remainder of the chapter.

TREATING THE SYMPTOMS

Bipolar illness is often a hidden disease that is recognized only in retrospect, after the symptoms escalate and become more pronounced. One man who was diagnosed in 1978, at age 33, said, "I'd been having episodes all my life but the frequency began to increase in 1978 because I was in a lot of stress." Initially, during a greater or lesser period of time before diagnosis, some people treat their bipolar symptoms with physician-prescribed medications. Self-medication with alcohol and drugs is extremely common and often propels people with bipolar illness into Alcoholics Anonymous (AA). A context of confusion surrounds those who, through trial and error, search for relief of symptoms. No one, including health care professionals, seems to understand what is happening. One 40-year-old woman recounted:

I started ten years ago with a real high, a super high. I thought I could do anything and I was sleeping maybe one or two hours a night. I didn't know what was going on with me at all. I had no earthly idea.

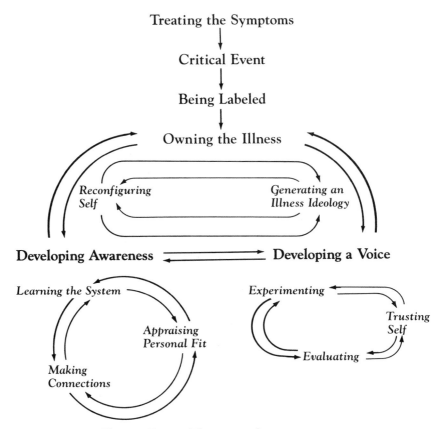

Figure 7–1.   The quest for equanimity.

A man said:

> *I think that I was for a very long time a bipolar and they just didn't recognize it. I covered it up with drinking and drugs pretty much or I was able to fight it through . . . until six years ago when I just had a slam dunk depression. . . . [It was a] fetal position type thing and [I was] totally psychotic. I just didn't remember, literally didn't remember six days there. It was classic because I had stayed up four or five, six days complaining of no sleep and all of a sudden just complete—BAM—totally reversed out in depression.*

These people saw psychiatrists and therapists, and were often hospitalized with varying psychiatric diagnoses; a few were even put in jail, yet were never diagnosed as bipolar. Years of turmoil and fractured lives result from this symptomatic treatment, even if relief is obtained for periods of time.

CRITICAL EVENT

Eventually, as symptoms increase in frequency, intensity, or duration, a critical event occurs in each person's illness trajectory and results in the diagnosis of bipolar disorder. The critical event frequently involves dramatic behavior such as aggression, mania, or attempts at suicide. One woman overdosed and was diagnosed in the hospital she was taken to. Another woman threatened violence toward men, and another was diagnosed after spending 23 days in jail. One man attempted to rob a bank; another embarked on a spending spree that put him thousands of dollars in debt.

BEING LABELED

The diagnosis of bipolar disorder often evokes feelings of relief because the mere naming of the problematic behaviors and painful symptoms permits a conversation about what the illness is and how it can be treated. Chaos is given a name. A pattern emerges, and the pattern provides meaning for what previously was meaningless.

A woman who had "been through hell," which included batteries of physical and psychological tests and numerous hospitalizations, said, upon learning her diagnosis, "I was relieved because I thought I was dying. You feel like you'll get better once you get a correct diagnosis." A man who had treated himself for years with alcohol and drugs said, "I was relieved that there was a diagnosis and medications." For one woman, "being diagnosed saved my life." When manic, she had experienced numerous altercations at work and, at one time, had written a disparaging letter about her boss to the local newspaper. The label provided a defense for her antagonistic behavior. In contrast, one man "ran like a rabbit"

upon hearing the diagnosis "because my mother was manic depressive and I watched her life become a living hell and felt the
effects of her illness on my family."

In all cases, being labeled had a profound effect. Participants
agreed, as one woman said, "It's hard to carry a label around. It's
hard to accept what might be true."

Stigma

Although labeling may bring initial relief, "with the label comes
social stigma. It takes one episode to label you and with it you get
a whole new set of stresses. It's enough to set you on another trip."
A man said, "Once you're labeled, that's it; you lose 85% of your
friends." Another man laughed sardonically, implying that 85%
was a gross underestimate. Being labeled, "You no longer fit . . .
unless you keep it to yourself." "Once people know your history
they back off. I love going to reunions because I can always tell by
people's behavior if they've heard about me or not."

One man shared a story about a job interview. After he had told
the employer he was bipolar, the employer laughed and said he had
known a man who was bipolar and killed himself. "I guess it was
for the best," the employer said.

Participants noticed that if they were depressed, no one with-
drew ("We just don't talk about it"), but if they were manic, "We
scare people." "Even the police think manic means maniac. By being bipolar you are open for arrest." One woman talked about performing her job and having people say within earshot, "Oh here's
that crazy bitch"; they acted afraid of her long after her last manic
attack. A woman said, "I think it's going to kill me in the end if I
keep worrying about what other people think." Many agreed with
one man's comment, "The stigma's the worst part of the disease."

Consequences of labeling are also financial. Once a person is
given a psychiatric diagnosis, insurance carriers may choose not
to insure him or her.

Self-Disclosure

As soon as they are diagnosed, people have to make a decision
about self-disclosure—whom to tell and what to tell about their

illness. One young man said, "I told nobody except my therapist and my wife. That's it." Others are more willing to reveal their diagnosis, especially if the awareness may benefit them. People change their minds about self-disclosure over time; depending on their experiences, they may become more secretive or more open about their illness.

OWNING THE ILLNESS

Owning the illness refers to a lengthy process people go through as they gradually integrate the illness into their image of themselves (reconfiguring the self) and as they develop beliefs about the illness (generating an illness ideology). Owning the illness requires much time and is extremely difficult. It occurs by degrees, beginning with a verbal admission of illness and progressing to an integration of the illness, as interpreted, into one's mental conception of the self. The owning process is always fluid, and people revisit the issues over the years, often reconceptualizing their beliefs about the nature of the illness and its relation to how they think about themselves.

Until people own their illness, there is no hope of equanimity. People who avoid taking an active look at their "ceaseless undulations" appear unprepared for each new emotional storm and describe feeling totally out of control of their lives. Owning the illness helps prevent feeling victimized.

Reconfiguring the Self

Once labeled, a person, over time, reconfigures the self as a person with mental illness. People's personal gestalts change; they enlarge to include their new sense of self. This is a slow and difficult process. One woman said, "The hardest point for me was admitting I was bipolar. To really recognize the nature of the disease is very very difficult." Another woman said, "I went through the denial stage. Once you get over the denial stage you can go on. That's what I did."

Whether an individual has reconfigured the self and owned the illness is clear in his or her conversation and behavior. One man who came briefly to the support group did not identify himself as having bipolar disorder, as the other group members did. He described the usefulness of attending encounter and educational groups, making it clear that he did not interpret his problems as a result of being bipolar but rather as a result of childhood psychological trauma.

With diagnosis comes a new understanding of family and personal history. Upon reflection, people often recognized that their family members also suffered from bipolar illness. They remembered their past vividly and redefined their personal histories: "I never felt right since age seven. I'd tell my dad and he'd say, 'You're just having growing pains. They'll go away.'" A man said, "I always kept to myself a lot. I had to do that to stay out of trouble." Recognition of family history and an increased understanding of their own past will influence a gradual reconfiguring of the self.

Generating an Illness Ideology

Over time, as people read about bipolar disorder, listen to the comments of others, and live with their illness, they formulate their beliefs about bipolar disorder. Although their beliefs are subject to change throughout their lives, at any one point an experienced person does have beliefs about causation and treatment of the illness. The majority ascribe to the biochemical theory and also recognize contributing factors from the family environment. However, some espouse other ideologies. One woman believed that vitamin B12 deficiency caused depression. Another said, "My first two psychiatrists said that sudden pain or trauma can cause manic depression . . . sudden blows to the head, automobile accidents." In the support group, a man changed, in a period of 7 months, from owning his bipolar illness to "trying to relate my problem to a neck injury" sustained during an inverted spin in a plane when he was a Navy pilot. He reinterpreted his mood swings as energy swings. "I'm trying to find a solution other than the name bipolar manic depressive. Manic depressive is a description of the symptoms. It can't tell you the cause." If he were misdiagnosed as he proclaimed, he would be a candidate for a pension, and he would no longer have to live with the stigma that was so painful. His escalating mania may also have contributed to his changed views.

DEVELOPING AWARENESS

As people struggle with their illness, they develop awareness of the health care system, the subtleties and ramifications of their illness, and their own responses to the illness and its treatment. Awareness develops over time and continues throughout the person's life.

Learning the System

People learn about the mental health system from experience and, if they are in a support group, by hearing others' stories. Because of their experiences, they become aware of how they feel about hospitalization and different physicians. They compare doctors and hospitals to each other and to their beliefs about what a "good" doctor or hospital should be like.

One young man with previous hospitalizations in numerous cities found a hospital he liked "because I can go outside to smoke, the doctors and nurses are really caring . . . I know I can come and go if I want (it's an open unit)." He described care at another hospital as "Neanderthal" and felt that the horrible hospitalization experience had prolonged his illness. After he found the hospital he liked, he moved within commuting distance and will now see only the doctors at that hospital. Another man said, "I learned I need a psychiatrist for my medications and a therapist who is not a medical doctor. I don't think I can be totally honest with a doctor who could admit me to a hospital and regulate my moods. I tend to hold back." This young man had a history of being hospitalized against his will by several physicians.

Doctors gained reputations that were discussed freely in the support group. "Doctor Shock" was the name given to a physician who frequently prescribed shock therapy. "Mr. Chemical" referred to a physician who "plies you full of drugs." "Power trippers are doctors who try to control people and do not listen."

Many people are forced to seek social security disability and/or to deal with Health and Rehabilitative Services (HRS). Support groups are especially useful in teaching people how to obtain social security, disability, and HRS housing. Learning the system is critical, because many bipolar people need multiple types of assistance. People who are new to the illness and the local resources have to cope not only with their out-of-control symptoms, but also with the confusion that comes from lack of knowledge.

Making Connections

As people live with their illness, they begin to make connections between their symptoms and illness, symptoms and treatment, and symptoms and consequences. This pattern recognition heightens their awareness and permits personal choices. One woman said, "Get in tune with yourself. Pay attention to what's happened to you. Keep a journal so you can start to see patterns. I did that for a long time. The more you know yourself, the more in control you are of it. That's my best piece of advice."

Between Symptoms and Illness. As these people continued to suffer mood fluctuations, some began to recognize the cause and context of their symptoms and to connect their symptoms with environmental conditions or with life events. Several people described being very excited "on the full moon," called PMS (premoon syndrome) by one woman. Some described being more manic during the summer months and more depressed during the winter and "on grey days." For many people, manic episodes were precipitated by stress. Each person decided how stress was manifesting itself and eventually made personal accommodations such as choosing to retire early, choosing a job that was low-stress, or getting divorced.

For some people, the connection of mood swings to external occurrences was not possible. Some experienced severe mood changes almost daily, leading one participant to label his illness DMS—daily mood swings. Others said, "I cycle like clockwork, every six months. It doesn't make sense"; or, "I have very long swings, so if I'm in a swing I need to be eased down to neutral. I don't want real rapid up or down swings. I don't want to 'sling-shot' to the top and have so much velocity that I'll go through the roof."

Learning personal rhythms of illness was helpful in avoiding certain people, situations, or places, or in anticipating and even planning for the next manic. One man gave strict instructions to his wife and left a signed affidavit with the police that permitted them to pick him up if he drank even an ounce of alcohol. Alcohol inevitably triggered psychotic episodes that resulted in a wake of violence and subsequent depression.

Participants also learned the symptoms of their illness that fore-shadowed a breakdown. "The key indicator to whether I was going on a manic or not was whether I was sleepy." If this man couldn't sleep, he was "on the upswing." He takes thorazine every night "to defeat the manic cycle."

Embodied listening is the process that allows people to learn to connect symptoms to context and to behavior. Levin (1985) ad-vised: "[W]e should listen in silence to our bodily felt experience. Thinking needs to learn by feeling, by just being with our bodily being" (p. 61). As people learn to listen through their bodies, they become attuned to the nuances, the more subtle undulations, of their own personal rhythms. Such bodily awareness is critical to learning to predict and attempting to alleviate one's moods. One woman described her feelings:

> *I feel at the moment I'm stable. I'm not having the nervous-ness. I'm not having the tension. I'm not having the heart racing. None of the things that would tend to make me feel like I'm on an up. I'm not having any of the crying con-stantly. I still seem to want to sleep a lot but I can't because my mind is alert. I think a lot of that is either whatever is going on with me or I'm not quite adjusted to the medicine dosage yet because the doctor totally changed my medicine.*

Learning embodied listening requires many years of concerted effort. Participants described "going up" as "insidious" because it made them less likely to recognize their gradual mood escalations.

"If you feel down I think you know it. But sometimes when you feel up you don't realize you're up until after the fact." Feeling good feels good, to a point, but these people recognized that when they started feeling good they were likely to "go over the edge." "I get scared when I start feeling good," said one woman. Fear derives from the hyperagitation, panic, and paranoia often associated with mania and also from the painful consequences that frequently result from manic attacks.

Between Symptoms and Treatment. Medication is the main treatment for bipolar disorder, and individuals' responses to medication are quite idiosyncratic. Among the support group, lithium dosages ranged from 300 to 2,700 mg. Learning about one's responses to medication is crucial to achieving equanimity because frightening and dramatic responses are not uncommon. Much of the group's time was spent discussing different drugs—their side effects, interactions, and usefulness for different problems. Personal horror stories were legion. One involved a woman on an MAO inhibitor who was not told of the necessary diet alterations. She ended up in an intensive care unit and almost died of a hypertensive crisis. One man's uncontrollable repetitive grimace dramatically revealed a permanent side effect of neuroleptics. Others described experiences that ranged from extreme psychomotor retardation to agitation, nightmares, and suicidal ideation. Participants worried about long-term effects such as kidney, brain, and thyroid damage and about the side effect of "sudden unexplained death" that is described in the Haldol insert. Over time, these people learned what drug(s) worked for their specific symptoms. They recognized clearly, however, that any drug's effectiveness was limited and that "many symptoms can only be alleviated by medication." "In spite of what they [physicians] tell you, this is an uncontrollable illness."

Changing medications was always problematic. "We are all very fearsome—and fearsome is the word—of having to change drugs. You have to withdraw slowly, then have an extended period of time with no chemical defense where you have to change your life because you probably can't function and then you start all over." One woman said angrily, "This whole process of finding a drug that may work can take up to one to two years. That's one to two years wasted." She was referring to being miserable and dysfunctional for those years.

Between Symptoms and Consequences. Participants learned early that bipolar illness has devastating and far-reaching consequences. Loss was the theme that most clearly reflected what people who had experienced psychotic highs had felt: loss of money, loss of friends and family, loss of jobs, and loss of self. One man lamented, "I've lost several jobs. Twenty years ago I was driving a Mercedes, I was wearing a Rolex watch, Palm Beach suits. I was working for *New York Life.* I was pretty well off then." In the course of one year, I watched a 26-year-old man move three times, declare bankruptcy, change jobs three times, alienate friends and family. His disease literally assaulted him.

Loss of friends and family because of recurrent manic episodes and depression leads to social isolation:

If they don't know what you have and they see you go for a long period of time, being up and bubbly and what they consider to be the normal you, and then suddenly you go down, it's like they think you don't like them anymore. You don't hang around them, you don't go places, you don't do things and the friendships tend to dissolve from it. And it is a feeling of forever starting over again. For me there is also an intense feeling of embarrassment. I am very embarrassed about it.

One man incisively and expressively summed up his rejection by friends and family: "I don't get many hugs these days."

A woman, describing her transformation after taking lithium, said, "I'm glad to be diagnosed but I miss me. I miss the good part of the mania. Since lithium I have boring ideas, less energy and I'm no longer decisive." Kate Millet refused her medication because "lithium makes you a little fuzzy around the edges (1990, p. 46). Both expressed a loss of self.

Participants poignantly described the humiliation that is the aftermath of manic attacks. "When I see people afterwards I can tell by the way they act that something uncomfortable occurred." Typically, when participants reflect about what has occurred, they think, "God, I hope it was a dream . . . it turns out it was reality. It's really humiliating." Because of these varied losses, they always seem to be starting over, and each time is a little more difficult.

Appraising Personal Fit

As participants learned the system and began to make connections, they simultaneously appraised the "fit" of their treatment, including medications, psychiatrists, psychotherapists, hospitals, and clinics. They also appraised the fit of their life-style and work routine.

Because this illness has a long and turbulent path, these people inevitably are exposed to a variety of health care agencies and staff. Participants judged their experiences and began to think about what types of treatment they preferred. One man said, "I avoid hospitals like the plague. I'm petrified what they can do to you." Another recounted:

> *Going into a crisis stabilization unit (CSU). It's just assholes to elbows. Somebody's always going to be there trying to be a total nut case. CSUs are always very stressful. It depends on how crowded they are. Graduate on out of there as quickly as possible . . . no one wants to be there. If you're a manic you're labeled a troublemaker from the word go. The drugs that they give you are bad drugs. It's a death trip . . . they overload you . . . you get a vegetable, zombie effect.*

Another said, "Doctors want to test drugs on people. They don't really listen to your history or to what you feel." One doctor had not believed that this man had a chemical problem. When the man requested a medication change, the doctor told him he was trying to test authority. "The doctor called it an authority problem. I really wasn't thinking about his authority. I was really thinking about how I felt." Physicians' behavior such as this was harshly criticized by the group. "Get a doctor that you can work with" was a common refrain. A therapeutic alliance in which doctors and patients negotiate with each other was the goal.

At the same time, participants were thinking about their life-styles, including their work, family, and social relationships. These issues were reappraised with each new crisis.

DEVELOPING A VOICE

Gradually, as these people struggled with owning their illness and becoming aware of what it is like to live with it in all its ramifications, they developed a voice. Initially, the voice was internal. It gathered strength as they crystallized their beliefs about their illness. Over time, it became external: they began to speak out for themselves to employers, doctors, and family. The people in the group spoke forcefully and articulately. The group modulator was proud of a new group that had formed in another area of town: "They are speaking up. They are not letting the doctor speak for them." A woman said this may require "being dirty, nasty, and mean instead of being too nice." Over time, these people developed a voice by experimenting, evaluating, and learning to trust themselves.

Experimenting

When living was painful, feeling bad was tiresome, and doctors and medications were not helpful, some people experimented with their treatment and their life-style. They thought about their work—whether they should work, the type of work they do, and their working conditions; about their marriage—whether they should stay married; about their treatment—whether they should be hospitalized when illness strikes again, who the physician should be, what the medications should be. The support group provided a forum for discussion of these issues.

People conducted experiments to see "what happens if I do xyz," in the hope of finding equanimity. For a period of one week, I had almost daily phone contact with a young man who had suffered increasingly frequent and lengthy hospitalizations for mania. The consequences of his psychotic attacks were devastating. He called to talk about his escalating mood and what he was doing about it: "I'm experimenting on myself through this period. I want to see what conclusions I can make." His aim was "to cut my losses." He altered his medication, attempted but failed to reach his doctor, cut down on his night life, and increased his fluid intake because he was working outside in very hot conditions. A woman, tired of feeling depressed and sluggish, stopped all medications. One man who nurtures and cultivates an acre of diverse and unusual plants learned, through experimentation, that he has to drink a lot of Gatorade when he's working outside in the summer or he will "go toxic" from his Tegretol. He also learned to come in at noon from mid-May through September or he'll be too manic and sweat too much. His alarm wrist watch reminds him to take his pills. He has also learned to stretch in the morning "to center myself," to eat a good breakfast, and "to not schedule too full of a day which would be overstimulating."

Evaluating

As people experimented, they evaluated their results. They actually felt the results via embodied listening. The young man who tried to prevent a manic attack said:

> *I'm starting to identify patterns. I've learned I can party or I can work but I can't do both at the same time. I have to temper my business because when things go well I have to watch myself. If I'm running on high octane I have to be doubly careful. In terms of my medications if I double my Stelazine for a short period of time I'm okay. The Mellaril didn't do it.*

A young woman who suffered daily mood swings recognized that she was highly intelligent, skilled in several areas, and had no problems getting good jobs. However, she consistently got fired (she had 32 jobs in 11 years) because she frequently had "trouble getting through the day . . . to talk to someone, even to just say, 'Hello, how are you?' requires incredible effort." After evaluating her job history and stress level, she chose to work at a job with minimum wage. She continued to refuse promotions and opportunities for consultant work.

Trusting Self

As these people began to make decisions, they learned to trust themselves— if not always to make good decisions, at least to make the best decisions they could at the time. One man said, "We know ourselves better than anybody does. We've done the research."

In spite of physicians' admonishments and occasional skepticism from the support group, people made their own decisions, often with far-reaching consequences. For example, a man incurred familial wrath by refusing to go to his parents' fiftieth wedding anniversary party, planned by his siblings. A woman decided that she will no longer permit her family to come to her birthday celebration. "I will not put myself out again to have them knock me down again." Several people smoked marijuana for various reasons but said it did not affect their illness in a negative way. Some claimed that it helped the manic. A man said:

> I hate the hospital. I work hard to keep my bubblings [referring to his manic] to myself but I went to the doctor as pretty radically high, manic manic as opposed to hypomanic. He was flat ready to put me in the hospital. I practically begged. It got real quiet. I was just lucky I took my yoga before I went to see him. So instead of putting me in the hospital he put me on lithium.

Another man didn't want to quit work "but I did what I had to do because I didn't want to continue getting arrested and beat up. I have my own little system and it keeps me out of the doghouse. You have to become an expert. You have to become a PhD in your illness."

Developing a voice is necessary for self-care and is essential to the quest for equanimity. As participants became aware of and knowledgeable about their problems, the limitations of treatment, and their personal responses, they recognized clearly that they

were the only ones who knew their illness and that no one would
care about them as much as they cared about themselves. Thus,
they experimented, evaluated, and learned to trust themselves.

SUMMARY AND IMPLICATIONS

This chapter has presented a grounded theory on the quest for
equanimity by people with bipolar disorder. Severe and often
frequent mood undulations ranging from mania to depression,
and their self-destructive consequences, propel these people to
strive for a level of equanimity that affords them a measure of
self-possession and self-confidence.

Implications for Clinical Practice

Interviews with and participant observation of people with bipolar disorder permitted me to learn from them what it is like to live
with their illness. Such awareness provides clear directives to
health team members as they plan patient-centered care.

Equanimity cannot be bestowed on people, no matter how
benevolent or knowledgeable health care providers are. Equanimity is learned and earned through trial and error, accompanied by introspection. The ongoing, fluctuating, and interrelated
processes that are requisite for equanimity—owning the illness,
developing awareness, and developing a voice—can be facilitated by health care workers who actively work toward those
aims.

Learning to understand the illness and its personal manifestations takes much time and is integral to owning the illness. Care
providers need to appreciate and respect this, working with the
person to assess the variables that seem to affect his or her illness
response. Careful history taking and attentive listening should accompany "medication management" appointments. Providers can
help the person make connections between symptoms and illness,
symptoms and treatment, and symptoms and consequences. They
can facilitate the need to learn the mental health system and to discover individual responses to and preferences for treatment.

People with bipolar disorders want a voice. They want to experiment with different styles of treatment and different ways of living and to feel free to evaluate their responses. They want to learn to trust themselves, which they must do if they are to acquire any degree of equanimity. Providers can support their struggle and join hands with them in a therapeutic alliance. Issues that inevitably arise in this "roller coaster disease"—medication, hospitalization, work/family/social relationships—need to be discussed openly and honestly between client and health care provider. If this occurs, the issue of "compliance" that is discussed so frequently will become obsolete. Knowledge of this theory and a commitment to therapeutic alliance should enable providers to facilitate equanimity and adaptive functioning in their clients.

Implications for Research

The proposed theory is, as all grounded theories are, "hypothetical generalization." Validity assessments are necessary. The responses of people in the bipolar support group, psychiatric nurses, and nurse therapists at local, state, and national presentations support the accuracy and utility of this theory. It may be worthwhile to test further the validity of the theory by interviewing others with bipolar disorder and ascertaining whether their experience supports the theory. If differences become known, modifications can be made to alter or extend the theory so that it explains all behavioral variation.

The present theory can benefit from more extensive data analysis. Use of the coding paradigm, axial coding, and theoretical sampling (discussed in Chapter 6) with each category (e.g., learning the system, making connections, experimenting) will densify and expand the theory. Future research publications that focus on specific categories should review relevant literature, thereby enhancing the breadth and depth of our knowledge in the chosen area.

The present study can be improved by a more extensive literature review that demonstrates correspondence with the theory and its concepts. If space were not limited, extant literature that focuses on the categories/concepts in the theory (e.g., stigma, the labeling phenomenon) and other relevant issues would be integrated in this report. Grounded theories are best suited for monographs that allow for lengthier manuscripts.

A study of the social structural processes relevant to the present study is important. Such a study will provide a more comprehensive perspective by contributing a macroanalysis of the local mental health system, and/or of the larger society that influences these people's lives, to the present interactional microanalysis.

Numerous issues in this study require additional data and further examination. For example, we need to learn more about the meaning of psychiatric hospitalization for different groups of people. When is hospitalization helpful or not helpful? What qualities make it so? Suicide is a vital concern for clients, family members, and health care professionals. We need to know more about how people with bipolar disorder think about suicide. How is their thinking similar to or different from that of people with fatal illnesses? Issues of self-disclosure are complex and have far-reaching consequences for people with many different illnesses. How do people with different types of illnesses decide to disclose or not disclose their illness? To whom do they disclose? What do they disclose? When and where do they disclose?

Case histories in nursing are rare, yet they provide wonderful insights into human experience and, if done well, can demonstrate the relevance of theory for understanding and predicting human behavior. Because of the masses of interview data they collect, grounded theorists often can write a case history based on some of the data used to generate their theory. A case history that illuminates one person's experience with living with a bipolar disorder enables the researcher to "depict a type, an average, an extreme, or an exemplary case" (Strauss, 1987, p. 221). In a case history, the person becomes alive, and the context of the illness is established. Substantive theory is applied to the case, vividly revealing the concepts and constructs as they are used to interpret a person's life. The theory relates the particular to the general, providing an enlarged picture of the case. For an example of a case history that illustrates their theories on pain, awareness contexts, and dying trajectories, see Strauss and Glaser's

(1970) poignant description of a 54-year-old woman with cancer who experienced a lingering death in a hospital.

The present theory can be built on and expanded. For example, is this theory or any part of it relevant for people with other types of mental illness, or for people with other types of chronic illness? Although the basic social problem of mood undulations will be different, the phases of owning the illness, developing awareness, and developing a voice may be useful sensitizing constructs.

Qualitative studies frequently are considered precursors to quantitative research. Experts in instrument development could develop an instrument, based on this theory, that aims to predict where a person is in the process of the quest for equanimity. Experts in quantitative methods can test the theory for predictability, reliability, and validity. However, the purists among qualitative researchers would disagree as to the value of this testing, for they would believe that the theory speaks for itself and should not be deconstructed for quantitative measurements.

REFERENCES

Brown, R. (1989). U.S. experience with Valproate in manic depressive illness: A multicenter trial. *The Journal of Clinical Psychiatry, 50,* 13-16.

Calabrese, J. & Delucchi, G. (1989). Phenomenology of rapid cycling manic depression and its treatment with Valproate. *Journal of Clinical Psychiatry, 50*(3), 30-34.

Duke, P., & Hochman, G. (1992). *A brilliant madness.* New York: Bantam Books.

Egeland, J. (1988). A genetic study of manic-depressive disorder among the Old Order Amish of Pennsylvania. *Pharmacopsychiatry, 21,* 74-75.

Fawcett, J. (1989). Valproate use in acute mania and bipolar disorder: An international perspective. *Journal of Clinical Psychiatry, 50*(3), 10-12.

Fieve, R. (1989). *Moodswing.* New York: Bantam Books.

Fox, H. (1988). Convalescent phase of bipolar disorder. *Journal of Clinical Psychiatry, 49*(11), 452-454.

Goodwin, R., & Jamison, K. (1990). *Manic-depressive Illness.* New York: Oxford University Press.

Leedy, P. L. (1989). *Practical research planning and design* (4th ed.). New York: Macmillan.

Levin, D. (1985). *The body's recollection of being.* London: Routledge & Kegan Paul.

Logan, J. (1976). *Josh, my up and down, in and out life.* New York: Delacorte Press.

McElroy, S. (1989). Valproate in psychiatric disorders: Literature review and clinical guidelines. *The Journal of Clinical Psychiatry, 50,* 30-34.

McEnany, G. (1990). Psychobiological indices of bipolar mood disorder: Future trends in nursing care. *Archives of Psychiatric Nursing, 4*(1), 29-38.

Millet, K. (1990). *The looney-bin trip.* New York: Simon & Schuster.

Molnar, G., Feeney, G., & Fava, G. (1988). Duration and symptoms of bipolar prodromes. *American Journal of Psychiatry, 145*(13), 1576-1578.

Ragucci, A. T. (1972). The ethnographic approach and nursing research. *Nursing Research, 21,* 485-490.

Schou, M., & Weeke, A. (1988). Did manic-depressive patients who committed suicide receive prophylactic or continuation treatment at the time? *British Journal of Psychiatry, 153,* 324-327.

Schou, M. (1988). The integrated approach. *Acta psychiatr. scand. suppl, 78,* 119-123.

Silverstone, T., & Romans-Clarkson, S. (1989). Bipolar affective disorder: Causes and prevention of relapse. *British Journal of Psychiatry, 154,* 321-335.

Strauss, A. (1987). Qualitative analysis for social scientists. New York: Cambridge University Press.

Strauss, A., & Glaser, B. (1970). *Anguish: A case history of a dying trajectory.* Mill Valley, CA: Scientology.

Strober, M., Morrell, W., Lampert, C., & Burroughs, J. (1990). Relapse following discontinuation of lithium maintenance therapy in adolescents with bipolar I illness: A naturalistic study. *American Journal of Psychiatry, 147*(4), 457-461.

Van Gent, E., Vida, S., & Zwart, R. (1988). Group therapy in addition to lithium therapy in patients with bipolar disorders. *Acta psychiat. belg; 88,* 405-418.

Wulsin, M., Bachot, M., & Hoffman, D. (1988). Group therapy in manic-depressive illness. *American Journal of Psychotherapy, 42*(2), 263-271.

8

Ethnography: The Method

Carol P. Germain

*T*he central concept in ethnography is culture, broadly defined as the learned social behavior or the way of life of a particular group of people. Ethnography provides knowledge (theory) that can be used to help us understand our own culture(s) and those of others, and also provides a basis for planned culture change. The many varieties of ethnography make a singular definition impossible, but there are shared components that this chapter will address. As a product, conventional or classical ethnography is a factual description and analysis of aspects of the way of life of a particular culture, subculture, or subcultural group. As a research process, ethnography is the traditional approach to the development of theories of culture by the anthropologies that deal with living people, including cultural, social, and educational anthropology. Ethnography has been associated traditionally with remote, foreign, or primitive cultures such as those studied by the early cultural anthropologists. One purpose for studying such cultures, beyond theory development, was to enable the researcher to acquire a perspective beyond his or her ethnocentric one so that later analysis of the subcultures of the researcher's own society could be accomplished more objectively. Today, the emphasis has shifted from the study of foreign or exotic cultures to the importance of obtaining cultural knowledge of one's own society.

Patton (1990) stated that every human group that is together for a period of time will evolve a culture. Cultures and subcultures in American society may be found in rural and urban ethnic and racial enclaves; nonethnic groups such as those located in prisons and bars; complex organizations; factories; the social institutions of education; the military and military bases; health care institutions such as nursing homes, hospitals, or shelters for the homeless or the abused; community-based groups of various types such as street gangs, motorcycle gangs, and teenage groups such as jocks and skinheads; religious communities; and disciplines such as nursing and medicine. Thus, for example, nursing is a professional culture, a hospital is a sociocultural institution, and a unit of a hospital can be viewed as a subculture.

Cultural groups have characteristics such as beliefs, values, ideals, norms (rules of behavior), controls and sanctions for social deviance, language, dress, rituals, interaction patterns, artifacts (technology), sociopolitical patterns, structure and function, and many others. Structure refers to the social structure or configuration of a group, such as the organizational structure of a modern organization or the kinship structure of a tribal group. Function refers to the patterns of social relations among members of a group, for example, hierarchical or egalitarian.

Although originating in anthropology, ethnography is part of the cultural research of other disciplines including social psychology, sociology, political science, education, and nursing. It is also used in feminist research. Leininger's (1985) ethnonursing research method, derived partly from ethnography, focuses on nursing phenomena from a cross-cultural perspective.

In addition to the explicit cultural emphasis of ethnography, the major ingredient of the research process is that one becomes part of the subculture being studied by physical association with the people in their setting during a period of fieldwork. Through the essential data collection methods of participant-observation in selected cultural activities and in-depth interviewing of the members of the subculture, the researcher learns from informants the meanings they attach to their activities, events, behaviors, knowledge, rituals, and other aspects of their life-style. Ethnography also shares certain general characteristics of qualitative research, namely context preservation rather than context control, thus providing for a holistic perspective; an emic perspective that elicits and addresses data from the perspective of cultural insiders; a dominantly inductive approach to data analysis and theory generation; and an interactive approach that recognizes members of the culture who provide data (informants) as co-participants in the research process.

It should be remembered that participant-observation is a method of data collection. Although all ethnography involves participant-observation to varying degrees, not all participant-observation research aims at producing ethnography. Likewise, whereas all ethnography deals with culture, not all cultural research need be, nor is, ethnography. The adjective "ethnographic" refers to culture in a general sense, including the gathering of cultural data that can occur in very brief encounters with individuals or communities—for example, in the ethnographic exercises of fieldwork students. "Doing ethnography" refers to prolonged, systematic, in-depth study. Gehring (1973) described ethnography as:

> *The art and discipline of watching and listening and of trying to inductively derive meaning from behaviors initiated by others. One must see the general in the rich, particularizing detail of good ethnography. To watch and to listen must come before interpretation and analysis. (p. 1223)*

As the major research instrument, the ethnographer seeks *emic* or insider answers to research questions and aims to capture the cultural context in rich, particularizing detail by observing and participating in the events of the subculture. With the help of the culture's members, the ethnographer looks for themes, patterns, connections, and relationships that have meaning for the people in it. This thick description of the culture, including the interpretive verbatim data from informants, becomes a major part of the ethnography and eventually permits others to assess the analysis and conclusions of the ethnographer, who brings an etic or scientific/theoretic perspective to bear on the final analysis of the cultural data.

Because of the value of context preservation, ethnographies are lengthy and are often presented as books or monographs, or on film or videotape. Journal articles that provide a condensed summary of a full ethnography are referred to by Werner and Schoepfle (1987a) as "sketch ethnographies" (p. 47). These reports can be found in such journals as *Human Organization, Journal of Contemporary Ethnography, Qualitative Health Research,* and *Sociology of Health and Illness,* as well as the nursing research literature.

Liebow's (1967) *Tally's Corner,* and Gans's (1962) *The Urban Villagers* are examples of ethnographies of subcultures of American society. Examples of nursing ethnographies in books are Germain's (1979) *The Cancer Unit: An Ethnography;* Kayser-Jones's (1981) *Old, Alone, and Neglected,* a comparative study of a nursing home in Scotland and one in the United States; and Wolf's (1988) *Nurses' Work, The Sacred and the Profane,* a study of nursing rituals in a large, urban hospital. The book edited by Kay (1982) contains multiple ethnographies of human birth in one volume. Morse (1992) edited a book containing several examples of traditional and ethnoscience ethnography.

Valuable information about cultures and subcultures may also be obtained from the works of novelists, journalists, and missionaries. However, the differences between these ethnographic accounts and ethnography are in the rigor of the research process and in the goal, which for ethnography is a contribution to science through emphasis on theory development.

ETHNOGRAPHIC PARADIGMS

Lett (1987) pointed out: "The majority of anthropologists are generally comfortable operating within an unspecified and largely implicit paradigmatic framework" (p. 83). The paradigm level of anthropology requires considerable refinement although some attempts at clarification have been made. For example, Sanday (1979) explained that current anthropological ethnography is governed by a continuously developing paradigm and described the evolution of the holistic, semiotic, and behavioristic "styles," as well as the internal theoretical differences of the holistic and semiotic "styles" (p. 23). The holistic (traditional, classical, or conventional) paradigm is represented in the works of Boas, Malinowski, Radcliffe-Brown, Benedict, and Mead. The semiotic approach has two prongs. The first is ethnoscience ethnography, also called componential analysis, cognitive anthropology, or the "new" ethnography. This view holds that culture is located in the minds of people, is expressed in a group's language or semantic system, and is analyzed in domains of cultural knowledge. The works of Spradley (1970) and others reflect this view. The second prong is symbolic anthropology in which culture is viewed as a symbolic system made up of shared, identifiable, public symbols and meanings, and which posits that cultural knowledge is embedded in thick description provided by culture members. This view is represented in the interpretive work of Geertz (1973) and others. The behavioristic approach departs from the inductive framework and tests predetermined deductive propositions, although some observational data on preselected categories may be included. In her analysis, Sanday (1979/1983) pointed out that most anthropological fieldworkers have been trained by scholars who employ some combination of these "styles," and which mode one adopts depends on one's goals and one's tastes.

Lett (1987) explained that, although certain features of the concept of culture are accepted by all anthropologists, there is no standard, accepted definition. He presented his interpretation of four recent approaches to the study of culture derived from Keesing (1974), and further defined and critiqued these later in the text. The first approach is culture as an adaptive system of learned beliefs and behaviors that help human societies adjust to their environments. This view is associated with cultural ecology and cultural materialism. Its problems for study are significant social issues. The second approach views culture as a cognitive system composed of whatever one needs to know to operate acceptably in a culture and is associated with the paradigm known variously as ethnoscience, cognitive anthropology, or the "new" ethnography, as described above. A third approach, structuralism, maintains that structures of human thought processes determine culture and that emic cultural data are collected for intellectual, not social, purposes. The fourth approach, symbolic anthropology (referred to above), is described as the interpretive study of culture that deals with questions of meaning, that is, ". . . shared patterns of interpretation and perspective embodied in symbols by means of which people develop and communicate their knowledge about and attitudes towards life" (p. 110).

Lett prefaced his definitions of eleven anthropologic paradigms, some no longer in use, by stating that ". . . most anthropologists rely heavily upon the concept of 'culture' as an explanatory mechanism" (p. 85). Lett specifically critiqued the paradigms of cultural materialism, structuralism, and symbolic anthropology. Although describing these paradigms as incommensurable because they identify different problems for investigation, Lett also suggested that when problems overlap between the paradigms of cultural materialism, which addresses problems associated with the maintenance of human life, and symbolic anthropology, which addresses problems associated with human identity, ". . . a very purposeful and deliberate kind of eclecticism" (p. 124) can offer complementary explanations.

Probably the most frequently used approaches to ethnography in nursing are the varieties of the holistic (classical or traditional) approach, which views cultures as wholes with interacting component groups (Jacob, 1988); ethnoscience ethnography, which looks at culture as the ideas, beliefs, and knowledge that a group of people hold and that are expressed in language (ideational culture); and cultural materialism and cultural ecology, in which culture is viewed as an adaptive system and is considered in terms of a group's observable patterns of behavior, customs, and way of life (materialist culture). Fetterman (1989) noted that ethnographers need to know about both cultural behavior and cultural knowledge to describe a culture or subculture adequately: "Both material and ideational definitions of culture are useful at different times in exploring fully how groups of people think and behave in their natural environment" (p. 27).

Ethnography and Theory Development

Ethnography contributes descriptive and explanatory theories of culture and cultural behaviors and meanings. Each ethnography is itself a descriptive theory of culture, broad in scope. An ethnography may generate other middle-range theories such as taxonomies and hypotheses for further study. Successive levels of explanatory theory generated from holist research are presented by Reason (1981) as derived from Diesing (1971). In this pattern model of explanation, fieldwork data are analyzed and resultant themes are connected empirically in a network or pattern that, in turn, explains the human system in its context. The account, then, describes and explains the kind of relations the various parts have for each other.

One alternative model of theory development is Diers's (1979) presentation of levels of scientific inquiry. Ethnoscience ethnography can yield descriptive theory in the form of taxonomic analyses of particular domains of meaning or other types of classification theory. This type of research answers the question "What is this?" and is at the factor-searching level of inquiry (level I). Exploratory, descriptive, relation-searching studies at the second level of scientific inquiry (level II) answer the question "What's happening here?" The search for themes or patterns through the study of the parts of a culture, the relationship of the parts to each other, and the relationship of the parts to the whole cultural context would result in descriptive and explanatory (factor-relating) theory. Traditional or conventional ethnography generally incorporates both these levels of inquiry, but its mode of relation-searching is qualitative rather than quantitative. Thus, ethnography is theory-generating and in the context of discovery, as contrasted with studies that are theory-testing and in the context of verification. The theory produced is grounded theory in that it is grounded in or derived from the empirical data of cultural description.

Classifications of Ethnography

Anyone who examines a program of a meeting of the Society for Applied Anthropology or the American Anthropological Association can attest that anthropological research is classified in largely nonparadigmatic ways. Werner and Schoepfle (1987a), proponents of ethnoscience, acknowledged the complexities of any classification system for ethnography due to all the possible subtypes and the cross-cutting of classificatory principles. Nevertheless, they identified several ways of classifying ethnographies. The first taxonomy consists of three types: processual or social process ethnographies; photographic and film ethnographies; and encyclopedic ethnographies, in which the unit of study is usually an entire language community such as the Navajo language. Processual ethnographies include eight subtypes. The holistic approach, the hallmark of classical or traditional ethnography, has been contemporarily extended to any isolatable human group. Germain's (1979) ethnography of a cancer unit in a community general hospital was placed in this category. The microethnography of small groups (fewer than 15 members) is addressed within the holistic subtype as well. Spradley's (1970) *You Owe Yourself a Drunk* and Goffman's (1961) *Asylums* are classified as cross-sectional ethnography. The distinguishing characteristic of a second classification system is its binary feature, for example, urban/rural, and full description/sketch. A third classification is based on major streams in anthropological theory—including cultural materialism, structuralism, and symbolic anthropology—and the encyclopedic focus of traditional ethnoscience, among others. A final classification system is according to the unit of analysis. This may include the group involved (the social dimension) such as street drug sellers; the space occupied by a group (the geographic dimension) such as a village or school; the knowledge system or cultural domain such as how people define medical emergencies (Evaneshko & Kay, 1982); and the time or temporal unit in the interactional focus such as the life history.

Critical ethnography, according to Thomas (1993), is a variation of conventional ethnography but has the avowed political purpose of changing existing oppressive social circumstances. Thomas stated that critical ethnography is not related to the Frankfort school of critical theory.

THE RESEARCH PROCESS

Basic components of the ethnographic research process are presented below as they apply to ethnography in the holistic (or conventional) tradition. These guidelines are, of course, modifiable for contemporary variations. The processes by which cultural data are obtained, analyzed, and interpreted share some components with other qualitative designs. However, certain distinctions are important for those who wish to do or to critique ethnography.

Aims

People's cultural knowledge is often unknown to them or taken for granted, and they do not get the opportunity to stand back from the exigencies of everyday life to examine pertinent aspects. Ethnographers seek answers to significant research questions that are aimed at explicating aspects of culture in context. The answers eventuate in cultural theory grounded in the knowledge people use to organize their behavior and interpret their experience. Thus, ethnography aims to get at the implicit or latent (backstage) culture in addition to the explicit, public, or manifest (frontstage) aspects of culture.

The Research Problem

The problem is one that can best be addressed through descriptive analysis of a particular culture or subcultural group. The researcher will be guided initially by specific research questions addressing the ethnographic focus. Initial questions will take the general form of "What is this?" or "What's happening here in this subculture?" The direction of the research and the research questions is not as fixed ahead of time as it is with the more linear quantitative research designs. There is a degree of flexibility with ethnographic research that permits the revision of questions as new discoveries lead to new directions for cultural understanding. Initial questions may change after immersion in the field because cultural informants may provide data that lead to more meaningful questions or that help the researcher sharpen the initial ones.

Review of the Literature

Because ethnography involves exploration, an extensive data-based literature is not expected to be available on the particular research focus. In fact, as Spradley (1979) stated: "Ethnography starts with a conscious attitude of almost complete ignorance" (p. 4). However, a critical review of sources that led to the selection of the problem to be studied at this exploratory level should be provided, although this literature may be largely conceptual rather than data-based. The pulling together of threads or themes from a number of diverse sources may provide the framework for examining the complex human situations for which ethnography is most appropriate.

The Setting

For nursing, the setting for ethnography can be wherever there are people and activities that give rise to cultural questions related to nursing and health care that need to be addressed in holistic context, including people's homes. The researcher must know that significant data are obtainable in a particular setting but pilot studies are not a characteristic of ethnography. Meanings are emphasized rather than surface data, and trust needs to be built over time with informants, to get meaningful data in context. Entering the field as a stranger limits bias and also allows for a degree of culture shock. This, in moderation, is not negative, for it allows the ethnographer to get the feel as well as the facts of the cultural scene.

Gaining Access

It is very helpful to know at least one insider who can provide initial access to the setting. However, several levels of clearance and consent may be required before an ethnographer can enter a sub-culture to initiate field study. The prefieldwork phase is time-consuming but essential so that the members of the subculture can become aware of, and supportive of, the primacy of the research role of this stranger to their setting. Access rules, such as the frequency and hours of coming and going, the means of identification of the ethnographer, permission to use technical recording devices or camera, and determination of what data sources are absolutely off limits must be worked out in advance insofar as possible. A private place, however small, to which the ethnographer can withdraw to write field notes should be sought. Role negotiations regarding the range of participant-observation activities are especially important when the ethnographer is a nurse in a health care setting.

A liaison person, or key informant, may be identified at this time to guide the researcher's entry and orientation to aspects of the culture, to fulfill the gatekeeper role for the duration of the study, and to introduce the researcher to other key informants who can serve as guides and provide crucial data. A key informant can also assure members of the culture that the researcher is safe to have around.

All who provide data are informants. However, in ethnography, the term informant does not carry the sometimes pejorative connotation of the common use of the term. Key informants and other informants are culture bearers who are very much a part of the research process. Because the ethnographer is interested in the people's perceptions of their own situation, members of the subculture who provide such data are viewed as co-participants in the research process. These people are selected because they know well the citizens, language, history, rituals, and backstage data of their community and can teach the researcher about them. It is essential to get as much informant description as possible and to cross-validate informants' perceptions. The researcher should validate his or her own perceptions with key informants as well.

Informants have various motivations for participating in a research enterprise that involves a time commitment and possibly some risks. These motivations may include pride in sharing aspects of one's culture, curiosity, commitment to science as an enterprise, the opportunity to share feelings and concerns, or a break from the routine aspects of their life-style.

Ethical and Legal Considerations

Possessing a nursing license may give greater access as a participant-observer in a health care setting to a nurse ethnographer than to other social scientists but it carries particular ethical and legal obligations. The ethical principles of respect for persons, beneficence, and justice, which are incorporated in the Belmont Report (Department of Health, Education and Welfare, 1979) must be adhered to in all research involving human subjects. However, the application of these principles is necessarily different in each ethnography, because the ethnographer interacts as a participant with live persons in constantly evolving, unpredictable human situations. Ethical issues will undoubtedly arise. Although general issues may be surmised, one does not know the specific issues in advance. In general, ethical considerations in ethnography by nurse researchers involve:

1. Obtaining initial informed consent from informants and renegotiating consent throughout the period of fieldwork. Specific written permission is usually required for tape recordings and photographs. In some states, recent laws related to the HIV/AIDS epidemic require explicit permission to read patients' records and to speak to patients' visitors. Finding out about such rules from the institution's research review board or an equivalent is essential.
2. The protection of privacy, anonymity, and confidentiality of members of the subculture during the period of data collection and at the time of publication of the report, while still maintaining the scientific integrity of the report.
3. Objectivity versus subjectivity with regard to selection, recording, and reporting phenomena.
4. Decisions regarding intervention versus nonintervention in the activities of the subculture.
5. Professional accountability for the legal and ethical components of the assumed participant-observer activities. This

sometimes means walking a tightrope with regard to weighing the potential long-range benefits of the research vis-à-vis potential early termination from the setting if issues surrounding the protection of human subjects arise and cannot be resolved.

6. Potential use of findings due to power relationships among various levels of the study population.

Germain (1985), Tilden (1980), and Munhall (1988) offered more detailed sources for examination of ethical issues in ethnography and other empirical, qualitative research.

With regard to legal aspects, nurse ethnographers planning field research in a clinical setting should check to see that their professional liability policy covers them in a research role. The potential ethnographer is advised that field data in some jurisdictions are subject to subpoena. Thus, notes and tape recordings must be safeguarded, and the anonymity of the subjects and locations must be provided for through the use of pseudonyms in field notes and in the final report. On the other hand, in some jurisdictions, one's scholarly status as a researcher makes some data legally privileged.

Sampling

No ethnography is ever a complete picture of a subculture. The sample is that part of the reality that is observed and recorded. Sampling is done of events, activities, informants, documents, and other data sources. Because the best cultural informants are sought, that is, those who can "tell it like it is," random sampling or systematic sampling are not appropriate. The sampling principle is not based on numbers of interviews or events but rather on the richness of the data, that is, how accurately they portray the full context of the culture as well as answers to the research questions. These research questions provide direction for the ethnographer's selection and involvement in the scenes of the subculture.

Informant (participant) sampling and event sampling are initially purposive and opportunistic. Fetterman (1989) called this type of sampling stratified judgment sampling. The ethnographer seeks out persons, events, places, documents, and other sources that provide the greatest opportunities to gather the most relevant data. Sampling becomes, however, increasingly theoretical, that is, directed by logic and aim (see below).

Data Collection Methods

Because data for ethnography are obtained primarily through the human senses, the ethnographer is the primary research instrument. There is triangulation of data collection methods in order to obtain the widest range of perspectives on issues as well as to obtain a complete data set. Knafl and Breitmayer (1991) addressed triangulation in detail.

Participant-observation is the major data collection method of ethnography, and because actively participating in some way in the experience and actions of others to find meaning necessitates interpersonal and group interaction, interviewing members of the subculture is likewise an essential component. Other methods of data collection such as documentary analysis supplement these major ones. Because the ethnographer accumulates a very large data set, it is wise to seek grant funds for the study, if only for transcription of tape-recorded data.

Participant-Observation. Participant-observation means immersion of the researcher in the cultural data of the field. The researcher attempts to become a part of the subculture being studied by participating in a low-keyed manner so as to induce as little change as possible. The stance is one of a listener and learner. Participant-observation allows the researcher to look beyond statements of ideal behavior (cognitive conceptualization of culture) to observe behaviors directly (behavioral conceptualization of culture) so that the correspondence or the discrepancy between the real and ideal cultural statements can be described, assessed, and explained.

Data obtained through participant-observation are recorded in field notes as close to verbatim as possible and in specific, concrete, and particularistic detail. Using a laptop computer in the field can save transcription time because data can be entered directly onto disks. If a laptop computer is not available or cannot be used and taking notes during an event is impossible or inappropriate, brief notes may be jotted down (condensed notes) and, as soon as possible, expanded to include a full description of the participant-observation or interview experience, taking care not to rephrase the local language or to move to higher levels of abstraction.

Junker (1960, pp. 35–38) described a continuum of participant-observation and noted that the practicing fieldworker oscillates through this range during the course of the study. Major points on the continuum, adapted from Junker on the basis of the author's experiences as a nurse ethnographer, are:

- Complete observer. In this role, the fieldworker may be visible but does not interact with those being observed—for example, in a meeting of a board of directors, or when professionally "hanging around" (nonparticipant observation). Invisible observation may be accomplished through a one-way window or a hidden vantage point (the potted palm technique) or through the use of cameras, ethics permitting. It may be necessary for a nurse ethnographer to figuratively sit on her hands so as not to intervene when observation is in order. On the other hand, to continue only to observe, without interaction or participation, assumes that the researcher can interpret the experiences of others without their input.

- Observer-as-participant. The research role of the observer is publicly known at the outset and the research is intentionally not kept under wraps. This role may provide access to a wide range of information, and even secrets (or backregion data) may be made available when the researcher becomes known for guarding confidential information. The researcher can be selective with regard to observation and participation and has the flexibility to move about opportunistically as the research demands.

- Participant-as-observer. The research role is not wholly concealed, but the research activities are subordinated to the person's primary role in the setting, which may be as an employee. This role may limit the researcher's flexibility in movement to events that maximize data collection and may also limit access to certain kinds of information, especially backstage or backregion information, which fellow workers might be reluctant to share.

- Complete participant. When this role is deliberate, the participant-observer's identity as a researcher is intentionally concealed as he or she attempts to become a full-fledged member of the group under study. In today's research scene, this deceptive role is considered by most to be unethical, because it violates the principle of informed consent of study subjects. However, this role is sometimes inadvertent, such as when some noncentral and anonymous persons in an isolated event or activity in the subculture do not realize that they are part of a study, and when it is not wise to interrupt such activities to explain the study. It may also be used when the subjects' identities are not in jeopardy, for example, in a study of gambling behavior when no individual and no specific location can be identified.

Leininger (1985) and Spradley (1980) offered variations on the above version of the participant-observation continuum.

The ethnographer must work out a participant role that enhances data collection and blends in with the life of the people being studied. The data collection focus guides movement on the continuum of participant-observation, which is also influenced by the design of the study, the research purpose and problem(s), the aspect of the culture being studied, and the background and ability of the ethnographer to assume tasks that are a natural part of the subculture.

Engaging in the activities of another culture or subculture through participant-observation and trying to find meaning in the behaviors of others demand considerable introspection on the part of the ethnographer, who, by the accumulation of education and professional and life experiences, brings his or her own cultural perspectives (etic) to the field. Quint (1968), a nurse sociologist, acknowledged that biases exist but emphasized that, when doing participant-observation, it is necessary to identify one's own inner conflicts and biases and use them as an essential part of the data being collected. Thus, in addition to field notes of participant-observations and written or taped records of interviews, it is recommended that participant-observers keep a personal field journal to record feelings, reactions, biases, and other results of introspection. This process is sometimes referred to as reflexivity. A different section of the field journal is devoted to memos related to theoretical insights, ideas for theoretical sampling, further questions, and the like.

Good fieldwork relationships call for some kind of reciprocity on the part of the ethnographer. This reciprocity can take many forms, such as being a volunteer driver for residents of a shelter for abused women (Germain, 1984). Role reciprocity enhances data collection and need not interfere with objectivity if change induced by the researcher is minimal. Bruyn (1966), a sociologist, pointed out:

> While the traditional role of the scientist is that of a neutral observer who remains unmoved, unchanged, and untouched in his examination of phenomena, the role of the participant-observer requires sharing the sentiments of people in social situations; as a consequence he himself is changed as well as changing to some degree the situation in which he is a participant. (p. 14)

For the researcher, the important point is to record these changes and use them as part of the data being analyzed. Agar (1986) stated that "ethnography is neither 'subjective' nor 'objective.' It is interpretive, mediating two worlds through a third" (p. 19).

Interviewing. In-depth interviewing—formal and informal; structured, semistructured, or unstructured—of individual or group informants is essential to grasp the native's point of view, as well as to clarify discrepancies among members of the subculture or between the researcher's perceptions and members' perceptions. Probes are used to get responses to specific questions, to encourage the sharing of detailed information about specific events, and to further clarify certain topics. Taylor and Bogdan (1984) noted that qualitative interviews are flexible and dynamic. In-depth interviewing has the added dimension of repeated face-to-face encounters, modeled after a conversation between equals.

Some interviews are formal, having purpose, structure, and appointed times, but qualitative (ethnographic) interviews often contain less structure than is contained in the use of formalized open-ended questions. This permits the researcher to get essential questions answered but also allows for unanticipated or serendipitous data. As Evaneshko and Kay (1982) noted: "Ethnographic inquiry is different from open-ended interviews in that the latter is structured to stay within pre-established general guidelines, while the former is more free roaming and pursues promising avenues of cultural knowledge suggested by the informant's remarks" (p. 53). Many interviews are "on the hoof," that is, questioning of informants takes place while the ethnographer accompanies them during the natural pace of cultural activities.

Supplementary Data Sources. Because ethnography frequently embraces change over time and across situations, past events may require analysis to determine their influence on current behaviors. Thus, archival data, oral life histories, and personal diaries may be used. Documentary analysis of such materials as minutes of meetings, policies and procedures statements, newsletters, newspaper articles, or patient records may provide supplementary data. Examining formal hierarchical or kinship structures, language, cultural artifacts (technology), photographs, or films may add to the understanding of the culture under study. Some demographic data are collected as well, in order to describe relevant characteristics of the members of the subculture.

Although some ethnographers may choose to employ closed-ended data collection tools such as questionnaires or personality inventories, there are limitations to the use of these when a sole researcher studies a complex part of society. A team of ethnographers would facilitate intercoder reliability and mutual support, but teams are expensive and, with a team, there is a risk of loss of the intimate, trusting relationships that are built up over time and are an essential part of the ethnographic process. Moreover, the essence of ethnography is the discovery of a way of life and the meaning of events and relationships to the people studied, from their point of view, rather than through the use of tools developed from a priori assumptions, although these may supplement fieldwork methods.

Phases of Fieldwork

Being in the field may mean that a researcher actually lives for a period of time with the people being studied or spends a certain amount of time in the subculture as a participant-observer on a regular basis such as two or three hours, three times a week, with flexibility in scheduling to maximize data collection. The data collection phase is often exciting and intriguing, and fieldworkers are attracted to spending considerable time in the field. However, Berg (1989) noted that two hours of data collection may require as long as eight hours to expand into comprehensive field notes.

Trips to the field should be goal-oriented, but goals may be suspended temporarily if more significant opportunities arise. Depending on the researcher's focus, which is guided by the research questions and ongoing data analysis, the researcher takes samples from the total scene or population of data. The occurrence of significant cultural events and the amount of time demanding the researcher's presence to obtain a valid sample of the scene are very important considerations in planning time in the field. For example, an ethnography with a focus on registered nurse role behavior in the subculture of a hospital acute care unit would necessitate sampling all three shifts, probably over at least a one-year period, because there are notable seasonal variations in hospital life.

The actual length of time needed for the fieldwork phase of a study varies according to the research questions, the complexity of the subculture, the building of relationships with key informants, access to significant data, and seasonal or cyclic variations that influence the subculture. Generally, one year has been considered a reasonable time to be accepted by persons in a relatively complex subculture, to learn its manifest and latent aspects, to attend to a wide variety of the subculture's activities, to see members in various contexts, to conduct theoretical sampling, and to follow certain events to their conclusions. In-depth knowledge of the subculture rather than surface familiarity with it is the goal.

During the initial phase of fieldwork, the ethnographer learns about the culture by asking questions and seeking clarification and explanations from cultural informants. He or she obtains a broad overview of the situation, writing detailed field notes or descriptive accounts of what goes on there, the characteristics of the people, what they say and how they act, their cultural artifacts, and the structure, function, and sociopolitical system of the group. Necessary demographic data are obtained. The setting is mapped, and spatial, physical, and other characteristics of the environment are recorded. Because historical data may be relevant to the current context, access to archives may be necessary.

Building trusting relationships is essential during this period so that, over the long term, quality data may be obtained. It has been suggested that ethnographers might distort events by their mere presence, because people may act guarded and reserved, but the experience of ethnographers has been that, after a few days, the people of the subculture must focus their energy and attention on the events of their usual life-style. The ethnographer who enacts the agreed-on participant-observer role competently and provides appropriate reciprocity tends to blend into the background, so to speak. After this initial period of general observations and involvement in the activities of the subculture, the researcher may note the need for refining or revising the research questions.

Collection of data and preliminary data analysis proceed simultaneously. This process of data collection and analysis in ethnography has been described as dialectical or cyclical, as compared with the linear model of hypothetico-deductive studies. As coding of data and categorization proceed (see below), persons, events, and other sources are more deliberately chosen (theoretical sampling) based on the data analysis. The ethnographer's cultural inferences, formed through observing, participating, listening, and analyzing, are working hypotheses that must be tested repeatedly until there is validation that people share a particular system of meanings. Although general descriptive observations continue until the end of the study, deliberate or focused sampling is necessary to validate or compare data, to cover the entire range of the phenomena under study, to fill in gaps in the data, and to seek negative cases, that is, those that do not support or that refute the developing theory.

There is a search for patterns; these are gradually discovered and then interrelated with other patterns. When no new data add to the emergent themes or patterns and no new dimensions or insights are identified that can shed light on the research questions (data saturation), the active fieldwork phase ends. Although the study of complex cultures could go on and on, pragmatic considerations may be the determining factors in the cessation of data collection. Finances, the demands of other types of work or life activities, the end of a sabbatical, and a dissertation deadline are examples of such considerations.

Role disengagement must be incorporated into the final phase. Termination of fieldwork means terminating relationships built over a long period of time. The members of the subculture, as well as the fieldworker, need preparation for this departure. Whenever possible, arrangements should be made by the researcher to continue contact in some way with informants or to make some forays back into the field during the final analysis and writing period for clarification, verification, validation, or closure on certain issues. Also, the members of the subculture and the ethnographer need to develop a plan for sharing the outcomes of the study.

Data Management

All data from all sources make up the ethnographic record. Processing one's field notes immediately after each visit is time-consuming but important, because it allows for ongoing review of data and assists the researcher in establishing goals for subsequent visits. The time-consuming and tedious tasks of storing codes, cutting, sorting, indexing, cross-referencing, filing, and other aspects of data management can be greatly reduced with modern computer technology, including qualitative data management software (Tesch, 1990; Walker, 1993). As soon as possible, it is wise for the fieldworker to type data into a word processor (or to have an assistant do this) and to guard against loss by storing one hard copy in a confidential but secure and separate location. Another intact set provides a working copy. Typing field notes double-spaced on one-half or three-quarters of the horizontal measure of a page leaves room in the wide margin for codes and for jotting down memos or questions. Each page of field notes should be numbered and should contain the date, time, and location of the observations or interview.

If a computer software package for qualitative data management is not used for enhanced data management, additional copies of field notes are useful for cutting and sorting into file folders or some other convenient cross-referencing system after coding and categorizing of data have been done.

Data Analysis

The entire ethnographic record is subjected to analysis. The ethnographer uses primarily qualitative content analysis to inductively derive patterns or themes from the data. Although there is no single way to conduct content analysis, there are basic guidelines.

Coding of data from the seemingly immense volume of qualitative information contained in field notes and interviews is the first step in the process of content analysis and is essential for moving from the concrete to higher levels of generalization. Codes are labels assigned to units of meaning. These units will vary with the type of data. A meaningful unit may occur in a line, a sentence, a paragraph, or a larger section of data. Initial codes, especially of interview data, are frequently repeated from the raw data itself. Coding is critical because it provides a direct link with the concrete data of the cultural reality. Overcoding may occur in the early stages of analysis, in an effort to retain as much relevant information as possible. Recoding may be necessary as data accumulate and new codes are compared with early codes.

When codes are compared, similar codes are grouped into categories. Categories might be, for example, responses of a particular type, systems of relationships, stages of a process, types of behaviors such as gestures of deference, and so on. Although the phrase "categories emerged from the data" is often used with regard to the outcomes of qualitative content analysis, in fact, categories do not emerge spontaneously. They are identified by a careful mental process of logical analysis of content from all data sources. Categories are compared and clustered. Care must be taken that leaps are not made from codes or categories to clusters or concepts based on the prior knowledge of the researcher. It takes conscious and continued mental effort to avoid imposing etic knowledge on the data. The field journal can assist in managing intellectual and emotional biases.

The processed data are reviewed periodically for emergent concepts, typifications, themes, and patterns. Theoretical memos, kept in the field journal, assist this movement from the concrete to higher levels of abstraction. Variations that are meaningful but atypical must be accounted for as well. Every culture has occasional aberrations that may prove to have future relevance.

Qualitative researchers resist imposing an a priori theoretical schema on the data. This imposition is more aligned with a quantitative research approach rather than induction from the data. However, as an alternative coding system, some ethnographers use the codes of the Human Relations Area Files (HRAF) (Lagacé, 1974), which comprise both a major cultural data archive or worldwide, ethnographic data bank and a system for the rapid and accurate retrieval of data on specific cultures and topics for hologeistic studies. Over 310 cultural units are represented in files arranged according to a special subject classification system consisting of over 700 numbered subject categories grouped into 79 major topical selections. The HRAF are located at several major universities throughout the country.

Writing the Report

Although coding, categorizing, and questioning the data take place throughout the data collection phase, the major work of analysis and interpretation takes place after leaving the field and is guided by the assumptions and research questions. As long a period of time may be needed for the final intensive analysis, synthesis, and writing of the ethnography as was spent in the field.

Werner and Schoepfle (1987b) estimated that a one-year ethnographic field study may generate 3,000 pages of transcription and an ethnography drawn from this data base may have 300 pages or a 1:10 data reduction.

Comparing, contrasting, analyzing, and synthesizing take considerable time and mental effort. Subjective meanings of members of the subculture, verified through the observer's work, serve as a basis for the drawing of cultural inferences, which, it should be remembered, are the researcher's meanings of the meanings communicated by informants. That is, although the descriptive data are provided by members of the subculture and can be validated by them, the final analysis and conclusions are the researcher's, guided by his or her own theoretical perspectives. Several graphic display devices presented by Miles and Huberman (1984) may be useful as aids in data reduction, analysis, and conceptualization. During the final analysis, comparisons with existing ethnographies and middle-range theories are made. Existing theories may be supported or refuted, and new middle-range theories, in addition to the descriptive and explanatory theory of culture, may be induced.

Ethnography is usually reported in narrative, literary style in order to preserve the flavor and nuances of the cultural scene. This style allows expression of the world of meaning. Each ethnography contains multiple levels of abstraction, from raw data providing the native's point of view to constructed taxonomies, cultural inferences, analysis, conclusions, and problems or hypotheses for further study. Maps, diagrams, and tables of demographic data may be included to enhance the narrative.

Basic researchers who study cultures or subcultures may intend to make a contribution to knowledge for its own sake. In this case, making recommendations for cultural change within the report may be inappropriate. However, applied anthropologists and applied ethnographers from other disciplines not only may aim to make a theoretical contribution to the understanding of the human species but also will ask themselves how this knowledge advances the cause of or serves the needs of humankind (Spradley, 1980, p. 19). Thus, some ethnographies may contain the researcher's recommendations for change, and some applied anthropologists may actually engage in a cultural change project through applying an intervention, collecting data throughout, evaluating outcomes, and including these in the ethnographic report.

Styles of reporting ethnography vary as do styles of doing ethnography. Some analysis, for example, may be incorporated within the thick description and more completely emphasized in a separate, final section. This opportunity for creativity and flexibility in reporting style compared with the usual style of quantitative research reports is what makes ethnography challenging to write and, if well written, easy to read. If an ethnography reads easily, it is not because the study and the writing of the report were easy to do; rather, it is a mark of the ethnographer's ability to synthesize and write in a style that facilitates reading while preserving scientific adequacy. Bruyn (1966) suggested that "the participant-observer must remain a scientist with the insights of a Shakespearean dramatist" (p. 253).

The nature of the final report is affected not only by the background and style of the ethnographer and the group described but also by the intended audience. The ethnographer must decide, for example, whether the ethnography is intended primarily for other scientists, a dissertation committee, an employer who commissions a study, the educated lay public, or a combination of these. In addition to the descriptive analysis of the culture, each presentation of an ethnography should include a description of the methodology as well as changes that occurred in the ethnographer as a result of the research enterprise.

Criteria for Scientific Adequacy

Ethnographers are as concerned as other scientists that their work meet criteria for scientific merit, or trustworthiness, appropriate to the level and type of inquiry. Explicit standards for assessing the scientific adequacy of ethnography have changed over time. For example, Bruyn (1966) cited six criteria of subjective adequacy for making interpretations in community studies:

1. The time a researcher spends with a group;
2. Place, or actual observation of subjects in their everyday lives;
3. Social circumstances, or the variety of social settings, roles, and activities witnessed;
4. Language, or the understanding of different connotations, phrasings, and sentence structures in daily use;
5. Intimacy of the encounters;
6. Consensus, or "confirmation-in-the-context" that the meanings interpreted by the observer are correct.

Germain (1979), in her ethnographic study of a cancer unit, provided an example of how these criteria were addressed.

Traditional criteria for ethnography include a qualitative interpretation of the quantitative terms *validity* and *reliability*. In the
following treatment, traditional criteria are first presented and
then fused with the more contemporary generic criteria of Lincoln and Guba (1985). The Sandelowki (1986) and Catanzaro and
Olshansky (1988) modifications of Lincoln and Guba's criteria follow. This sequence is used because some nursing research proposal review groups seem to prefer the more generic criteria for
all qualitative studies.

Validity.   Validity is the primary criterion of good ethnography. The test of validity in ethnography is how accurately the instrument (the researcher) captures (measures) the observed
reality and portrays this reality in the research report. Face validity is established by the assumption that members selected as informants to represent the subculture have expert knowledge in
certain cultural components. Content validity is established
through verification with as many cultural informants as possible.

Sample selection bias, observer bias, accuracy in recording field
notes, analytical accuracy, and bias in reporting affect internal
validity, as do historical and maturation factors. During a study,
for example, the motives of informants may change, their positions or statuses may be altered, or their commitment to the project may wane.

External validity or generalizability of ethnography is sometimes criticized by those who regard its contribution to be a study
of a single case. A response to this is that an in-depth study of a
situation over a long period of time is more generative of insights
than broad surveys or the experimental study of variables in isolation from meaningful context. Burgess (1966) cited in Denzin
(1978, p. 197), explained that, in the sense that a single specimen
is representative of its kind or species and is typical (belonging
to a type), a case may be made for some degree of generalization
to other specimens of a similar type or class of units. Benoliel
(1984) noted that two important assumptions underlying the qualitative paradigm are the importance of understanding the situation
from the participants themselves and believing that truth ultimately rests on the direct experience of individuals.

External validity, or transferability, or "fittingness" occurs when findings fit other contexts as judged by readers, or when readers find the report meaningful in terms of their own experience. Thick description and verbatim quotations in the report increase transferability.

Internal validity, credibility, or truth value is enhanced by the ethnographer's direct and repeated involvement in the scenes of the culture, the selection of key informants who have cultural expertise, the testing of inferences (working hypotheses) until there is validation that meanings are shared, and the verification of information with as many informants as possible. Validity can be affected by the researcher's sample selection bias, observer bias, accuracy in recording field notes, bias in selecting what to report, and ability to assess whether informants are accurate portrayers of their culture. The researcher's field journal is examined by an auditor for evidence of biases made explicit. In addition to prolonged engagement and persistent observation in the field, validity, credibility, or truth value is also established through triangulation processes for completion; peer or colleague debriefing whereby the ethnographer's analyses and interpretations can be challenged and the soundness of working hypotheses and future plans can be assessed; and negative case analysis in which there is testing and refining of working hypotheses until the final version is consistent with all observations of the phenomenon without exception.

Reliability. Traditionally, reliability is the consistency of both the sources of data, including participants and the researcher, and the methods of data collection. One cannot literally replicate an ethnography, because there is no way to capture time, but a good ethnography presents what can be expected to occur. Frake (1964) (cited in Spradley, 1980) stated that the adequacy of ethnography is to be evaluated "by the ability of a stranger to the culture (who may be the ethnographer) to use the ethnographer's statements as instructions for appropriately anticipating the scenes of the society" (p. 10).

Reliability, dependability, consistency, or auditability is enhanced by asking the same questions of different informants over a long period of time and in different circumstances; obtaining repeatability of data over time from each key informant; carefully matching what informants say with their observed behavior; and seeking explanations for discrepancies. In interviewing, the researcher purposely varies approaches with individual informants in order to enhance credibility of data. Reliability, dependability, or consistency is also established through peer debriefing over time, and referential adequacy, in which some raw data are stored and later retrieved, analyzed, and compared with previously analyzed data for consistency.

Inquiry audits are formal assessments of all processes by an expert. These are conducted on all field notes, field journals, and products of analysis at several points during the data collection and analysis stages. Confirmability audits are conducted when the project is nearing completion and at its completion, to determine whether the findings and conclusions are supported by the data. Guidelines for inquiry and confirmability audits have been presented by Lincoln and Guba (1985).

Preparation for Ethnography

Researchers contemplating ethnography must like to learn about the culture and life-style of others and be comfortable in the learner's role of asking many questions in settings where the action is, such as in the real world of the multiple varieties of clinical nursing practice. It helps to have a high tolerance for uncertainty and ambiguity as well as an ability to withstand the cultural shock, including actual symptoms of illness, that occurs to some degree when entering a new territory. A nurse standing back and observing the cultural scenes of nursing practice is not immune to culture shock. A somewhat laid-back personality that enables one to develop and maintain a stance of detached involvement—that is, being authentic and identifying with the community but still maintaining professional distance from it—is crucial. Flexibility and a sense of time appropriateness regarding asking questions of individuals or rescheduling interviews are essential to obtaining significant data. The ethnographer must be able to build trusting relationships with informants by keeping data confidential. And, following the excitement of data collection in the field, patience is essential for the lengthy and often tedious final analytic process. Not only must the ethnographer like to collect and process data; an ability and interest in writing a research report in a more stylistic literary fashion, that is, primarily in word symbols rather than numeric symbols, is a must.

Doing ethnography is often a lonely, though very rich and growth-producing experience. There are threats to physical safety, as well as physiological, emotional, and potentially legal and ethical risks involved. Informants in the field may be friendly and helpful, but they cannot provide the necessary kind of ongoing support that is necessary on such an adventurous undertaking. A personal and collegial support system outside the field, a sense of humor, and a great deal of work space in one's home or office (for stacks of field notes and resource materials) are necessary. To prepare for such a peak experience, one can use course work, supervised fieldwork exercises, peer/colleague support, an experienced ethnographer-adviser, and a habit of reading ethnographies. From the plethora of methods texts, selecting a few favored guides for the journey is important. The Council on Nursing and Anthropology (CONAA) provides colleague support for qualitative nurse researchers in addition to its primary scientific mission. Many of the current members are ethnographers.

Being a nurse ethnographer in a health care setting has advantages: it enables the capturing of nuances and the selection of data that may be missed or deemed insignificant by a non-nurse ethnographer. Nurse ethnographers also have the advantage of having been trained in interviewing skills, being accustomed to entering different subcultures for clinical experiences, knowing the language of health care, and having a degree of comfort in health care situations that may ease (but not entirely eliminate) culture shock.

Relevance for Nursing

Besides contributing descriptive and explanatory theory and possibly hypotheses for further study, ethnographic nursing research can promote understanding of the meaning of health and illness experiences to clients and providers, and can yield insights useful for promoting cultural change to improve nursing practice systems, for presenting nursing practice realities to the scientific and lay communities, for influencing health policy, and for addressing a wide range of human problems in our society and its health care systems. Multiple, comparative, transcultural ethnographies of nursing situations having a similar focus would contribute to a worldwide ethnology of nursing. And each ethnography of nursing, with its culture-preserving, vividly detailed description, becomes a piece of nursing history.

REFERENCES

Agar, M. (1986). *Speaking of ethnography.* Newbury Park, CA: Sage.

Benoliel, J. Q. (1984). Advancing nursing science: Qualitative approaches. *Western Journal of Nursing Research, 6*(3), 1–8.

Berg, G. (1989). *Qualitative research methods for the social sciences.* Boston: Allyn & Bacon.

Bruyn, S. (1966). *The human perspective in sociology.* Englewood Cliffs, NJ: Prentice-Hall.

Burgess, E. (1966). "Discussion." In C. Shaw, *The Jack Roller* (pp. 185–197). Chicago: University of Chicago Press.

Catanzaro, M., & Olshansky, E. (1988). Evaluating research reports. In N. F. Woods & M. Catanzaro (Eds.), *Nursing research: Theory and practice* (pp. 469–478). St. Louis: Mosby.

Denzin, N. (1978). *The research act* (2nd ed.). New York: McGraw-Hill.

Department of Health, Education and Welfare. (1979). The Belmont Report: Ethical principles and guidelines for the protection of human subjects of research (GPO 887-809). Washington, DC: U.S. Government Printing Office.

Diers, D. (1979). *Research in nursing practice.* Philadelphia: Lippincott.

Diesing, P. (1971). *Patterns of discovery in the social sciences.* Chicago: Aldine.

Evaneshko, V., & Kay, M. (1982). The ethnoscience research technique. *Western Journal of Nursing Research, 4*(1), 49–64.

Fetterman, D. (1989). *Ethnography: Step by step.* Newbury Park, CA: Sage.

Frake, C. (1964). Structural description of Subanum religious behavior. In W. Goodenough (Ed.), *Explorations in cultural anthropology* (pp. 111–130). New York: McGraw-Hill.

Gans, H. (1962). *The urban villagers.* New York: Free Press.

Geertz, C. (1973). *The interpretation of cultures.* New York: Basic Books.

Gehring, F. (1973). Anthropology and education. In J. Honigman (Ed.), *Handbook of social and cultural anthropology.* Chicago: Rand McNally.

Germain, C. (1979/1982). *The cancer unit: An ethnography.* Wakefield, MA: Nursing Resources, Inc./Rockville, MD: Aspen.

Germain, C. (1984). Sheltering abused women: A nursing perspective. *Journal of Psychosocial Nursing, 22*(9), 24-31.

Germain, C. (1985). Ethical considerations for the nurse ethnographer doing field research in clinical settings. In A. Carmi (Ed.), *Medicolegal library: Vol. 4. Nursing law and ethics.* Germany: Springer Verlag.

Goffman, E. (1961). *Asylums.* Chicago: Aldine.

Jacob, E. (1988). Clarifying qualitative research: A focus on traditions. *Educational Researcher, 17*(1), 16-24.

Junker, B. (1960). *Field work.* Chicago: University of Chicago Press.

Kay, M. (Ed.). (1982). *Anthropology of human birth.* Philadelphia: F. A. Davis.

Kayser-Jones, J. (1981). *Old, alone, and neglected.* Los Angeles: University of California Press.

Keesing, R. (1974). Theories of culture. *Annual Review of Anthropology, 3,* 73-98.

Knafl, K., & Breitmayer, B. (1991). Triangulation in qualitative research: Issues of conceptual clarity and purpose. In J. Morse (Ed.). *Qualitative nursing research: A contemporary dialogue* (pp. 226-239). Newbury Park, CA: Sage.

Lagacé, R. (1974). *Nature and use of the HRAF files.* New Haven, CT: Human Relations Area Files Inc.

Leininger, M. (1985). Ethnography and ethnonursing: Models and modes of qualitative data analysis. In M. Leininger (Ed.), *Qualitative research methods in nursing* (pp. 33-69). Orlando, FL: Grune & Stratton.

Lett, J. (1987). *The human enterprise: A critical introduction to anthropological theory.* Boulder, CO: Westview Press.

Liebow, E. (1967). *Tally's corner.* Boston: Little, Brown.

Lincoln, Y., & Guba, E. (1985). *Naturalistic inquiry.* Beverly Hills, CA: Sage.

Miles, M., & Huberman, A. M. (1984). *Qualitative data analysis: A sourcebook of new methods.* Beverly Hills, CA: Sage.

Morse, J. (1992). *Qualitative health research.* Newbury Park, CA: Sage.

Munhall, P. (1988). Ethical considerations in qualitative research. *Western Journal of Nursing Research, 10*(2), 150-162.

Patton, M. (1990). *Qualitative evaluation and research methods* (2nd ed.). Newbury Park, CA: Sage.

Quint, J. (1968). Role models and the professional nurse identity. *Journal of Nursing Education, 6*(2), 11-16.

Reason, P. (1981). Patterns of discovery in the social sciences. In R. Reason & J. Rowan (Eds.), *Human inquiry* (pp. 183-189). New York: Wiley.

Sanday, P. (1983). The ethnographic paradigm(s). In J. Van Maanen (Ed.), *Qualitative methodology* (pp. 19-36). Beverly Hills, CA: Sage. (Original work published 1979, in *Administrative Science Quarterly.*)

Sandelowski, M. (1986). The problem of rigor in qualitative research. *Advances in Nursing Science, 8*(3), 27-37.

Spradley, J. (1970). *You owe yourself a drunk: An ethnography of urban nomads.* Boston: Little, Brown.

Spradley, J. (1979). *The ethnographic interview.* New York: Holt, Rinehart & Winston.

Spradley, J. (1980). *Participant observation.* New York: Holt, Rinehart & Winston.

Taylor, S., & Bogdan, R. (1984). *Introduction to qualitative research: The search for meanings* (2nd ed.). New York: Wiley.

Tesch, R. (1990). *Qualitative research: Analysis types and software tools.* Bristol, PA: The Falmer Press, Taylor & Francis, Inc.

Thomas, J. (1993). *Critical ethnography.* Newbury Park, CA: Sage.

Tilden, V. (1980). Qualitative research: A new frontier for nursing. In A. Davis & J. Krueger (Eds.), (pp. 73-83). *Patients, nurses, ethics.* New York: American Journal of Nursing Co.

Walker, B. L. (1993). Computer analysis of qualitative data. *Qualitative Health Research, 3*(1), 91-111.

Werner, O., & Schoepfle, G. (1987a). *Systematic fieldwork: Foundations of ethnography and interviewing: Vol. 1.* Newbury Park, CA: Sage.

Werner, O., & Schoepfle, G. (1987b). *Systematic fieldwork: Ethnographic analysis and data management: Vol. 2.* Newbury Park, CA: Sage.

Wolf, Z. (1988). *Nurses' work: The sacred and the profane.* Philadelphia: University of Pennsylvania Press.

9

Nursing Rituals: Doing Ethnography

Zane Robinson Wolf

*I*n almost every culture known to us, health and illness are symbolically located in the sacred domain (Zerubavel, 1979). Many of the attitudes and behaviors formerly viewed as sinful and associated with the domain of religion have been incorporated within the jurisdiction of medicine and health care (Fox, 1979).

The status of the American hospital suggests that its social significance is that of a partially sacred institution. Because the hospital is associated with a sacred quality, and sacred institutions have rituals, it could be expected that a system of rituals would develop within this modern, formal organization of American society. Nurses play an integral role in the rituals of the hospital, specifically those involved in the caring role of the nurse and including "laying-on-of-hands" behaviors.

Although nurses may seek a scientific explanation for their routines, procedures, and reports, rituals may, in fact, serve to fill gaps where scientific rationale fails. Nurses have not often studied nursing practices and procedures for ritual content. Moreover, many have condemned rituals as being without worth. Determining the existential meaning of nursing rituals may uncover the function of these rituals for nurses. Therefore, the purpose of this study was to describe and analyze the nature of nursing rituals during an ethnographic study.

To investigate nursing rituals, the definition of ritual proposed by DeCraemer, Vansina, and Fox (1976) was used: ritual is patterned, symbolic action that refers to the goals and values of a social group. The beliefs, values, and patterns of rituals present in the practices and procedures of a group of nurses working on a medical unit were examined. The questions posed by this study were the following:

1. What actions, words, and objects make up nursing rituals?
2. What are the types of nursing rituals demonstrated by professional nurses caring for adult patients on a hospital unit?
3. What explicit or manifest meanings and implicit or latent meanings do these rituals have for nurses, patients, families, physicians, and other hospital personnel?
4. How are nurses, patients, families, physicians, and other hospital personnel involved in these rituals?
5. How do nursing rituals emerge in the context of the routines, procedures, and reports of the nursing unit?

Specifically, the investigator examined postmortem care, medication administration, patient admission to and discharge from the hospital, change-of-shift reports, and the bath and other medical aseptic practices. (Descriptions of patient admission and discharge are not included in this chapter.) A review of the literature indicated that these nursing practices and procedures are situations in which nursing rituals could be identified and analyzed. The work of Turner (1957, 1967, 1969), Malinowski (1954), Douglas (1963, 1966, 1970, 1975), Van Gennep (1960), Bosk (1979,

1980), Zerubavel (1979), Walker (1967), and Fox (1979) framed the study.

Participant-observation, semistructured interviewing, and document and event analysis were the data collection methods used during the investigation. Detailed, textual data recorded in field notes provided descriptions of the actors and naturalistic context of an urban hospital's medical unit, 7H. Change-of-shift reports were audiotaped, transcribed verbatim, and included in the field notes. Data were collected over a twelve-month period during day, evening, and night shifts.

Informants included 7H nursing staff, patients and family members, and other hospital personnel, including escort staff, laboratory technicians, and physicians. Three members of the nursing staff who were key informants reviewed the results of the study and attested to the validity of the description.

7H AND THE 7H NURSES

7H was a unit in a large teaching hospital located in a run-down neighborhood of a major American city. The medical unit was sandwiched between an orthopedic unit above and a cardiac step-down unit below. 7H was adjacent to three other units on the same floor level: another medical unit to the right, and two small units to the left—an isolation unit and a psychiatric unit. 7H nursing staff maintained a good-neighbor policy with these nearby units. Staff visited the other units to "steal" linen, to beg for ice, and to borrow medications and central supply items when warranted by patient need. Staff from the other units reciprocated with forays into 7H's caches of hospital goods. Requests for permission almost always accompanied "begging, borrowing, and stealing" expeditions.

At the time of year when the study began, new graduate nurses and new resident physicians were arriving. The hospital was engaged in a major construction project, but it had little effect on 7H. The most direct benefit of the construction for the 7H nursing staff was a new parking garage, which eased the process of getting to and from work.

7H consisted of patient rooms with adjoining bathrooms, a large central corridor, the nurses' station, the utility room, and two offices. The nursing staff typically began each shift from the central location of the utility room and the nurses' station. From here they moved into the corridor and then to the sixteen patient rooms of the medical unit.

The patient rooms were semiprivate; at most times, the two beds were occupied. The rooms were small and had pastel painted walls. Each room had closets and a bathroom with a sink and toilet. A television was mounted on the wall, and the usual furniture—a bed, bedside cabinet, overbed table, and large chair—made up a patient unit. A large window brightened each room. Patients in the window beds enjoyed the distraction of the views outside the hospital; those in the door beds enjoyed the diversion of the corridor traffic. Traffic was brisk during the early part of the day shift and reached its peak from 8:15 A.M. until after 11 A.M. The 7H nursing staff walked in the corridor, speaking to each other about a call to a physician, a request for a laboratory study or another diagnostic test, or a request for change of diet to be sent to the dietary department. In the midst of this activity, a medical clerk sat at the desk in the nurses' station making telephone calls and doing paperwork for patients' charts.

Teams of physicians moved through the corridor, going in and out of patient rooms and animatedly discussing the progress and therapy of patients. Many patients with cardiac disease were admitted to the unit, most spending about three days on the unit. The turnover rate for patients was very rapid.

When 7H ran smoothly, the RNs, GNs, LGPNs, and nursing assistants moved in an almost serene fashion from checking patients, to calling on the telephone, to pouring their medications. Nurses joked with each other. But when the unit was "jumping," the nurses told anyone who listened that the pace was very hectic.

Nurses' Station

The nurses' station was located at the center of the unit, adjacent to the utility room and visible to patients, visitors, staff, and all hospital personnel having business on 7H. The chest-high counter was always deliberately littered with essential chart forms, booklets, and other printed material important to the unit's work flow, such as specimen slips and a sign-in sheet.

Along with the utility room, the nurses' station was a central coordination point of the activities of 7H. Hospital personnel, visitors, and patients went to the desk for help, information, and directions. Physicians' orders were written and transcribed there. Telephone calls were placed to request information and to identify and resolve problems. The station was also the central depot for incoming and outgoing mail. During the day shift, staff scattered charts on a desk within the nurses' station. Charts that were being worked on were piled high on the front desk.

On the walls of the nurses' station were two bulletin boards covered with printed information and an occasional thank-you card from a patient or a family. The printed information included notices about meetings or policy and procedure changes, time charts, and memos.

Utility Room

The utility room, adjacent to the nurses' station, was roughly halfway between the last patient rooms on either end of the unit. 7H nursing staff used the utility room to take coffee breaks or time-out from nursing activities, to read charts and articles about patient problems, to look up medications, to wait for change-of-shift report to begin, to converse, and to complain. When staff waited in the utility room for change-of-shift report to begin, they exchanged accounts of patients' experiences in the hospital or on 7H. Most of the time, change-of-shift report took place in the utility room.

Conversations about the nurses' personal lives frequently took place in the utility room. No nurse sat there very long during a shift, unless she was charting nurses' notes or eating lunch.

7H: The Work

As soon as change-of-shift reports and planning sessions were completed, nurses scrambled to begin the work of the shift. The most experienced RN on each shift distributed patient assignments among the staff and wrote these with an erasable magic marker on the primary board. The board was fastened to a wall opposite the nurses' station. Nursing staff names were written beside patient names and room numbers. The names of physicians assigned to patients also appeared on the primary board. All information was written in large print so that the hospital staff could easily identify staff who were caring for 7H patients. The distribution of patients on the board helped to organize the day, evening, and night shifts. Nurses knew their own patients as well as those of other nurses.

Patients were assigned using different nurse-to-patient ratios on each shift. Nevertheless, nursing responsibility flowed smoothly from nurse to nurse as district assignments were made. After the report was given, the cycle of work resumed with the administration of medications, treatments, baths, and other direct patient care activities as well as with the completion of paperwork and the preparation of patients for diagnostic tests and procedures.

Unanticipated patient problems arose during the shift and affected the division of work. Patients' conditions worsened and unit activity accelerated. Nurses answered questions from doctors and other hospital personnel. Patients accompanied by escort staff left and returned from hospital departments.

Frequent observations on patients continued throughout each shift as nurses checked IVs or bathed, medicated, and comforted their patients. Nurses continued to share nursing work and information about patients throughout the twenty-four-hour nursing day.

The Nursing Staff

From July to April, the permanent nursing staff of 7H consisted of twenty-nine people classified according to different nursing categories. The six RN members of the staff consisted of Deidre, nurse manager; Kate, assistant nurse manager; Miriam, primary nurse or charge nurse on night shift; Beth, primary nurse on day shift; Sarah, per diem nurse and primary nurse on day shift; and Tammy, primary nurse on day shift. The nine graduate nurses were Colleen, Sharon, Ann, Pamela, Loretta, Chris, Suzanne, Cecile, and Meredith. Some of the new nurses came to the unit in May or June;

others started late in the summer and in the early fall. After passing state board licensing examinations, all graduate nurses became RNs while working on 7H. Most passed by mid-September. The few who failed the examination on the first try in September passed in the February sessions.

The eleven LGPN staff included Marie, Dotty, Camille, Denise, Nancy, Mary, Wanda, Pat, Elsie, Leslie, and Mabel. Marie, Dotty, Camille, and Elsie worked the day shift most often. Nancy and Wanda worked the evening shift, and Denise and Mary, the night shift. Leslie and Mabel were awaiting positions on another unit and were transferred during the year. Rachel, Caroline, and Betty were nursing assistants, and Kathy was a nursing student extern who worked during the summer and on weekends when her college schedule permitted.

THE NURSING RITUAL OF POSTMORTEM CARE

7H nurses cared for patients both before and after death; because they had known the people before death, they did more than merely administer postmortem care to dead bodies. The resuscitation dilemma, or code/no code decision, provides a context for the discussion of postmortem care.

Dying and the "Do Not Resuscitate" Dilemma

7H nurses confronted dying and death as they worked, but dying and death disturbed them and disrupted the patterns of the unit. The nurses participated in the dying and deaths of some of the patients who came to their unit. They often predicted death, but some deaths surprised even the most experienced staff member.

Patients, families, and nurses shared the death crisis. Physicians arrived when called; they confirmed the death event and departed. Nurses anticipated, confirmed, and participated in the after-the-end activities. Families suffered throughout the dying and deaths of their loved ones.

All of the deaths that occurred on 7H involved the dilemma of whether "to resuscitate." The category III, DNR (do not resuscitate) predicament appeared innocuously in this change-of-shift report:

751W. Mr. Price with septic shock. Category III, DNR. Vital signs X 3. No problems on him. Venti-mask. The man is NPO, changed to liquid. No gag reflex yesterday. IV 80 drops per minute. 450 credit till 9 A.M. Another bag in back. Had a culture of his decubiti in E.R. Attempted to suction him. He fought it. He has a deviated septum. He's pinky. He has a mini neb. Check start date on his Sustacal. He's so thin, he has no meat. I've never seen anyone so thin in my life.

The category III, DNR phrase refers to a decision made by a patient and family to prevent resuscitation efforts by hospital staff in the event of cardiac or respiratory arrest. Because the phrase usually occurred with other abbreviations and with the contracted language used by nurses during change-of-shift report, it was difficult to detect from the reports the struggle that always accompanied the patient and family decision of Do Not Resuscitate.

The nurses on 7H wrestled with resuscitation decisions. Without a physician's order not to resuscitate, the nurses were afraid not to act. They equated inaction with letting someone die without nursing care. The basic rule followed by nurses in events that called for resuscitation—cardiac and respiratory arrests—was: Resuscitate everyone who does not have a Do Not Resuscitate order.

When a patient was classified as a DNR, certain therapeutic actions were abandoned. Blood sugar coverage with insulin was stopped along with other blood studies. However, the more basic life support measures of nutritional and fluid intake were maintained with a Sustacal feeding through a gastrointestinal tube and through IVs that were restarted after other "lines" infiltrated. Doctors continued to "round" on dying patients and to write orders. Nursing care continued. Nurses bathed, fed, checked breathing, monitored IVs, watched, and talked to the patients who waited for death.

Some patients were aware that death was imminent; others were not. When one of these slowly dying patients was "dumped" by his or her family, the 7H nurses became the most frequent source of contact with other people. For several weeks, a dying man, Irving Stern, was cared for almost exclusively during the day shift by Marie, LGPN. Beth, RN, was also a major caregiver. The patient, who was ninety years old, lay in bed with his eyelids half-closed. Aware of no one, he was sometimes restless, occasionally "rammy," but he hardly ever moved and he seldom moaned. His face was a reddish-blue color.

Mr. Stern breathed "on his own" without a ventilator. Members of his family agreed to make him a category III, DNR. Marie had not seen them visit during the day and did not know whether they visited in the evening. She resented their absence and disapproved of their behavior, especially that of his daughter.

Mr. Stern had been admitted to 7H with a stroke. He had come from a semi-independent residence for the elderly. Recently, he had experienced several episodes of fluctuating low blood pressures and some apneic periods that had led the nurses to conclude: "Oh, God, he's gonna go!" Despite these problems, he had lived and was able to take a small amount of nutrition by eating a pureed diet and receiving "keep open" IV fluids. He stopped eating; he received no medications except an occasional injection of Haldol. His respiratory rate was erratic at times. Rapid mouth breathing dried his lips and tongue. The physicians inserted a nasogastric tube for feedings and arranged for his discharge to a nursing home.

Both Marie, LGPN, and Deidre, RN and nurse manager, were surprised by the early arrival of the transport personnel. Marie was outraged, and had not enough time to stop his discharge. Mr. Stern made it to the nursing home, but was returned to the hospital and died on another unit. 7H nurses were sad, feeling guilty, and disgusted that a ninety-year-old man was shuttled back and forth between the hospital and a nursing home just before his death.

Marie interpreted Mr. Stern's discharge as an indication that optimum bed use was a higher priority than patient comfort. The "nothing much" that was being done for him was the nursing care 7H nurses gave on a twenty-four-hour basis. They bathed, fed, turned, and talked to Irving Stern while waiting for his death. They were unable to care for Mr. Stern after death, and regretted the way he died.

A Dying Patient, the DNR Dilemma, and His Postmortem Care

Harry Bowman had COPD (chronic obstructive pulmonary disease); a tracheotomy and oxygen helped him to breathe. He was in his 60s and had been in the hospital for several months. Most of his hospital time was spent in and out of the ICU. The nurses considered Mr. Bowman "a lovely man." He endured his chronic suffering. Often, he turned his face away from the door to his room and looked toward the window. He was alert to his situation and to his surroundings, a fact that made his lingering death seem particularly hard for him, his family, nurses, and physicians.

Mr. Bowman made an "active" decision to die. Over several days, Mr. Bowman, his family, the nurses, physicians, and respiratory therapists engaged in decisions and actions that eventually culminated in his death. With his consent, he became a DNR. Later, he had the ventilator disconnected, went back on the ventilator, and came off of it again. His nurses offered him food and pain medication, and kept oxygen/air flowing into his tracheotomy. He continued to decline for the next several days. The nurses and physicians waited patiently, and witnessed a sad and exhausted family watching a much loved man's end.

After Mr. Bowman's family left, Chris, GN, Beth, RN, and another nurse performed postmortem care. Chris had never done it before, so Beth saw her through it. "It was a joint effort." Beth described the events before and after his death.

I remember telling them to be careful about the way they turned him. He exsanguinated. The blood would just pour out of his mouth. I was with him. He was foamy, just brand new blood. It clotted just there. It just happened quickly. The wife was glad he waited until she came. It was a long time before we did the postmortem care. The son and wife were there. His breathing changed, so I got the doctor before he expired. The family stayed a while. They had a hard time let-ting go. . . . A lot of times when I do postmortem care, I treat them as if it's my family. . . . The spirit of whoever is there is in the room. The spirit stays by the body a while. He's too nearly gone. As though he's still there . . . I always cover the head last. It's the center of who the person was, the most distinguishing part. There's a reluctance to cover the face, putting off accepting death.

Postmortem Care of Mrs. Windrim, DNR Patient

Betty Windrim had been coming to the hospital for many years. She had been admitted to 7H about ten months earlier and was back again. Tired of her chronic disease and ready to die, Mrs. Windrim signed her own DNR permission in the doctors' progress notes.

Afternoon Report:

(7)49 Door: Betty Windrim . . . sixty-eight years old. She came in on the 23rd. On the 27th she arrested. She extubated herself on the 30th. She's here with CHF, end stage, CAD (coronary artery disease), and HTN (hypertension). She made herself a DNR. She is awake, alert, and oriented, but won't do diddle for herself except feed herself. She was kind of malnourished, I think. . . . She went into pulmonary edema over the weekend. Right now she's on a venti-mask for 50 percent (oxygen) which she takes off when she feels like it.

Mrs. Windrim surely was planning to die. She was annoyed with oxygen, and other hospital therapies. Talking was a great effort for her. She remained on bedrest for weeks until her death, too weak to get out of bed to a chair with the nurses' help. She lived for two and one-half months after her DNR decision. Living every day was a chore, because it was difficult to eat, breathe, and talk. She died in early February at 5:30 A.M. Cecile, a new RN, felt guilty because she was not with the patient when she stopped breathing and re-ported: "She coded at 5:30 A.M." No resuscitation attempts were ini-tiated on the woman who had signed her own DNR permission.

Postmortem Care of Mrs. Windrim

Betty Windrim was pronounced dead by the resident at 5:56 A.M. By 8:15 A.M., Mrs. Windrim's family had come to 7H to see her. Deidre went into room 749 to give postmortem care; Colleen, GN, and two nursing students were also in the room.

Mrs. Windrim's body was naked and lying flat in bed. Deidre and Colleen washed her skin. Deidre washed her face, arms, chest, and legs on the left. Colleen washed on the right, and she also washed the genital area. Mrs. Windrim's eyes were fixed. She was blue-tinged around her mouth and nose, and she did not move. The reality of her death was confirmed by the ever-increasing coldness of her skin and her lack of respiratory movement.

Colleen washed the unhealed antecubital cutdown incision, which leaked serous fluid. She did this gently, as if Mrs. Windrim could feel her touch on a painful, never-to-heal incision. Deidre and Colleen turned the patient over onto her left side, toward Deidre. Colleen cleaned all traces of the bowel movement and urine from Mrs. Windrim's skin. It was obvious that more stool would leak. Colleen placed the shroud under the patient's back, and later turned her onto the shroud.

Colleen tied the toe tag on the patient's right great toe, crossed her legs at the ankle, and tied them together with the shroud pack tie. Deidre tied the arms together at the wrists, padding them in between with a soft abdominal (ABD) pad. She covered the patient's naked body with the plastic shroud, after propping her chin with a rolled towel. She wrapped the left side of the shroud over first, the right side over second, folded up the ends of the shroud at the feet, and tied another shroud cord at the ankles over the shroud. She then tied the shroud at the waist and, finally, flipped the shroud at the patient's head over her face and tied it with a cord at the neck.

Deidre finished the postmortem care alone because Colleen had left with a nursing student to check on another patient's "funny" breathing. Deidre taped the shroud to ensure its closure. She said that she did not like to cover the patient's face. "I take a deep breath; it's almost as if they are still breathing." Deidre said that she was fanatical about cleaning the room before the arrival of the family. She explained this by associating it with a "calm and a sense of peace" in the room. Later, two male escort staff members came to the room and moved the body to the cold, stainless steel of the special litter and covered it with a green sheet. The body was taken to the morgue.

Postmortem Care of Mrs. Fanelli

Mrs. Fanelli was admitted to 7H after coming through the Emergency Unit and the Admissions/Discharge Unit. She was hyperglycemic and in a diabetic coma. Mrs. Fanelli coded six days after admission to 7H. A graduate nurse called the code; the resuscitation team arrived rapidly.

Code efforts progressed in a slow, uneven way for over an hour and a half. Eventually, Mrs. Fanelli went into a complete heart block, but the residents thought that a pulmonary embolus had caused the respiratory arrest. Despite resuscitation efforts, Mrs. Fanelli's pupils were fixed, dilated, and nonreactive to light, a universally ominous sign. A few minutes later, Mrs. Fanelli died. Her EKG was flat for several minutes.

Chris, GN, Dotty, LGPN, Jamie, LGPN (p.r.n. pool), Sharon, and Lynne, the neighboring unit's assistant nurse manager, were working on Mrs. Fanelli. Lynne got a suture removal kit to cut the sutures holding the subclavian catheter in the patient's skin. Jamie used a 5-cc. syringe to deflate the Foley balloon so that the urinary catheter could be removed. Jamie also obtained a towel and washcloth, then filled a basin with water and began to wash the patient's face after she touched her teeth to determine "if they were dentures or originals."

Jamie rapidly and efficiently washed the patient's chest, breasts, arms, and legs "just like A.M. care." Next she washed the perineal area. There was a small amount of blood present. Dotty helped Jamie turn the patient over. Jamie washed the patient's back, now bluish-purple, and said, "Oh really" in a disgusted voice. There was a large amount of odoriferous stool present at the patient's anus. Dotty said to Jamie in reproach, "What do you expect, she's dead."

Mrs. Fanelli's eyes were open, their glistening moisture gone in her death. Her blueness, paleness, and lack of movement dominated the scene. Jamie asked for sheets, because all the nurses in the room wanted to help her. Sheets were brought from a chair in the corridor. With Mrs. Fanelli turned onto her left side toward Dotty, Jamie placed a clean sheet with the plastic shroud on top, under the patient. In order to help Dotty turn the body, Jamie rolled the plastic shroud up with the sheet. Jamie gestured for Dotty to turn the patient over toward her. Jamie put the cellulose pads in place at the anus. Dotty helped by pulling out the dirty sheets and pulling through the clean bottom sheet and shroud. Mrs. Fanelli was then turned flat in bed. Jamie put a clean gown on her, shielding her nakedness. After stamping the toe tag, total body tag, and personal belongings tag with Mrs. Fanelli's Addressograph plate at the nurses' station, Sharon reentered the room and tied the toe tag onto the patient's right toe. Jamie was ready to tie the patient's arms together with the shroud pack cord at the wrists. Dotty stopped her. "Don't do that," she said. She wanted the family to have the opportunity to touch untied hands when they came to see Mrs. Fanelli. Jamie said that she always tied the wrists together when she did postmortem care. Jamie went along with Dotty, saying, "We'll do whatever you want." Jamie and Dotty tucked the shroud underneath the mattress as if it were a bottom sheet and pulled the top sheet over the patient up to her neck. Dotty combed Mrs. Fanelli's shoulder-length hair.

Interspersed with the washing, tagging, and tying of postmortem care were the nurses' rapid efforts to tidy up the room for the family's arrival. They threw away disposable trash into the waste basket and saved the patient's powder and brush for the family. Mrs. Fanelli looked clean after death. Her sheets were spotless, and her side of the room looked neat, orderly, and clinical. No traces of the code or postmortem materials were visible. The door to the room was left open, the curtain around her bed was partially closed.

Around noon, a middle-aged man and woman, a son and daughter-in-law, came to see Mrs. Fanelli. Dr. Francis spoke to them. Both seemed very upset. Sharon, GN, came out of another patient's room and talked with them. She accompanied them into the room, paused a few seconds, and then left them alone with Mrs. Fanelli. After ten minutes, they left the room. Because the patient was lying on the shroud but not wrapped in it, Sharon wrapped the patient with another nurse's help. She put the ties in place at the neck, waist, and ankles. The patient's body and face were covered, and the shroud was tied at the neck, waist, and ankles. Next, escort staff lifted the patient onto the large stainless steel tray on the litter and brought the patient to the morgue.

Postmortem Care: Therapeutic Nursing Ritual

On the basis of the definition of DeCraemer, Vansina, and Fox (1976), postmortem care performed by nurses for their dead patients is a nursing ritual. The ritual is comprised of patterned symbolic actions that represent the values and norms of 7H nurses. Postmortem care is seldom, if ever, witnessed by other hospital personnel and patients' families. Thus, its character is not known. Postmortem care as a therapeutic nursing ritual improves the condition of patients and it removes the traces of suffering even after death. Postmortem care holds latent meaning for nurses as they can continue to provide therapeutic nursing interventions to patients who have died. The symbolic meaning of the postmortem ritual lies in the need of nurses (1) to remove the manifestations of suffering, (2) to purify the patient's body and the hospital room of the soil and profanity of death, and (3) to gradually relinquish their tenure of responsibility for the patient, given up only as the escort personnel transport the dead patient to the morgue. In other words, postmortem care helps nurses make their dead patient presentable for family viewing. It is part of nursing's long tradition of laying-on-of-hands. Even after patients die, nurses care for them, touching them with gentleness.

THE NURSING RITUAL OF MEDICATION ADMINISTRATION

Medication administration is a nursing function that requires special knowledge. 7H nurses took their responsibility for medication administration seriously and resented intrusion into what they perceived as their domain.

The nurses did not like to have patients identify and request medications that they thought they should receive while in the hospital. They could not accept the idea that a patient knew best about medications. They resented, for example, a patient who stayed in the hospital for two months and decided that he should get Dilantin. He persistently requested Dilantin from the nurses and doctors. Although the doctors were lukewarm toward his request, they finally prescribed the medication. During change-of-shift report, the day shift primary nurse, smiling sarcastically, said, "Mr. Sparks was thrilled at getting his Dilantin." The nurses disagreed with the patient's request and the doctors' decision. They felt that they knew better about this medication than did the patient and his doctors.

The nurses had acquired basic information about medication administration in their preservice educational programs, before they began working on 7H as GNs. They learned much more about the details of medication administration after coming to 7H.

Procedure

While the Hospital Policy and Procedure Manual contained many pages devoted to the administration of medications, 7H nurses seldom referred to it. The details of medication administration were often passed from an experienced nurse to an inexperienced nurse by verbal exchange or by demonstration. For example, when a Z-track, intramuscular injection of Imferon was ordered, the nurses discussed the technique of the injection procedure in detail; they did not consult the Policy and Procedure Manual. Nurses on the evening and night shifts consulted the manual most often, probably because fewer nurses were available to answer questions.

The Policy and Procedure Manual contained a large subsection entitled "IV and Medication Administration." Many topics were included, such as General Administration of Medication; Preparation and Administration of Oral, Parenteral, and Rectal Medicines; Administration of Post-Op Narcotics; and Blood Transfusions. These written procedures served as guides, even though they were consulted infrequently. A system of checks was outlined in the Policy and Procedure Manual:

Select the correct drug and read the label three times:
1. When selecting the drug.
2. When comparing the label with the data on the Kardex.
3. Before returning the drug to the patient's drawer.

This system of checks has persisted for nearly a century. A similar three-part system of checks was described in a pre-1900 American nursing journal. The purpose of the three-time check, then as now, was to help the nurse avoid error and to maintain accuracy.

Although 7H nurses seldom consulted the Policy and Procedure Manual, they knew and used the system of checks as a behavioral code. In describing their customs of medication administration, they acknowledged their use of this system. However, they used it silently, as an almost magical protection against medication errors.

Routines

As soon as change-of-shift report ended, the primary nurses made rounds on all of the patients in their districts. Medications were well-integrated into the fabric of these nursing activities. For example, during rounds, nurses discovered that patients needed pain medications. Most medications were given at regular times, except p.r.n. and one-dose medications. Generally, fewer medications were given in the afternoon than in the morning.

The afternoon pace began to accelerate after 1:45 P.M. when all of the staff had finished their lunch breaks. The work to be completed by the nurses on the day shift included administering treatments, taking afternoon temperatures (and other vital signs), checking IVs, moving patients back to bed, and dispensing 2 P.M. medications. Most of the time-consuming work of the day shift, such as bathing patients, was completed before 2 P.M.

During the evening shift, the staff divided 7H into three geographical districts. Ann, GN, reported that most of their time on the 4:00 to 12:00 shift was spent on pouring medications and taking off doctors' orders. The 6:00 P.M. medications were poured from 5:15 P.M. to about 6:15 P.M., at the time when patients ate or were being fed dinner. The 10:00 P.M. medications were poured from 9:30 P.M. to about 10:10 P.M. Midnight medications were started at 11:00 P.M. because night change-of-shift report almost always started promptly at midnight. Pam, GN, Ann, GN, and Nancy, LGPN, were usually assigned to one district each to give medications.

With a smaller staff on the evening and night shifts, administering medications and monitoring IVs exhausted much of the nurses' time. The heaviest times for medications on the night shift were 2:00 A.M. and 6:00 A.M. IVs were watched and replaced when "low." One RN gave most of the medications during this shift. The two LGPNs were assigned to one district to give p.r.n. medications.

There were days when the nurses on each shift were unable to maintain the scheduled times for medication administration. Patients may have been absent from rooms, perhaps to have a diagnostic test; medications may not have been "back" from the pharmacy; or there may have been an excessive number of p.r.n., preoperative, and prediagnostic test medications. At times, it seemed that the nurses were never finished. On busy weekends, it was at the time of administering medications that the RN saw all of the patients during the shift, except for the quick morning rounds after shift report.

In addition to time spent in actually administering medications, considerable time was spent stocking the medication cart with straws, juices, syringes, souffle cups, plastic medicine glasses, a small trash bag, and reminder notes on 3" × 5" cards, before beginning the rounds to give medications to patients of each district. Nurses also periodically ran to the medication refrigerator in the nourishment area of the nurses' station to obtain refrigerated medications or IVs.

The nurses had to consider numerous details concerning medication administration. Nurses used various devices to help them recall the detail of a one-dose or "single-dose" medication (red stickers on the Kardex), or the fact that a patient was not in his or her room during routine medication times (one of the reminder notes on 3" × 5" cards on the medication cart). Identibands on patients' wrists were supposed to be checked to ensure that the right patient received the right drug. The most annoying interruption of the medication routine occurred when newly ordered drugs did not come from the pharmacy when expected.

The Art of Medication Administration

The art of medication administration was revealed at the patients' bedsides. Nurses adjusted sluggish IVs; coaxed weak, nauseated, and querulous patients to take their medications; and almost painlessly gave injections to patients. At times, it was difficult for the nurse to get a weak patient to swallow an oral medication. For example, Beth prepared a medication dosage for Ellen Paul by crushing the medications at the medication cart with a mortar and pestle. She went into Mrs. Paul's room and put the medications into a tablespoonful of Cream-of-Wheat cereal. The patient did not want to take the medicine. She resisted gently, but only with the tenacity of an ill, long-suffering woman who could die at any time. "There'll be pills in there," Beth said to the patient. "I'm hiding them in the cereal; she had such a hard time swallowing. I'm doing one at a time." "I'll give you some orange juice so you can wash them down," Beth said to Mrs. Paul. "Oh my God, I'm too sick," she replied. Beth fed Mrs. Paul the cereal mixed with crushed medication one spoonful at a time. She helped the patient drink some juice. Slowly, Mrs. Paul managed to take her medications and eat a little breakfast.

Kate bargained with Irving Mann, a confused seventy-nine-year-old who was considered to be a difficult patient. She poured Mr. Mann's tablets into a souffle cup. She left the medicine cart in the hall and entered the patient's room. Mr. Mann repeatedly muttered to himself that he needed an "enemy" (enema). As Kate told him to take his pills and put the souffle cup to his lips, he pushed her hand away. Kate managed to tip the pills into his mouth. He removed the pills from his mouth and threw them to the floor. Later, he swallowed his newly poured morning medications. His nurse was finally successful on the second attempt.

In the next patient room was an alcoholic patient who had been recently admitted with ketoacidosis. Mabel was giving the patient a bath because Kate was occupied with medications. Mabel asked Kate if she could get the patient out of bed to change the linens; he had wet his bed. Kate said "Yes." Kate poured three tablets for the patient and poured water for the patient to drink with his medications. Kate poured the tablets from the souffle cup into the patient's hand, after she had asked him whether he was ready to take his medications. She told him that he was taking Decadron, Dilantin, and a multivitamin. The patient swallowed the Dilantin but dropped the other two pills in his lap. He told Kate that he "lost two." She carefully looked into the folds of his patient gown, found the pills, and watched as the patient took them. Kate then interrupted her medication duties to answer a telephone call.

A Highly Valued Nursing Function

The importance of medication administration was illustrated at mealtime, when nurses gave regularly prescribed medications before they fed patients who needed help with eating. They worried about the patients who were waiting to eat. They knew that helping people to eat was an important nursing duty but that it was more important to give patients their medications on time. In fact, giving medications had a higher priority than feeding patients.

In comparison to the rest of nursing care, Tammy ranked medications a high eight on a ten-point scale: "I try to do my teaching (about medications) along with other teaching. Meds predominate." Sarah agreed, emphasizing that knowledge of the use of medications in relation to a disease process is important. So also is the fact that patients need to be informed about their medications. "The teaching part of meds is more the domain of the RN."

The nurses agreed that medication administration was very time-consuming and at times it dominated their care, but they did not want to abandon it. In emphasizing this, Sarah said that, as medications were dispensed during medication rounds, "the patients will sometimes tell the RN about something they will not tell the physician."

Medication administration represented the seriousness and responsibility with which the nurses regarded their patient care duties. Medications were dangerous; errors could have catastrophic results for patients. Side effects of drugs could also be harmful. Nurses were accountable for their mistakes.

The dispensing of drugs with its concomitant nursing functions served as a visible focal point that emphasized, on a symbolic level, the seriousness of the nurses' duties regarding medications as well as the care of patients in general. Nurses wanted more experience with medications and they expected accuracy when medications were given. They assumed responsibility as they dispensed medications to their patients. Sarah spoke for all nurses when she commented about the seriousness of medication administration from the nurses' point of view: "You cannot cut corners on meds. It could hurt the patient."

Medications were recorded specifically, in greater detail than bed baths and other nursing care. Medication administration may have been more highly valued than other nursing priorities because this function represented a shared domain of responsibility with the doctors. Nurses and physicians shared the responsibility for observing the effects of medications on their patients. Both professional groups evaluated serum chemistry values carefully. For example, when a "K level" fell or rose beyond normal limits, the nurses called the doctor who then ordered appropriate medications.

RNs saw the administration of medications as their responsibility. They did not resist this, even though they complained about "heavy" shifts when medications and intravenous solutions kept them busy. RNs looked up medications in the "P.D.R." (Physicians' Desk Reference) more frequently than did the LGPNs. Often, RNs were observed teaching patients about their medications during routine rounds and upon discharge.

RNs assumed overall responsibility for medication administration during each shift and shared the dispensing of medications with LGPNs. LGPNs who worked on the day shift often gave oral medications to patients. During the evening shift, the LGPNs gave drugs without prodding from the RNs. LGPNs on the night shift reluctantly dispensed medications, most often giving p.r.n. medications.

RNs checked that doctors' orders were transcribed correctly from the order sheet by medical clerks. RNs signed physicians' verbal orders and either administered the medication immediately or asked another nurse to do so. LGPNs and the medical clerks did not have the responsibility of checking the accuracy of doctors' transcribed medication orders, either written or verbal. The RNs countersigned the orders as did any medical clerk who transcribed them to the Kardexes. The RNs, not the LGPNs, directly shared the responsibility of medication administration with the doctors.

Medication Errors

Mistakes happened on 7H, as they do when human beings are involved in any activity. RNs, GNs, and LGPNs made medication errors. GNs, the neophytes of the 7H nursing staff, made medication errors more often than the other members of the nursing staff. Nurses worried about the results of medication errors. They knew that serious medication errors could cause harm to patients. Seasoned RNs still recalled serious medication errors years later. Describing her most serious medication error, Sarah stated that she had been working on the cardiac step-down unit. After realizing that she had given a patient eight medications intended for another patient, she became very upset. She called the physician to report the error, cried, and wrote an incident report to document the error. Later, after going home, she called the unit during the evening shift to ask whether the patient was all right. She confessed her guilt and repeated the story of her most serious medication error twice. She blamed the error on the fact that, when she gave the medications, she had started with the patients in the last or highest numbered room in the unit instead of the lowest numbered room. She had violated the nursing routine of giving medications from the lowest numbered room in the unit to the highest. Although the patient was unharmed, Sarah still felt guilty about the medication error years later.

7H nurses verbally acknowledged making less serious errors. More serious medication errors were "written up" on incident reports. Other admissions of errors were made during change-of-shift reports and staff meetings. Through public confession, nurses shared both the error and guilt of these mistakes. Guilt, blame, and punishment were shared by nurses as a group. Guilt spread beyond the specific nurse who was directly responsible for the error to those nurses who had failed to detect the error rapidly. The open acknowledgment of error seemed to diffuse the blame among the nurses. All of the nurses, whether directly or indirectly involved, participated both in the guilt and in the confession of guilt. Medication errors symbolized failure in responsibility and betrayal of patient trust; they harmed those who had come for help.

The patterned actions of medication administration represented the responsibility toward their patients that 7H nurses accepted and assumed. Medication administration was a therapeutic nursing ritual; nurses gave medications to improve their patients' health. In order to avoid error and harm, 7H nurses practiced many routines, customs, and procedures. When error occurred, they confessed it publicly.

Patients, nurses, and physicians were convinced of the therapeutic benefits of most medications. Some drugs had obvious, immediate, and measurable effects. Occasionally, patients complained, along with nurses and doctors, that a drug did not work as expected. Nevertheless, hospital employees and patients expected most drugs to work and seemed to invest almost magical powers in the capabilities of medications. 7H nurses believed in the therapeutic power of medications with regard to potent and less potent drugs. They attested to the effectiveness of drugs during change-of-shift reports and during verbal exchanges throughout their shift.

Patients looked at medications magically or religiously. Patients became particularly upset if they did not receive their medications at the exact time. The timing of medications was important for members of the hospital staff as well as the patients. In fact, excessively late or early times of drug dispensing were considered medication errors.

Medication Administration: Therapeutic Nursing Ritual

Medication administration was a clearly identifiable, highly visible, and time-consuming part of nursing care on 7H. It constituted a therapeutic nursing ritual. Medications were healing objects, given to improve patients' conditions. Medication administration symbolized the reciprocal relationship between patient trust and nursing responsibility.

During the hospitalization experience, patients, nurses, doctors, and pharmacists were the chief actors involved in the dispensing of drugs. It was the nurses, however, who finally and most often gave drugs to patients in the hope of "doing good" and helping. In the end, the nurses bore the chief responsibility for medication administration.

The seriousness with which 7H nurses viewed medication administration was demonstrated most clearly when medication errors were identified. Nurses openly admitted their own guilt and attributed blame to others in the public arenas of staff meetings, change-of-shift reports, and incident reports. Through public confession, the nurses were able to share both the error and the guilt engendered by their mistakes. The character of these confessions emphasized the ritual nature of medication administration.

NURSING RITUALS IN MEDICAL ASEPTIC PRACTICES

Medical aseptic practices are the hygienic routines that nurses go through as they care for patients and perform some of the more profane aspects of their work. For 7H nurses, hospital work involved frequently bathing patients and handling their excreta, secretions, and bodily products.

Bathing and the Bed Bath

The bath often competed for time with other nursing activities. However, for 7H nurses, bathing patients was a rule. The whole tone of the eight-hour shift could be disturbed if linens were unavailable to finish bathing patients and changing beds. Nurses on the day shift required able patients to "get washed up now." Their insistence was hard to ignore. Even the most bath-resistant patients usually complied.

The Complete Bath

One morning, Kate was the primary nurse of a district. She walked into Joe McGuire's room. She was worried about this patient, because she had discovered during report that his abdomen was distended. After listening to his abdomen with a stethoscope and palpating it, she asked him if he had pain and whether he had "passed his water." Mr. McGuire said that he had, but could not find his urinal. Kate discovered it under the bed, empty.

She found that his bed sheets were wet. He had been incontinent of urine. She said, "That's good, because I was worried about you," indicating that she was relieved that his kidneys and bladder were working. Her patient replied, "The days are long but the nights are twice as long." He had been in the hospital three weeks. When Kate told him that she wanted to bathe him, he replied, "I think they bathed me ten times in one day." Kate replied, "Were you wetting yourself? Was it your bowels?" He answered, "I think they just like to wash me."

As Kate talked to her patient, she systematically collected a plastic basin, soap, a soap holder, lotion, and a disposable washcloth and towel from his bedside cabinet. She started to wash his face with water from the basin, talking to him about what she was doing. When she finished his face, she washed his left arm, right arm, his chest, and his abdomen with soap and hot water, rinsed them with water, and dried them with a towel. She then asked, "When was the last time you moved your bowels, Joe?" as she stood by the right side of the bed washing and drying him. He did not answer.

Kate next asked, "Joe, do you sweat a lot? Let me see your armpit. Joe, you have a good grip." Her patient nodded, not answering, but looking quite comfortable. Kate next uncovered him, washing his genitals with soap and water. After rinsing and drying him, she covered his genital area with a sheet. After this she changed the water in the basin, threw out the disposable washcloth, and used a fresh washcloth to wash his right and left legs. She turned Mr. McGuire onto his left side with his help. The side rail was up, so he could hold onto it. She washed his back and dried it. Finally, she washed his buttocks and perianal area. When she noticed an area of reddened skin over his sacrum, she told him about it, and instructed him to turn from side to side while in bed. After drying him, she massaged his reddened skin with lotion. Kate helped Mr. McGuire get out of bed and sit in a geri chair. Suddenly, he became dizzy. He did not respond to Kate for a few minutes. She discovered that his blood pressure had dropped and it was fluctuating. Kate, with the help of Gloria, the staff development instructor, moved Joe back to bed. Throughout her time with Mr. McGuire, Kate assessed his condition, and she was able to plan her care for him for the rest of the shift.

During the evening shift, 7H nurses had a scheduled time to bathe their patients. But they were also obligated to keep their patients clean before the scheduled time to begin P.M. care (8:00 P.M.). The nurses arranged their duty of bathing patients around their other duties of dispensing medications, replacing IVs, and so on. During the night shift, the bathing of incontinent patients was a priority, as it was on the evening shift. On all shifts, bathing an incontinent patient meant bathing his or her back, buttocks, and other body parts soiled by the stool, urine, or other discharge. Linens were changed and patients were repositioned on their sides or backs. On the evening and night shifts, nurses moved a cart with supplies from room to room so that they did not have to go back and forth to the supply closet. Keeping patients clean or "changing" them was seen by the LGPNs on nights as an unavoidable part, or the "bottom line," of their work on that shift.

Baths helped nurses show concern for their patients. "Respect is shown. If a patient is smelly and dirty, they would be embarrassed if they had visitors," Beth said about the necessity of the bath. She thought that giving a bath to patients was evidence that the nurse cared. "Not giving a bath might mean that you don't care enough." Her view of bathing patients each morning included a litany of descriptors: a way of caring for someone, like a mother cares for a child; loving care; in between toes and behind ears; a loving attitude while you did it even if rushed; a great deal to do with the way the patient sees the rest of the day; a good time for assessment; a quiet, uninterrupted time when they let off steam or just relax after not sleeping; and therapeutic touch. She pointed out that if a nurse neglects other details when caring for a patient, these are forgotten, "because of the care" involved during the morning bath.

7H nurses thought that a fifteen-minute period was the maximum acceptable time limit for leaving an incontinent patient uncleaned. Longer than that was unacceptable. Nurses knew that they were never to leave a patient lying in stool or urine. If a patient slipped by the nurses' hygienic vigilance, the nurses considered this unusual, even disgraceful. Dying, being resuscitated, or experiencing severe pain were patient situations that temporarily altered the inevitability of nurses' bathing patients. If patients lived, survived resuscitation, or had less pain, nurses rapidly cleaned them if they were soiled.

At times, the strong value that nurses placed on cleanliness conflicted with their patients' values. Some patients failed to see the importance of the frequent bathings that were scheduled throughout the nurses' twenty-four-hour workday. Other patients expected nurses to bathe them, no matter how successfully they were recuperating, or how capable they were of bathing themselves. Nurses seemed to follow the unwritten law, "Every patient must be bathed daily." Whether they were able to bathe themselves or needed the nurses to bathe them, 7H patients were unable to avoid the daily washings.

The "washing up" of patients seemed to help nurses feel a sense of accomplishment about nursing duties. Nurses on the day shift would comment, "I've got the two easiest ones done. Now comes the hard one." They apologized during shift report if a patient's bath remained to be finished after noon of the day shift or after the end of the shift on which they worked. In the following example, the day shift nurse was upset that her patient's bath had not been completed during the day shift. The patient had severe, chronic pain from metastatic cancer. The nurses responded to the patient's wish by delaying the completion of the bath until the patient agreed that he was ready. His nurse said:

> *Sometimes he lets us do it later in the day. He hasn't had back care. And he's also lying on the sheets that he went down to X-ray therapy in, but he did not want us to move him. As soon as he got back, he got his morphine again and his nursing student just gave him his Percocets. So I don't know if the pain's ever gonna go away enough for him to want . . . the sheets to be taken off. . . . But he's on a draw, two draw sheets and two bottom sheets. They're not soiled, though.*

Showing Gentleness, Respect for Patient Decisions, and Consideration for Patient Privacy during the Bath

Besides shortages in supplies, the only factor that seemed to hinder the nurses' progress with bathing was a patient's refusal. Refusal usually came from patients suffering from the pain of metastatic cancer. The pain sapped their strength. It was difficult for them to endure the mouth care, hair care, and other exertions of bathing. When nurses could avoid bathing patients, that is, if incontinence did not force them to clean them, they complied with the patients' requests.

Chris's assignment provided an example of a patient who temporarily refused her bath. Chris carefully completed Amy White's mouth care. Mrs. White, emaciated from metastatic breast cancer, was barely able to endure the mouth care. She was so weak that she swallowed her mouthwash, unable to expectorate it into the emesis basis held by Chris. When Chris asked her if she wanted her bath, she said, "Wait." Chris went to get her pain medication. Later, with the help of the pain-relieving narcotic, Chris finished Mrs. White's complete bed bath.

Mrs. White did not often speak to her nurses, family, or friends about her pain. When the nurse moved her, she screamed. The patient moaned "quite a bit, frequently." Whenever the nurses discovered Mrs. White's incontinence, they had to bathe her, but they did this as gently as they could. "It's so hard. When you rub her, she screams," said Chris. The patient could never be left, neglected and dirty, lying in her own urine and stool.

Patients who required a complete bath were often very debilitated; some were near death. The gentleness with which the nurses bathed these patients was universal. The bath exposed both the nurse's skills and the patient's nudity. Nurses knew that patients were embarrassed when they had to be bathed. Nurses and patients had to deal with violations of the usual personal space boundaries. Nurses had to be simultaneously adept and comforting. Patients needed reassurance that their nudity, incontinence, and bodily characteristics were private matters and would be kept private by nurses.

Patients were embarrassed by their incontinence, by the exposure of their genitals, and by nurses' contact with their private parts. Their facial expressions changed or they groaned as their breasts, genitals, or anal area were washed. At times they apologized, wishing aloud that they could manage bathing themselves. The nurses often dealt with the embarrassment by carefully talking to the patient about other matters while efficiently and matter-of-factly bathing them.

Some patients managed their embarrassment by hiding for a time the fact that they could not bathe themselves. The nurses soon discovered that a patient had not been bathing, because they noticed the patient's body odor. Body odors, originating from urine, feces, or other sources, were systematically investigated and removed by bathing during each shift. Nurses went on "incontinence check" rounds, seeking to detect soil and the odors associated with soil. They energetically bathed their patients, cleaning and purifying, keeping clean and dirty separate.

Handling Clean and "Dirty" Body Parts during the Bath

Nurses classified their patients' body parts in various categories of clean and dirty. They always bathed the patient's face first and the perianal area last. They followed an unspoken rule when bathing patients: Always wash from the clean to the dirty. The face, the neck, the chest, the arms, the legs, and the back were among the clean body parts. The hands were less clean than these. Nurses often used more soap, more friction, and more frequent washings for the hands. Feet were considered by some nurses to be dirty; they were treated the same way as hands, and were scrubbed with the same amount of soap and enthusiasm. The buttocks seemed a bit cleaner than the feet, but were dangerously close to the perianal region.

In general, the genitals, including the perineal region, and the perianal area were considered the dirtiest body parts. Nurses signaled this difference by carefully changing the bath water in the basin after washing the genital area and by washing the perianal area of the patient last. They also discarded the disposable washcloths after washing the genitals and the perianal area. They were more vigorous in their cleansing of these parts and of hands and feet than of other body parts.

The nurses' bathing practices brought them into unavoidable contact with body parts that were explicitly and implicitly considered by them to be dirty. Checking on patients' hygiene and bathing patients made the nurses confront their own and their patients' feelings about exposure of the "private parts" of the body. However, when some aspect of the patient's behavior suggested to the nurses that the patient might be enjoying the exposure and the contact, the nurses reacted and aired the situation in discussion during change-of-shift report. At one level of meaning, "sexual" was equated with "dirty" by the nurses. They had to keep genitals clean along with the perianal body area. They accepted the fact that their work contained contact with the dirty or profane elements of human functioning.

The nurses knew that patients' ideas of clean varied. "Some patients want their hands clean after they urinate. Others can insert a (rectal) suppository and not worry about their hands. I take my cues from the patient," said Beth, who also asserted that she was careful to wash her hands. "I don't want to take infection home [to] either me or my children."

Excreta, Secretions, and Infection

7H nurses removed and washed away the traces of human soil on a daily basis. Their common experience with infected materials, excreta such as urine and stool, and secretions such as respiratory and wound drainage, was closely associated with the repeated washings of patients during each shift.

The nurses believed in the efficacy of hand washing in order to protect themselves from possible contamination and infection. As students, they were repeatedly reminded in nursing school that hand washing was the best protection against contamination from a patient's bodily products. Many nurses believed that hand washing took care of cross-contamination. But hand washing was not the only medical aseptic technique that they used to protect themselves and patients from contamination by potentially infected materials.

Nursing students who spent time on 7H were advised by seasoned nurses how to decrease direct contact with excreta. On one occasion, Rachel, a nursing assistant, advised a nursing student to use gloves when obtaining a "clean catch" urine specimen. The student had to help an elderly female patient with the collection, and she held the specimen jar close to the urethral opening. To reinforce her advice about wearing gloves, Rachel added, "Afterwards, the clean catch jar will be all peed on."

The plastic, disposable gloves were an added protection against pathogenic microorganisms, but scientific theories of microbial transfer were not offered to explain their use. Disposable gloves were routinely used to protect nurses from infection. They were used almost as a panacea or a magical protection.

Nurses were fastidious in their handling of excreta. If a confused patient was incontinent of feces and managed to smear the stool on himself or his bed, nurses used gloves to protect themselves from the uncontained soilage. They washed and dried the patient and changed the linens so that no trace of stool was evident. If a patient was incontinent of urine or stool, the nurse who discovered this bathed the patient and changed the linens as soon as possible. All of the nurses were careful when handling soiled bed linens. They were often able to predict episodes of incontinence, since they knew most of their patients well. Miriam, for example, predicted that her patient would have diarrhea when she came back from the Radiology Department. Miriam "double sheeted" the bed. When the patient returned, her diarrheal incontinence was rapidly taken care of. Miriam's knowledge of her patient and her strategic preparations helped her to remove stool and maintain order.

7H nurses used gloves, hand washing, and containment of excreta and secretions to reduce and eliminate the effects of soil and to return patients and themselves to a state of cleanliness. If they were involved in a nursing duty considered to be clean, such as administering medications, and if they discovered an incontinent patient, they avoided contact with the excreta. Another nurse was asked to clean the soiled patient, so that the nurse involved in the clean activity could keep clean and dirty separate.

Nurses' proximity to infection elicited various reactions. For example, during change-of-shift report, two nurses discussed a doctor's order in caring for an infected toe. "Please place cotton between the toes on the right foot. Culture any pus," was how the order was written as the nurse repeated it from the Kardex. "'Pus,' what a word!" She exclaimed. The other nurse replied, "Pus!" The word itself suggested contamination and infection, evoking fear and revulsion.

Despite the fact that they did not welcome the exposure to infected materials, the nurses often expressed relief at sending a specimen to the laboratory. At least they would know what pathogen, if any, they were dealing with. This awareness helped to dispel some fear.

Often, the nurses' fear of potentially infected excreta became secondary to their concern about another problem of their patient. For example, an elderly woman with congestive heart failure, diabetes, and a recently healed fractured lower leg had problems with low blood sugar and with severe diarrhea. Miriam said, "The patient had diarrhea—well, loose stools three or four times" during the night shift and once during the day shift. The stool was irritating her perirectal skin, which was being treated with cleansing and Mycolog cream. "She gets Mycolog cream to her perirectal area and that is so gross. . . . Oh, it is terrible. It's worse and worse every day. Red areas, the skin just peeling off of it." Despite the fact that the patient had diarrhea several times, the nurses' discussions focused on the patient's skin breakdown. Rather than discussing their contact with stool, they discussed the Mycolog cream, where to keep it, either at the bedside or in the medication cart, and the need to use it frequently because of the patient's skin problem.

Nurses feared becoming infected from patients who had or were suspected of having communicable diseases. Sometimes their fear of becoming infected overrode their scientific knowledge. When in doubt as to the handling of infected patients, they consulted more experienced nursing staff instead of the infection control manual, a source of scientifically based techniques.

Nurses responded to their contacts with profane materials in a matter-of-fact manner, with humor, complaining, tolerance, and magical thinking. At times, they expressed a fearlessness about handling infected materials, demonstrating a strong sense of responsibility, bravery, or denial. For the most part, they accepted personal risks, but openly acknowledged their fear of carrying infection to their families.

Nurses were experts at keeping the clean and the dirty separate. More than other hospital personnel, they cared directly for infected patients and handled their bodily products. They were afraid of infection, but upheld the standard that they were responsible for all patients, and that even infected patients deserved respectful care.

The Bath: Therapeutic Nursing Ritual

On an explicit level, the bath was used as an opportunity for cleansing, checking patients' skin, and assessing general condition. It also provided an opportunity to listen to, talk with, or teach patients. The value of "good" personal hygiene for patients was internalized by nurses. They resisted changing the daily baths of the day shift to bathing patients every other day. On an implicit level, bathing patients was a nursing ritual because it represented purification, care of the patient by the laying-on-of-hands, and the opportunity to heal by washing away disease, or at least some of its traces.

THE NURSING RITUAL OF CHANGE-OF-SHIFT REPORT

Change-of-shift report was a scheduled, three-times-a-day opportunity for nurses to come together to discuss nursing care and patient progress. It marked the twenty-four-hour cycle of events on the unit, and represented a temporal structure that was imposed by nursing on hospital time.

Nurses "gave report" in sequence, from the lowest numbered to the highest numbered patient room in the district. Although they followed Kardexes that were also arranged in this order, they found it necessary to apologize, somewhat profusely, when they had to stop the report and return to a previous patient in order to add another fact.

Characteristically, each of the three change-of-shift reports differed little in content during each twenty-four-hour period. The morning report seemed to set the stage for each twenty-four-hour cycle. Details of patient events during the night, such as the administration of pain medications, confusion of patients, preparations for diagnostic tests, and discharges planned for the day shift, were frequently mentioned.

Nurses often reported matter-of-factly. For example:

The reason that he has so much bleeding, too, is he was on Coumadin at home until about maybe two or three days prior to admission. His PT—or his PTT—is—both are really elevated.
Right.
So he's going to be getting Vitamin K for three days.
O.K.

For the most part, the exchange of information during report was quiet and uneventful. When problems persisted, however, the nurses' reactions covered a range of emotional expressions: anger, sarcasm, humor, impatience, sadness, pity, criticism, hopelessness, and exasperation. During one report, two nurses commented, "We have a lot of CA on this floor." "Yeah, I know. . . . It's so depressing." Change-of-shift report served many functions for nurses.

7H nurses valued report as a means of sharing their clinical acumen through the identification of signs and symptoms in patients. They reported the signs and symptoms to their colleagues as data to be further investigated on the next shift. The nurses who listened were alerted to changes in the conditions of their patients. Both the presence and the absence of signs and symptoms were significant. They often expressed relief when they were able to report that a patient did not have expected signs and symptoms. When signs and symptoms persisted despite hospitalization and treatment, the nurses noted this fact with misgiving.

Nurses reported specific laboratory studies that were ordered for their patients. "What's he out for today?" a reporting nurse asked herself. She immediately answered, "CBC, BUN, creatinine, K, phosphorus, calcium, magnesium." Laboratory studies of one kind or another were ordered daily for most 7H patients. Fasting blood sugars and serum K (potassium) levels were the studies that were most frequently mentioned during change-of-shift report.

During report, nurses noted with relief that a specimen, such as urine, stool, or sputum, had been obtained from a patient. "We did all that last night. I got all my samples. I was really proud of that." They also reported on missing a specimen, as when a patient flushed away a specimen. Nurses prepared patients for various diagnostic studies, including endoscopies, ultrasounds, and different cardiac studies. The preparations for the studies and the reactions of the patients were reported. They described their observations and nursing care of patients following diagnostic tests. For example, a nurse stated, "His arteriogram was through the right groin. That site looks real good. There's no oozing; it's dry, pulses are good."

In the safe forum of change-of-shift report, nurses complained about patients, hospital staff, each other, and their work. This act of complaining by 7H nurses about their work on the unit was a form of release. Thus, their anger, hostility, powerlessness, and frustration were diverted from seemingly fruitless and possibly harmful confrontations. Often, the complaints centered on physicians. They criticized physicians' skills, interpersonal relationships with patients and nursing staff, decisions about patient care, and inaction in response to patient situations. They criticized the pharmacy, the Radiology Department, the nurse manager, patients, and family members. Change-of-shift report also provided a forum for airing disappointment.

Chronically ill and terminally ill patients drained emotional and physical resources of 7H nurses. During change-of-shift report, the nurses were often serious and they expressed sorrow over the life crises of their patients. However, they also used jokes and sarcastic humor to help them deal with death and with the unresolvable nature of their patients' problems, as well as with the powerlessness of their position as nurses. Humor, like complaining, served a positive purpose.

7H nurses worried about their patients and about themselves. When surgical patients were admitted to 7H, the nurses repeatedly voiced their concern. The nursing care of medical patients was central to their practice, and the nurses knew the limits of their knowledge and skill. Surgical patients caused them anxious moments. Sharon wished aloud that a patient going to the Operating

Room or having a coronary artery by-pass graft would not return to 7H after surgery: "He better not come back here."

The nurses were concerned about their patients' symptoms and disability. As vital signs became unstable and abnormal, nurses who were reporting off their shift told the nurses on the incoming shift when the next measurement was due. As nurses mentioned the possibilities of an infection in a diabetic patient's toe, they alerted their peers to their concerns. At times, anxieties were recognized as premonitions; most of the time, the most experienced nurses reported their premonitions. When these intuitive experiences were confirmed as patients became sicker, nurses were encouraged to take their own and other nurses' premonitions seriously.

Nurses expressed their fears about their own safety while caring for patients. They were afraid of being injured by combative patients who "took swings" at them. They knew nurses who had been injured by combative, confused patients. They were also afraid of becoming infected by patients with AIDS, hepatitis, tuberculosis, and other communicable diseases. 7H nurses told "war stories" about their patients that were interspersed with other aspects of change-of-shift report and represented a special kind of nursing lore.

Nurses talked about their patients' lives, tragedies, and independent acts with enthusiasm. These stories added relish to the discussion of facts in shift report and revealed sympathetic and compassionate feelings, as well as tolerant and intolerant reactions of the nurses toward their patients. They told stories of "what I put up with this weekend" or "what I put up with this shift" as a means of reporting to the incoming nurses the perils they had recently experienced. Kate reported that the unit had been "bananas" over the weekend: a confused patient hit his roommate; an elderly, confused male patient wandered into the rooms of women patients and touched their breasts and genitals; and a confused man repeatedly insisted he should have certain medications.

Nursing stories told during change-of-shift report were important enough to the nurses who were reporting that they needed to share the accounts with several nursing staff. Based on fact, the nursing lore contained in these accounts helped seasoned and neophyte nurses learn about patients, their nursing care, and other hospital situations that a nurse might experience. Telling these stories provided an opportunity to teach and to socialize.

Change-of-shift report reflected the serious as well as the friendly nature of the 7H nurses' working and social relationships. For a new graduate nurse, particularly one who was weak and having difficulty adjusting to the complex role of the hospital RN, the change-of-shift report functioned as a mechanism whereby the graduate was tested, shaped, sanctioned, and accepted or rejected.

For example, Meredith's shortcomings became apparent early. During report, Meredith was sharply questioned about her pronunciation of words, her confusion about where to feel pulses after a renal arteriogram, her failure to report sufficient information about many of the patients for whom she cared, and her confusion about which IV fluids were infusing. Many incidents alerted the nursing staff to her weaknesses. Meredith's reports were tension-ridden and emotionally exhausting for participants. Although they were sometimes impatient with Meredith, most of the RNs and GNs were supportive of her; however, Pam and Ann, the other GNs permanently staffing the evening shift, ridiculed her. Meredith tried very hard to adjust to the rigors of being a 7H nurse. However, her insecurities prevailed even though she was preceptored and shadowed by RNs and helped by Gloria, the staff development instructor. Eventually, Meredith agreed with Deidre that she should leave 7H and the hospital and seek employment in a less demanding situation.

Nurses used change-of-shift report to review potential patient problems, to warn about problem situations, to share concerns about gaps in their knowledge base, and to acknowledge errors. Report helped them to take stock of the work that was in store for the next shift as well as to review the work of the previous shift. It served as an audit of the nursing care given during the shift, and it contained many acknowledgments of error. Report was like a confessional: it enabled them to receive the support of their peers and to confront their concerns about harm to patients.

They used change-of-shift report as a means to set and maintain standards of nursing care. During report, negative criticism prevailed, not praise for work well done. Competition among the three shifts was evident as nurses reported on their patients. If one shift was more skillful than another, this was proclaimed during shift report. Sarah stated with pride that the day shift nurses had no problem with a patient's tracheotomy tube. The night nurses had had to call the supervisor and the respiratory therapist for assistance with the tube because they were unable to get the troublesome inner cannula out for cleaning. The day shift nurses reveled in their success.

Nurses also reproached others when safe patient care had been violated. Beth questioned the previous shift as she listened to report on one of her patients. Her patient's casted arm had been restrained a few days before. After the cast was removed, Beth worried. "They didn't restrain the arm that was casted, did they?" She was interested in protecting the patient and maintaining safe nursing care. They alerted those listening to report that certain information had not been passed from shift to shift. For example, the day nurses were not notified that a patient refused to accept an Imferon injection. The primary nurse on the day shift complained. "No. It wasn't passed on to me. So this morning it took me half an hour to figure out why . . . it wasn't signed out." Time was wasted and worry prolonged because information about a medication was not shared during report. A night nurse criticized the fact that the evening shift nurses forgot to report that a patient had not urinated during the shift. "They didn't tell me that she didn't void all night on their shift." Both examples served as reminders to staff—including those who eventually heard the reminder through the "grapevine" of change-of-shift report—that important details were not to be omitted during report.

Report progressed despite the many distractions and interruptions of 7H unit life. The most obvious distraction during report was noise. For example, a nurse in the hall called to a confused and wandering patient: "Sam, don't go away"; another patient called: "Nurse, please help me." Patients' signs and symptoms interrupted reports. Often, this interruption was a fact-giving or fact-receiving incident. "Mary Crowley's 3 P.M. [blood sugar]?" asked Colleen. "688," replied Sharon. "Oh, definitely 688. No wonder the woman doesn't feel well." The most dramatic interruption occurred as the nurses reacted to a patient's chest pain. Sarah, who was giving report, stopped abruptly and left the utility room to check on her patient.

Change-of-shift report demonstrated that RNs occupied a higher status position than LGPNs. RNs were the main actors among the nursing staff. LGPNs and nursing assistants contributed occasionally to report, such as by asking whether a patient had had a diagnostic test or noting the recent appearance of a pressure ulcer. Most often, they quietly listened as the RNs exchanged facts and thoughts.

7H nurses used a hospital-bound and nursing-specific language during report. This language defied comprehension by uninitiated nursing students. Thoughts were often expressed with incorrect grammar, which further confused the uninitiated. Words were omitted as nurses rapidly exchanged the messages of report. "Push some Lasix on her tonight," "He's going for an echo," and "She's out for lytes," are a few examples. Abbreviations were the rule and not the exception. Acronymns became neologisms. CABG (pronounced "cabbage"—coronary artery bypass graft) was commonly used.

The hidden functions of change-of-shift report illustrate the importance of the report in socializing new nurses into their role, upholding nursing standards, and maintaining nurses' responsibility for the care of patients.

During report, nurses frequently identified unfinished work. A nurse reporting off occasionally offered to complete work even if the work had begun close to the time of change-of-shift report. During report, nurses questioned unclear physician orders, so the next nurse could clarify the orders after contacting the physician. They also anxiously awaited reports of laboratory study results and told incoming nurses of their concern.

Change-of-Shift Report: Occupational Nursing Ritual

On a symbolic level, change-of-shift report represented nurses' taking on the responsibility for their patients. Patients were "owned" by the nurses, and ownership was passed from shift to shift. Several nurses "owned" a patient during his or her hospitalization. Nurses spoke of "my patient" as they described their specific domain of responsibility.

Change-of-shift report emphasized the continuous, temporal nature of the hospital and the nursing unit. Patients were "covered" by means of reports and by the nursing staff's need to protect them with a blanket of twenty-four-hour responsibility and accountability. The nurses took their responsibility of caring for patients seriously and transferred this responsibility from shift to shift by the vehicle of report. Change-of-shift report helped the nurses to freeze or suspend time, so that they were able to focus on events and facts specific to their patients.

As an occupational ritual, change-of-shift report was a stage where nurses learned what it meant to be a nurse. Here, the goals and values of nursing were taught and reemphasized.

SUMMARY

Types of nursing rituals identified in this study include therapeutic and occupational rituals. Therapeutic rituals (Douglas, 1963, 1966, 1975; Turner, 1957, 1967, 1969) are identified as symbolic healing actions that improve the condition of patients. Occupational rituals or rituals of socialization include symbolic actions that facilitate the transition of professional neophytes into their professional role (Bosk, 1980; Fox, 1979; Zerubavel, 1979).

Nursing rituals fulfill an important although not highly visible function in a nursing unit of a modern American hospital. They enable nurses to carry out caring activities for patients who are acutely or chronically ill, old, and dying. Rituals help to reaffirm values and beliefs of nurses. Explication of the implicit meanings of nursing rituals illuminates nursing for nurses and others who seek to understand nursing services. Descriptive analyses of nursing rituals direct attention to the hidden work of the hospital staff nurse, work sometimes taken for granted by professionals and the public who fail to see the many difficult, intimate, and risky aspects of nursing work and how certain ritual behavior promotes its accomplishment.

Other studies on nursing ritual are needed to expand the theory of nursing ritual in this descriptive analysis, and to move it from descriptive to explanatory theory. For example, the transmission of the beliefs, rules of conduct, and customs that take place during change-of-shift report has not been extensively

investigated. Neither have the more practical aspects of shift report been studied, including the types of information exchanged
or the influence of shift report on planning and priority setting
for the nurses who work during the ensuing shift. Also, few empirical studies examine the effects of bathing on patient outcomes, such as skin integrity, cardiac function, and comfort
levels, and patient bathing preferences. This is surprising, because the bath is such an essential ritual for the nursing profession and is thought to help patients.

Nursing's close association with profane materials, including
excretions and secretions, has most likely affected society's perception of the role of nurse. Investigations about these influences
may reveal valuable insights into some of the status problems that
nurses have encountered for many years. Equally important is the
association of nurses with death. Although nurses are frustrated
with the intrusion of hospital technology on patients' deaths, they
have not yet established themselves as standard setters for helping
patients achieve tranquil deaths. Ways of dying and problems associated with repeated resuscitations, advance directives, and brain-
dead status need to be studied from the perspective of nursing and
in the context of the postmortem ritual.

Types of medication errors and methods of medication administration, such as unit dose systems, have been explored by nursing
and other disciplines in various studies, but little research has focused on the impact of systems of medication administration on
medication error rates or the effect of medication errors on the
nurses who make them. Because of fear of litigation, medication
error data are difficult to access. This fear has limited research opportunities. Additional efforts are needed to expand the research
literature on the complex practices of medication administration
and the ritual nature of some of these practices.

Finally, rituals illustrate the unity of nurses as a social group.
Rather than serving to support the status quo, nursing rituals com-
bine the practical and the symbolic and are meaningful to nurses
in specific situations. They may serve to sustain the social structure and order of nursing; if they do, they must be viewed with
interest and not purged from nursing merely because they are
termed mindless or obsessive.

REFERENCES

Bosk, C. (1979). *Forgive and remember*. Chicago: University of Chicago Press.

Bosk, C. (1980). Occupational rituals in patient management. *New England Journal of Medicine, 302*(2), 71-76.

DeCraemer, W., Vansina, J., & Fox, R. (1976). Religious movements in Central Africa. *Comparative Studies in Society and History, 18,* 458-475.

Douglas, M. (1963). *The Lele of the Kasai*. London: Oxford University Press.

Douglas, M. (1966). *Purity and danger*. London: Routledge & Kegan Paul.

Douglas, M. (1970). The healing rite. *Man, 5,* 302-308.

Douglas, M. (1975). *Implicit meanings: Essays on anthropology*. London: Routledge & Kegan Paul.

Fox, R. C. (1979). The autopsy: Its place in the attitude-learning of second-year medical students. In R. C. Fox, *Essays in medical sociology*. New York: Wiley.

Malinowski, B. (1954). *Magic, science and religion and other essays*. Garden City, NY: Doubleday.

Turner, V. (1957). *Schism and continuity in an African society*. New York: Humanistic Press.

Turner, V. (1967). Symbol in Ndembu ritual. In V. Turner, *The forest of symbols: Aspects of Ndembu ritual*. Ithaca, NY: Cornell University Press.

Turner, V. (1969). *The ritual process*. Ithaca, NY: Cornell University Press.

Van Gennep, A. (1960). *The rites of passage*. Chicago: University of Chicago Press.

Walker, V. (1967). *Nursing and ritualistic practice*. New York: Macmillan.

Wolf, Z. R. (1986). *Nursing rituals in an adult acute care hospital: An ethnography*. Ann Arbor, MI: University Microfilms International (8614888).

Wolf, Z. R. (1988a). *Nurses' work: The sacred and the profane*. Philadelphia: University of Pennsylvania Press.

Wolf, Z. R. (1988b). Nursing rituals. *Canadian Journal of Nursing Research, 20*(3), 59-69.

Zerubavel, E. (1979). *Patterns of time in hospital life*. Chicago: University of Chicago Press.

10

Case Study: The Method

Carla Mariano

*I*n the world of science, the term case study is an enigma. As Lincoln and Guba (1985) noted:

> *[W]hile the literature is replete with references to case studies and with examples of case study reports, there seems to be little agreement about what a case study is . . . there is no simple taxonomy within which various kinds of case studies might be classified. (pp. 360-361)*

Case studies are variously described as a research strategy/design (Bogdan & Biklen, 1982; Kratochwill & Levin, 1992; Yin, 1989); a reporting mode (Lincoln & Guba, 1985); a teaching technique (Christensen, 1987); and an evaluation method (Patton, 1990). The case study is used in a variety of settings—schools, health care, the military, business, and industry—and by numerous disciplines—psychology, sociology, anthropology, history, ethics, economics, medicine, psychiatry, law, nursing, education, social work, management, political science, and public administration, to name but a few. In addition, the unit of analysis varies greatly among case studies. The unit of analysis can be a person, family, group, community, organization, culture, event, movement, program, or process.

Case studies are conducted at "various levels of complexity—from a single, brief, trivial episode to a lengthy major life-event with multiple strands" (Bromley, 1986, p. 2). They also use differing levels of analysis: merely factual, interpretative, and evaluative/judgmental levels of analysis (Lincoln & Guba, 1985). Case studies can focus on a single case as the unit of analysis or on multiple cases which are then compared.

Within the research arena, case studies can be exploratory, descriptive, interpretative, or explanatory (Tesch, 1990; Yin, 1989). Designs range from purely qualitative naturalistic inquiries (Lincoln & Guba, 1985) to single-case experiments (Barlow & Hersen, 1985) and complex time series designs (Cryer, 1986). The case study approach can be used either for hypothesis/theory generation or for hypothesis/theory testing. An understanding of case study develops in one a genuine appreciation for a mainstay axiom of qualitative research: there are truly multiple realities.

Because the purpose of this book is the consideration of qualitative research approaches, the remainder of this chapter will focus on the case study method primarily within the naturalistic paradigm.

DEFINITIONS AND CHARACTERISTICS

A case study is an "intensive, systematic investigation of a single individual, group, community, or some other unit, typically conducted under naturalistic conditions, in which the investigator examines in-depth data related to background, current status, environmental characteristics and interactions" (Woods & Catanzaro, 1988, p. 553).

Bromley (1986) characterized a case study as "a general term widely used, especially in the social and behavioral sciences, to refer to the description and analysis of a particular entity. . . . Such singular entities are usually natural occurrences with definable boundaries, although they exist and function within a context of surrounding circumstances. Such entities also exist over a short period of time relative to that context" (p. 8). Bromley also contended that the case study method is a "basic form of scientific inquiry that underpins effective professional practice especially in relation to human problems" (p. 41).

Yin (1989) defined a case study as an empirical inquiry that "investigates a contemporary phenomenon within its real-life context; when the boundaries between phenomenon and context are not clearly evident; and in which multiple sources of evidence are used" (p. 23). Denny, as cited in Guba and Lincoln (1981) defined the case study as "an intensive or complete examination of a facet, an issue, or perhaps the events of a geographic setting over time" (p. 370). Tesch (1990) described a case study as an ". . . intensive and detailed study of one individual or of a group as an entity, through observation, self-reports, and other means" (p. 39).

Four elements typify case studies: context, boundaries, time, and intensity. Case studies are conducted in context. Bromley (1986) reminded us: "The proper focus of a case study is not so much a 'person' as a 'person in a situation'" (p. 25). This is equally true when studying an organization, an event, or a process. The case must be viewed in its "ecological context" (Bromley, 1986), that is, in its physical, social, cultural, and symbolic environment. Naturalistic ontology proposes that "realities are wholes that cannot be understood in isolation from their contexts, nor can they be fragmented for separate study of the parts" (Lincoln & Guba, 1985, p. 39). For thorough understanding to occur, the research must be conducted with the case-in-context. This is crucial for three reasons:

1. Because it must be determined whether the conclusions apply to other contexts;
2. Because of "the belief in complex mutual shaping rather than linear causation, which suggests that the phenomenon must be studied in its full-scale influence (force) field" (Lincoln & Guba, 1985, p. 39);

3. Because values are an integral element of context, defining and influencing behavior.

Hinds, Chaves, and Cypess (1992) suggested that phenomena are always embedded within four layers of context:

1. The immediate context—the present, the here and now;
2. The specific context—one's unique and individual perspective, incorporating both the immediate past and significant facets of the current situation;
3. The general context—an individual's "general life frame of reference" (p. 38); the present situation is often interpreted in view of this context;
4. The metacontext—a social construction representing a shared social attitude and viewpoint.

Hinds et al. (1992) noted that meaning originates from interaction with these various contexts.

In a case study, the researcher defines the boundaries of the inquiry. Stake (1983) noted that "The case need not be a person or enterprise. It can be whatever *bounded system* (to use Louis Smith's term) is of interest" (p. 283). The investigator delineates the issues and reference points. This characteristic distinguishes the case study approach; that is, boundaries are continually kept in focus with the emphasis on what is and what is not the case:

What is happening and deemed important within those boundaries (the emic) is considered vital and usually determines what the study is about, as contrasted with other kinds of studies where hypotheses or issues previously targeted by the investigators (the etic) usually determine the study. (Stake, 1983, p. 283)

Case studies are present-oriented. They examine contemporary experience rather than historic events. Although the investigator may use "historical" data about the person or organization, the investigation focuses on the here and now. Case studies can be differentiated from life histories, which chronicle the links and connectedness of an individual's or group's life occurrences.

The issue of data collection over time is another important consideration in case study research. This issue is discussed in a later section.

Case studies employ an intensive orientation to the phenomenon under study. A very close association between the researcher and the participant(s) usually occurs over a long period. The researcher immerses himself or herself in the setting or situation and collects extensive evidence to describe and/or explain the case. Understandings that develop as an outcome of the study are often powerful and profound.

PURPOSE AND RATIONALE

Case studies are conducted for several reasons. Guba and Lincoln (1981; Lincoln & Guba, 1985) identified four purposes of case studies:

1. To chronicle (recording facts or events temporally or in the order in which they occurred);
2. To render (describing, depicting, or characterizing);
3. To teach (instructing);
4. To test (using a case to test particular theories and/or hypotheses).

Table 10-1 presents a typology of case studies and indicates the four purposes, the corresponding levels of analysis, and the product of each type of endeavor.

Case studies are conducted when little is known about a phenomenon or situation or when the traits of an individual, organization, or event are unusual. They are very useful in the exploratory phase of an investigation when:

1. There is little prior research in the area;
2. There is a need for preliminary data and information for planning larger research studies;
3. The generation of hypotheses for further verification is desirable.

Table 10–1
Case Study Types

Purpose of the Case Study	Factual		Levels of the Case Study Interpretative		Evaluative	
	Action	Product	Action	Product	Action	Product
Chronicle	Record	Register	Construe	History	Deliberate	Evidence
Render	Construct	Profile	Synthesize	Meanings	Epitomize	Portrayal
Teach	Present	Cognitions	Clarify	Understandings	Contrast	Discriminations
Test	Examine	Facts	Relate	Theory	Weigh	Judgments

Note: From *Effective Evaluation* by E. Guba and Y. Lincoln, 1981. San Francisco: Jossey-Bass Publishers. Reprinted by permission of Jossey-Bass Publishers.

Another reason for using the case study approach is to illustrate, demonstrate, or test a theory; this was the goal with many of the psychoanalytic case studies. Yin (1981a) contended that "although case studies indeed can be used for exploratory purposes, the approach also may be used for either descriptive or explanatory purposes as well—i.e., to describe a situation . . . or to test explanations for why specific events have occurred. In the explanatory function, the case study can therefore be used to make causal inferences" (p. 98).

However, Stake (1983) noted:

When explanations, propositional knowledge, and law are the aims of an inquiry, the case study will often be at a disadvantage. When the aims are understanding, extension of experience, and increase in conviction in that which is known, the disadvantage disappears. (p. 281)

• • •

Although case studies have been used by anthropologists, psychoanalysts and many others as a method of exploration preliminary to theory development, the characteristics of the method are usually more suited to expansionist than reductionist pursuits. Theory building is the search for essences, pervasive and determining ingredients, and the making of laws. The case study, however, proliferates rather than narrows. One is left with more to pay attention to rather than less. The case study attends to the idiosyncratic more than to the pervasive. The fact that it has been useful in theory building does not mean that is its best use. Its best use appears to be for adding to existing experience and humanistic understanding. Its characteristics match the "readiness" people have for added experience . . . intentionality and empathy are central to the comprehension of social problems, but so also is information that is holistic and episodic. The discourse of persons struggling to increase their understanding of social matters features and solicits these qualities. And these qualities match nicely the characteristics of the case study. (p. 284)

Case studies are also the approach of choice when a particular problem has arisen and necessitates a solution. Problematic decision making in an organization, cases of child abuse and neglect, substance abuse in families, and so on—all require exploration from a case study approach. The results/conclusions of this type of case study often take the form of policies or recommendations for remedial or therapeutic action (Denzin, 1989; Majchrzak, 1984).

Ideally, a case study attempts to integrate theory and practice by applying general concepts and knowledge to a particular situation in the real world. (Bromley, 1986, p. 42)

In all of these situations, the distinctive need for case studies arises out of the desire to understand complex social phenomena. In brief, the case study allows an investigation to retain the holistic and meaningful characteristics of real-life events. (Yin, 1989, p. 14)

CASE STUDY RESEARCH PROCESS

Strategies used in data collection and analysis in a case study are similar to some of the techniques used in other qualitative designs. There are, however, specifics related to collecting, organizing, and analyzing data in a case study.

The process of case study consists of the following elements:

- Identifying the purpose and questions of the study;
- Identifying the theoretical propositions if appropriate to the type of case study being conducted;
- Determining the unit of analysis;
- Developing a case study protocol (the guide for carrying out the case study);
- Deciding on the most appropriate design;
- Conducting the case study—collecting, analyzing, and interpreting the data;
- Writing the case study report.

Purpose/Questions

The content, organization, duration, data collection points, and type of evidence of a case study are dependent on the purpose of the inquiry. Therefore, the aims and goals of the study should be explicitly stated.

Research questions best answered by case studies are *what, how,* and *why* questions. Powers and Knapp (1990) indicated that case studies are concerned with "discovering what the relevant variables are that may explain, for example, why a study subject thinks and acts in certain ways, how a program was implemented, or how and why a particular event took place" (p. 18). *What* questions lead to exploratory/descriptive case studies and *how* or *why* questions convey an explanatory case study approach. Because the potential number of factors and amount of data in any case study can be enormous, defining the research question becomes one of the most important steps in this type of research.

Theory

Depending on the purpose of the case study, a theoretical framework or theoretical propositions may guide the inquiry. These a priori propositions reflect the research questions, literature review, and researcher intuitions. They focus attention on what should be explored in the study. In explanatory or theory-testing case studies, this theoretical orientation shapes the analysis and the examination of alternative interpretations. With exploratory/descriptive case studies, the theoretical propositions or framework usually evolve from the data themselves.

Regardless of the question being asked, the investigator should clearly examine and specify his or her *assumptions* about the phenomenon of interest at the outset of the study.

Unit of Analysis

The unit of analysis (e.g., individual, family, organization, event) and the context in which the unit occurs must be clearly differentiated at the beginning of the inquiry. Clarity of focus is imperative to the appropriate collection of data.

Elucidating the unit of analysis also has implications for the study design. Case studies can be conducted as holistic or embedded case studies. A holistic design examines the phenomenon of interest as a totality, from a global perspective (a group as a whole). An embedded design examines multiple units or subunits within the case, even though the study may be about a single entity (individuals within a particular group). As one can see, the identification of the unit(s) of analysis would have many implications for whom to interview or what to observe.

Case Study Protocol

The case study protocol (Yin, 1989) serves as the researcher's guide in conducting the case study. It keeps the goal of the study in the forefront while defining the field procedures, the data collection procedures, and the analytic procedures. The protocol identifies how entré will be gained, what resources may be necessary while in the field, a preliminary schedule for data collection activities, and a consideration of unexpected happenings. It further defines what data need to be collected and why; the sources of information and evidence, e.g., which people need to be interviewed, which documents need to be examined, and which observations must be done; and the data collection strategies. Lastly, the study protocol identifies the beginning plans for the analysis and development of the case report. The protocol serves as a preliminary guide and may need to be modified as the research emerges. However, it does keep the investigator focused on the purpose of the investigation.

Design

Two basic designs are used when conducting case studies: the single-case design and the multiple-case design. Prior to data collection, it is important to decide which design will best answer the research question.

The Single-Case Design.   The single-case design is used when the case represents a typical case, a critical case, an extreme or unique case, or a revelatory case (Yin, 1989).

The use of a critical case is appropriate when the investigator wishes to test a well-formulated and pivotal theory. Theories specify interrelated constructs and circumstances in which these propositions are thought to be true. A critical case can be used to ascertain whether these propositions are accurate, or whether there are competing explanations that are more apropos. In this way, the theory can be confirmed, extended, or challenged. Use of the critical case can contribute significantly to knowledge generation and theory building.

When a case is unique, extreme, or rare (as when there has been no opportunity, in practice or research, to uncover and confirm common patterns), a single-case design is beneficial. It is used to document and analyze the precise nature of the phenomenon under investigation and to raise questions for further exploration.

A revelatory case is one in which the researcher is privy to a situation that heretofore had been unavailable to scientific inquiry. This inaccessibility can be due to the newness of a situation or can occur when a phenomenon is common but scientists have not had the opportunity to access that particular event or population (such as certain subcultures). Revelatory case studies enlighten us about phenomena obscurely understood, if understood at all, and stimulate further research in the area.

Single-case studies also are used to illustrate typical or exemplary situations that are representative of larger groups or incidents.

The Multiple-Case Design.   In the multiple-case design, inferences and interpretations are drawn from a group of cases. This type of design is appropriate when the researcher is interested in exploring the same phenomenon in a diversity of situations or with a number of individuals. It is used when the investigator desires to establish whether a proposed explanation is confirmed across a number of cases. The multiple-case design is particularly applicable when generating theory through the constant comparative method of grounded theory (Strauss & Corbin, 1990).

Schultz and Kerr (1986) discussed the use of two strategies for conducting comparative case studies: the "most-similar-case" and the "most-different-systems" approaches. The most-similar-case technique analyzes findings and characteristics across similar or comparable cases. The most-different-systems technique is somewhat akin to the use of the "negative case," that is, actively seeking variation and difference to add depth to our understanding. These authors suggested that comparative case studies can be approached from either an idiographic or a nomothetic perspective. An idiographic perspective focuses on the particulars of the case whereas the nomothetic orientation emphasizes generalizations based on laws or principles.

Data Collection

The case study approach requires the gathering of comprehensive, in-depth data about the case in point, to describe the phenomenon or to explain the "case." Although the unit of analysis may be only one case or a small number of cases, the number of variables of interest in each case is usually large, and all must be examined. The information for each case must be as thorough as possible.

The case study approach often uses both qualitative and quantitative evidence. This evidence may come from a variety of sources: fieldwork, focused and open-ended interviews, verbal reports, direct observation, participant observation, documents, questionnaires, measurement instruments, clinical or agency records, life profiles, pictures, "epiphanies . . . existentially problematic moments in the lives of individuals" (Denzin, 1989, p. 129), archival accounts, artifacts, or any combination of the above. Case data also can include impressions and statements of others about the case— "in effect, all the information one has accumulated about each particular case goes into that case study" (Patton, 1990, p. 386).

Principles of Data Collection.   Three principles of data collection (Lincoln & Guba, 1985; Yin, 1989) are helpful in increasing the trustworthiness and quality of a case study:

1. Using multiple sources of evidence;
2. Establishing a case study base;
3. Maintaining a chain of evidence.

The use of numerous sources of data provides for triangulation of data sources—multiple measures and appraisals of the same phenomenon. Triangulation can include comparing the perspectives of several participants, comparing interview with observational or documentary data, or comparing the consistency of responses over time. The technique of triangulating different data sources increases the accuracy and credibility (construct validity) of the findings. It facilitates the researcher's corroboration of the findings by using different but converging lines of investigation.

A case study data base consists of observational field notes, audio- or videotapes, case logs, documents, and narratives. In case study research, the case study report often is not distinguished from the case study data base. It is important that there be a retrievable data base so other researchers can examine the evidence without being restricted exclusively to the case report. This procedure substantially increases the dependability (reliability) of the entire project.

Maintaining a chain of evidence is similar to what Lincoln and Guba (1985) referred to as an audit trail. The principle is to permit an external viewer to follow the researcher's process and procedures from research question to evidence to conclusion and vice versa. This "chain of evidence" greatly enhances the confirmability (reliability) of the case.

An additional principle of good data collection is the gathering of evidence over time. The case study is considered by some to be a "slice of life." A particular quantitative approach is the one-time case study design. Nonetheless, the more appropriate precept in the naturalistic paradigm is prolonged engagement. The researcher needs sufficient time and opportunity to become familiar with and understand the context within which the person or event is embedded. A period of prolonged engagement promotes the researcher's understanding of the "culture" of the person or organization and the building of trust. It aids in recognizing and accounting for distortions of either the researcher or the participants. Prolonged engagement also provides the researcher with the opportunity to get to know the subtleties of the situation and have the time to "peel away" layers until the core of the phenomenon, the real meaning, emerges.

Persistence during observation focuses the researcher on details, characteristics, and factors that give relevance to the phenomenon being explored. "If prolonged engagement provides scope, persistent observation provides depth" (Lincoln & Guba, 1985, p. 304).

Analysis

Yin (1989) noted:

> *[T]he analysis of case study evidence is one of the least developed and most difficult aspects of doing case studies. . . . Unlike statistical analysis, there are few fixed formulas . . . and the strategies and techniques have not been well defined. . . . Instead, much depends on an investigator's own style or rigorous thinking, along with sufficient presentation of evidence and careful consideration of alternative interpretations. (p. 105)*

Basically, there are two strategies for analyzing case study data:

1. Developing a case description (whether purely descriptive or exploratory);
2. Employing the theoretical propositions on which the study is based to explain the case (Yin, 1989).

These two strategies are similar to Tesch's (1990) systems for interpretational qualitative analysis: creating an organizing scheme from the data themselves, or creating an organizing scheme from the adopted theoretical framework that has directed the inquiry.

A third strategy, the quasi-judicial (Q-J) method (Bromley, 1986), combines features of the judicial and scientific methods. It is frequently used in psychological case studies. The Q-J method attempts to solve scientific and practice problems by applying rigorous reasoning in the interpretation of empirical data that have been systematically collected.

Following are descriptions of each of these methods of analysis.

Exploratory/Descriptive Strategy. The early scientists and practitioners who conducted case studies did not describe their techniques for analysis. "They interpreted their observations in the very basic sense of reflecting on their data until they achieved a better understanding of what they meant" (Tesch, 1990, p. 69). Those pioneers of the case study method produced enlightened portrayals of the people and events that they studied.

Today, however, there are many approaches for analyzing qualitative data for exploratory/descriptive case studies. These include content analysis, analytic induction, constant comparison, and phenomenological analysis. (For details, the reader is referred to discussion of these approaches in other chapters.)

Although each of these modes of analysis is different, there are generic elements integral to all. Data analysis occurs simultaneously with data collection. In order for the investigator to determine whether evidence from various sources intersects on a particular set of facts, the researcher must integrate data collection with data analysis so each informs the other.

The analysis is comprehensive and systematic, but not inflexible. Data are divided into smaller units for analysis and then reintegrated into a conceptual whole. Various authors refer to this process as "de-contextualizing/re-contextualizing" (Seidel, Kjolseth, & Seymor, 1988); coding and categorizing/pattern, theme, thesis development (Bogdan & Biklen, 1982); and extracting/clustering/exhaustive description (Colaizzi, 1978). The outcome of any of these analyses is "some type of higher-level synthesis. While much work in the analysis process consists of 'taking apart' (for instance, into smaller pieces), the final goal is the emergence of a larger, consolidated picture" (Tesch, 1990, p. 97).

Interpretation of the data is the expectation. Patton (1990) defined interpretation as "attaching significance to what was found, offering explanations, drawing conclusions, extrapolating lessons, making inferences, building linkages, attaching meanings, imposing order, and dealing with rival explanations, disconfirming cases, and data irregularities as part of testing the viability of an interpretation" (p. 423). He furnished Schlechty and Noblit's (1982) description of the purposes of interpretation:

1. Making the obvious obvious;
2. Making the obvious dubious;
3. Making the hidden obvious.

There is an "interpenetration of data and analysis" (Lofland & Lofland, 1984, p. 146), or a "balance between description and interpretation" (Patton, 1990, p. 429). Interpretations and analytic text are directly supported (grounded in) description, documentary evidence, and direct quotations. A distinction is made between evidence and inference.

A variety of products emerge from these diverse analytic strategies (Tesch, 1990): a "composite summary" (Hycner, 1985); a description of "patterns and themes" (Patton, 1990); an "identification of the fundamental structure" of the phenomenon of interest (Colaizzi, 1978); a "creative synthesis" (Moustakas, 1990); a "personalized structure" (Denzin, 1983); a "provisional hypothesis" (Turner, 1981); a policy for alleviating fundamental social problems (Majchrzak, 1984); or a "formal or substantive theory" (Strauss, 1987).

The investigator uses three dominant processes in analysis: reflection, comparison, and creativity. Reflection is both personal and data-bound. By examining his or her own assumptions and intimate involvement with the case material, the researcher attempts to become aware of and suspend (bracket), to the extent possible, preconceived ideas. These preconceptions may unduly bias not only the investigation but also the understanding of the phenomenon. Through reflection on, dialoguing with, and critical appraisal of the data, the investigator develops a clarity of meaning and advances the descriptive evidence to a more conceptual level.

The case study researcher uses comparison in most phases of the analysis. From forming coding categories to designating data into specific categories to contrasting negative evidence, the investigator is attempting to discover conceptual similarities and differences. In cross-case analysis, the investigator conducts several individual case studies and compares explanations for each, in order to form a more general explanation. Case analysis also includes the development of themes and patterns within or across cases or sites. Association and contrast are the analytic processes utilized in both of these analytic strategies.

Creativity is the hallmark of qualitative analysis. Because there is no "one right way" to make meaning, the researcher must blend critical thinking and creative insight. The use of metaphor, analogy, and imagery is beneficial when generating this type of "creative scholarship" (Mariano, 1990). Patton (1990) provided some valuable advice for nurturing creative thinking:

> *Be open; generate options; divergence before convergence; use multiple stimuli, side-track, zig-zag, and circumnavigate; change patterns, make linkages; trust yourself; work at it; and play at it. (pp. 434–435)*

Theoretical Orientation Strategy.   In this approach, a predetermined theoretical perspective or framework guides the case analysis: The objective is the building and testing of an explanation. A variety of analytic modes is used (Yin, 1989).

Pattern matching is based on a procedure discussed by Campbell (1975). It compares an a priori predicted pattern derived from theory with an observed pattern to see whether the patterns conform. Another way to pattern-match is to articulate a number of mutually exclusive rival theoretical propositions and then compare the observed pattern with each of these competing explanations.

Explanation building is very similar to the grounded theory strategy. However, one again begins with an initial theoretical statement or proposition versus developing the theory derived from the data themselves. This procedure seeks to explain a phenomenon through the development of a set of causal links. An iterative process (Yin, 1989) is used. Explanation building consists of identifying an initial proposition, comparing findings from the first case with the proposition, revising the proposition, recomparing the case with the revised proposition, comparing the subsequent revision with additional cases, and repeating the process as necessary until a solid, uncontended explanation evolves.

The above strategies are analogous to the methods used by detectives in solving crimes. The goal is to achieve a single explanation for the crime by ruling out rival explanations. Yin (1981b) described this process as follows. The detective is presented with the crime scene, its context, and possible eye-witness reports. The detective must decide the relevance of various evidence. Some case facts will be unrelated; other clues, however, must be vigorously followed. "The adequate explanation for the crime then becomes a plausible rendition of a motive, opportunity, and method that more fully accounts for the facts than do alternative explanations" (p. 61).

When testing theory, it is important that the case be argued from different theoretical perspectives, thereby ruling out perspectives that fail to account for the available evidence (Bromley, 1986, p. 42).

Another technique, the time-series analytic strategy, compares changes or specific indicators of the case over time with a prespecified theoretically meaningful trend.

Miles and Huberman (1984) described two models for data analysis: the flow model and the interactive model. Each of these models requires the use of an extant conceptual framework prior to data collection. Four components comprise these models: data collection, data reduction, data display, and conclusion drawing/verification. These authors placed great emphasis on the value of display as an integral aspect of analysis and a mode for understanding case material.

The Quasi-Judicial Strategy.   The first step in the quasi-judicial (Q-J) method is to state clearly the problems or issues. Background information is gathered to provide the context within which the problem or phenomenon is to be understood. Prima facie explanations about the issue can usually be furnished based on the background information alone. These rather obvious answers should be examined first because they often guide the investigator's search for further evidence. If these original explanations do not correspond with the available evidence, alternative hypotheses are generated.

The investigator then collects sufficient evidence to eliminate as many of the proposed explanations as possible, continually looking for one that will account for all of the evidence and be countered by none of the evidence. The evidence, as well as its source, is closely scrutinized for explanatory power, relevance, and credibility.

A critical query is made into the internal congruity, logic, and validity of the entire argument that claims solution or explanation. Some lines of argument will be deficient and others will be convincing. The best interpretation compatible with the evidence is chosen. This process and its outcome should contribute to the "case-law" (patterns of meaning or abstract and general principles explaining the phenomenon) of the discipline.

Whatever the approach to analysis, the ultimate aim is "[to] treat the evidence fairly, to produce compelling analytic conclusions, and to rule out alternative interpretations" (Yin, 1989, p. 106). The goal is not to identify the "truth," but to eliminate erroneous interpretations so that one has the most feasible and compelling rendition of the case under study.

Reporting

Case study reports can be presented in written or verbal format or through more innovative means such as photographs or videotapes. Regardless of the format, the case report remains one of the most suitable means for relating the results of naturalistic inquiry. Because most case studies generate written products, I will focus on the written report.

It is not easy to articulate the methods for writing a case study report, because there are no rules or standardized procedures. At best, one can state that the researcher must become immersed in a process of composing and, often, of artistry. As Guba and Lincoln (1981) noted:

Probably not much more can be said than that the usual principles of good composition—the writing of understandable prose—apply. (p. 375)

The audiences of the case study report must be identified. Different constituencies have different needs and interests in the case being presented. These diverse audiences may require of the report different emphases, particulars, compositional style, and length.

Lincoln and Guba (1985, p. 362) suggested the following elements as the content of a case study report:

- An explication of the problem or issue;
- A detailed description of the context/setting within which the phenomenon occurred;

- A complete delineation of the processes and transactions in the setting/context that are relevant to the focus of the inquiry;
- A discussion of the results ("lessons to be learned") of the study that lend understanding to the phenomenon of interest.

In addition, they recommended a methodological section or appendix to detail the investigator's credentials, assumptions, and biases regarding the phenomenon of interest or the setting. This section would give an exact reporting of the data collection and analysis methods used in the study and it would furnish a precise account of the steps taken to ensure the quality and trustworthiness of the study.

There are several varieties of written case reports (Yin, 1989). One is the single-case study in which a lengthy narrative (often book length) is developed to describe or analyze the case. A variant of the single-case report is the multiple-case report. This form is comprised of multiple narratives (usually chapters) individually describing each of the cases in the study. One or more chapters then incorporates the cross-case analysis and findings (themes/patterns across cases). A third example of a written report describes or analyzes a single or multiple case; however, it does not use the customary narrative. This model incorporates a sequence of answers to a set of questions, usually those on which the study was based. A fourth type of written report is used exclusively with multiple-case studies. The entire report is devoted to the cross-case analysis; no individual cases are reported. Specific chapters focus on specific cross-case issues or themes. Individual case information is interspersed throughout each issue-chapter or it presented in highlighted vignettes.

EVALUATION OF CASE STUDIES

A number of criteria are used to evaluate case studies. These include criteria that establish the trustworthiness (Lincoln & Guba, 1985; Sandelowski, 1986) of the study as well as additional standards specific to case study.

Trustworthiness necessitates the achievement of four objectives: credibility, transferability, dependability, and confirmability. Credibility uses techniques that ensure that plausible interpretations and constructions will be generated. The techniques include prolonged engagement, triangulation, peer debriefing, negative case analysis, and member or participant checking of the researcher's interpretations. Transferability allows someone to decide whether the conclusions or findings can be transferred to another context. This is done by providing a detailed data base and thick description of the phenomenon. Dependability, which permits another to follow the process and procedures of the inquiry, is accomplished by incorporating an audit procedure in the study. Confirmability attests that the findings, conclusions, and recommendations are supported by the data and that there is an internal congruity between interpretations and actual evidence. This again is accomplished by the use of an audit process.

Burns (1989) identified additional standards for the evaluation of qualitative research: descriptive vividness; methodological congruence (rigor in documentation, procedure, ethics, and auditability); analytical preciseness; theoretical connectedness; and heuristic relevance (intuitive recognition, relationship to existing knowledge, applicability).

Yin (1989) identified what he saw as the characteristics of an exemplary case study. Primarily, the case study should be significant. It should make a significant contribution to the understanding of an unknown phenomenon; or compare two or more pivotal but rival theories in a discipline to explain the case; or incorporate both discovery and theory construction in the case study.

The case study must be as complete as possible. The evidence collected should be extensive and relevant. Critical pieces of evidence ought to be given thorough attention. Not all data are relevant, so the investigator must present *meaningful* information. The researcher needs to stay in the field as long as necessary to achieve "completeness."

An explanatory case study must examine the evidence from varying perspectives and viewpoints or consider alternative propositions. The investigator should anticipate what these alternative interpretations are and be able to demonstrate how and why these rival explanations can be rejected based on the facts of the case.

The case study report should present the most compelling data so the reader can independently come to a conclusion regarding the worth of the inquiry. The report should instill in the reader a confidence that the investigator has truly acted with scholarly and professional ethics. Evidence must be presented in a truthful, objective manner and must include both supporting and challenging information. The researcher must be selective in the inclusion of evidence. However, that selectivity refers to the relevancy of the data; for example, to the most critical evidence or the fair treatment of all cases, and not to the exclusion of any data that do not support the researcher's conclusions.

Review and validation of the investigator's interpretations should be done by the study participants. This minimizes bias in the presentation and ensures that the facts have not been misconstrued. In addition, it often gives the participants a better understanding of the whole phenomenon under investigation (Yin, 1981a).

Finally, it behooves the investigator to fashion the case study report in an engaging style. Through technique and form, it should captivate the audience and entice them to read or hear more. This requires an investigator who is enthusiastic about the study and strongly desires to communicate the findings of the inquiry.

ADVANTAGES OF AND ISSUES IN CASE STUDY RESEARCH

Stake (1983) noted that case study will often be the favored method of inquiry because it is "epistemologically in harmony with the reader's experience" (p. 279) and therefore provides a basis for natural generalization. Guba and Lincoln (1981) identified a number of reasons for the choice of the case study. A case study produces "thick description," which lets others in different settings decide whether the entity studied is applicable to their own situation or context. The case study is grounded, thereby providing a perspective that evolves directly from experience versus a priori hypotheses, assumptions, or instruments. Case studies are "holistic and lifelike"; they paint realistic pictures of actual participants in their own language. A case study report integrates a large and often diverse amount of information in a unified, focused manner. Unlike statistical scientific reports, case studies communicate to their audience in such a way as to illuminate meaning and increase understanding.

Lastly, a case study builds on the reader's "tacit knowledge" or that which is implicitly understood. Case studies provide others with vicarious experiences:

> *[P]laced in the actual situation, the reader of a case study would sense many things that he could not scientifically document but in which he would have a great deal of confidence. . . . We all know more than we can say; the case study provides a vehicle for the transference of that kind of wordless knowledge. (Guba & Lincoln, 1981, p. 377)*

There are, however, several issues associated with case study research that need to be addressed. The problem of generalizability of case study findings is often raised as a disadvantage of this method of inquiry. "It is difficult to argue with certainty that what is learned from a single case is representative of patterns or trends in the entire population" (Skodal-Wilson, 1985, p. 137). The question frequently arises regarding "truth." Does "truth" lie in general axioms or in particulars?

Stake (1983) contended that valuable understanding can come from a complete and detailed knowledge of the particular. He considered this knowledge to be a type of generalization, albeit not a scientific generalization. He used the term "naturalistic generalization," emanating from a recognition of similarities of entities in and out of context, to define this knowledge:

> *Naturalistic generalizations develop within a person as a product of experience. They derive from the tacit knowledge of how things are, why they are, how people feel about them, and how these things are likely to be later on in other places with which this person is familiar. They seldom take*

the form of predictions but lead regularly to expectation.
They guide action, in fact they are inseparable from ac-
tion . . . . (p. 282)

Case studies have unique issues related to ethics. These ethical
concerns can arise from inquiry "shaping" by the investigator, manipulation of the data, nonreporting of contradictory data, and
bias in interpretations. Use of the techniques identified in the section on evaluation of case studies (utilizing an external auditor,
member checking, grounding interpretations in evidence, and so
on) will help to ensure the integrity of the case study.

Another ethical dilemma in the case study approach is protecting the anonymity of the participant(s) or site(s) in the study. Assurance of anonymity is particularly problematic when the
researcher is investigating a unique situation. Guba and Lincoln
(1981) suggested following the principle that participants "own"
the data that apply to them. Data will not be reported without explicit consent of the participants after being fully informed about
anticipated use and potential risks.

RESEARCHER CHARACTERISTICS

A number of authors have expounded on the attributes and skills
required of researchers who conduct qualitative research (Bromley, 1986; Mariano, 1990; Yin, 1989). These characteristics are
equally applicable to the conduct of case study inquiry.

Case study investigators must be comfortable with ambiguity
and flexible enough to deal with the unexpected as an opportunity rather than a menace. A willingness to comprehend meaning
in context and to accept more than one "truth" enhances one's appreciation and ability to conduct case studies.

The case study researcher must possess good communication
skills. The art of listening and absorbing large amounts of data
without bias, an aptitude for observing with an inquiring mind,
and the facility for writing in an articulate and interesting style are
imperative for quality case study research.

The case study researcher must be mature, introspective, and
reflective. Awareness of one's assumptions, preconceptions, and

values is especially important when making inferences and interpreting phenomena; otherwise, a case study can be misused to support the researcher's preconceived position.

The ability to conceptualize is essential for the case study researcher. Using the vast amount of data amassed, patterns must be identified, themes discovered, connections made, propositions developed, and meaning abstracted. Imagination coupled with discipline is necessary for the case study investigator to produce creative scholarship.

THE FUTURE OF CASE STUDY RESEARCH

Case studies will continue to be essential in investigating certain topics of interest to nursing. Refinement and advancement will occur as investigators continue to analyze and share their own experiences with the method. The usefulness of the case study approach for all facets of inquiry (description, exploration, and explanation) makes it an invaluable strategy for understanding and for increasing knowledge about the human condition.

REFERENCES

Barlow, D., & Hersen, M. (1985). *Single-case experimental designs: Strategies for studying behavior* (2nd ed.). New York: Pergamon.

Bogdan, R. C., & Biklen, S. K. (1982). *Qualitative research for education: An introduction to theory and methods.* Boston: Allyn & Bacon.

Bromley, D. B. (1986). *The case-study method in psychology and related disciplines.* Chichester, England: Wiley.

Burns, N. (1989). Standards for qualitative research. *Nursing Science Quarterly, 2*(1), 44-52.

Campbell, D. (1975, July). Degrees of freedom and the case study. *Comparative Political Studies, 8,* 178-193.

Christensen, C. R. (1987). *Teaching and the case method.* Boston: Harvard Business School.

Colaizzi, P. F. (1978). Psychological research as the phenomenologist views it. In R. Valle & M. King (Eds.), *Existential-phenomenological alternatives for psychology.* New York: Oxford University Press.

Cryer, J. D. (1986). *Time series analysis.* Boston: Duxbury Press.

Denzin, N. K. (1983). Interpretive interactionism. In G. Morgan (Ed.), *Beyond method: Strategies for social work* (pp. 129–146). Newbury Park, CA: Sage.

Denzin, N. K. (1989). *Interpretive interactionism.* Newbury Park, CA: Sage.

Guba, E. G., & Lincoln, Y. S. (1981). *Effective evaluation.* San Francisco: Jossey-Bass.

Hinds, P., Chaves, D., & Cypess, S. (1992). Context as a source of meaning and understanding. In J. Morse (Ed.), *Qualitative health research* (pp. 31–42). Newbury Park, CA: Sage.

Hycner, R. H. (1985). Some guidelines for the phenomenological analysis of interview data. *Human Studies, 8,* 279–303.

Kratochwill, T. R., & Levin, J. R. (Eds.). (1992). *Single-case research design and analysis: New directions for psychology and education.* Hillsdale, NJ: Erlbaum.

Lincoln, Y. S., & Guba, E. G. (1985). *Naturalistic inquiry.* Beverly Hills, CA: Sage.

Lofland, J., & Lofland, L. H. (1984). *Analyzing social settings: A guide to qualitative observation and analysis* (2nd ed.). Belmont, CA: Wadsworth.

Majchrzak, A. (1984). *Methods for policy research.* Newbury Park, CA: Sage.

Mariano, C. (1990). Qualitative research: Instructional strategies and curricular considerations. *Nursing & Health Care, 11*(7), 354–359.

Miles, M. B., & Huberman, A. M. (1984). *Qualitative data analysis: A sourcebook of new methods.* Beverly Hills, CA: Sage.

Moustakas, C. (1990). *Heuristic research: Design, methodology, and applications.* Newbury Park, CA: Sage.

Patton, M. Q. (1990). *Qualitative evaluation and research methods* (2nd ed.). Newbury Park, CA: Sage.

Powers, B. A., & Knapp, T. R. (1990). *A dictionary of nursing theory and research.* Newbury Park, CA: Sage.

Sandelowski, M. (1986). The problem of rigor in qualitative research. *Advances in Nursing Science, 8*(3), 27–37.

Schlechty, P., & Noblit, G. (1982). Some uses of sociological theory in educational evaluation. In R. Corwin (Ed.), *Policy research.* Greenwich, CT: JAI Press.

Schultz, P. R., & Kerr, B. J. (1986). Comparative case study as a strategy for nursing research. In P. L. Chinn (Ed.), *Nursing research methodology: Issues and implementation* (pp. 195–220). Rockville, MD: Aspen.

Seidel, J., Kjolseth, R., & Seymor, E. (1988). *The ethnograph: A user's guide.* Littleton, CO: Qualis Research Associates.

Skodal-Wilson, H. (1985). *Research in nursing.* Menlo Park, CA: Addison-Wesley.

Stake, R. (1983). The case study method in social inquiry. In G. Madaus, M. Scriven, & D. Stufflebeam (Eds.), *Evaluation models: Viewpoints on educational and human services evaluation* (pp. 279-286). Boston: Bluwer-Nijhoff.

Strauss, A. L. (1987). *Qualitative analysis for social scientists.* New York: Cambridge University Press.

Strauss, A. L., & Corbin, J. (1990). *Basics of qualitative research: Grounded theory procedures and techniques.* Newbury Park, CA: Sage.

Tesch, R. (1990). *Qualitative research: Analysis types and software tools.* Bristol, PA: Falmer Press.

Turner, B. A. (1981). Some practical aspects of qualitative data analysis: One way of organizing the cognitive process associated with the generation of grounded theory. *Quality and Quantity, 15,* 225-247.

Woods, N. F., & Catanzaro, M. (1988). *Nursing research: Theory and practice.* St. Louis, MO: Mosby.

Yin, R. K. (1981a). The case study as a serious research strategy. *Knowledge: Creation, Diffusion, Utilization, 3*(1), 97-114.

Yin, R. K. (1981b). The case study crisis: Some answers. *Administrative Science Quarterly, 26,* 58-65.

Yin, R. K. (1989). *Case study research: Design and methods* (rev. ed.). Newbury Park, CA: Sage.

11

The Centrality of Caring: A Case Study

Charles J. Beauchamp

This chapter begins with a discussion of the case study method as it relates to this particular study. A brief introduction to the study is presented as a way of joining the previous chapter with this chapter. A background of the case that will be studied is provided so that, as the reader moves through the chapter, the context and situation of the design and methods can easily be followed. Next is presented the actual design of the case study, outlining the research aim, an explication of the phenomenon, the conceptual perspective, the data-gathering process, and a discussion of the presentation of the data. The narrative report of the data will give the reader an appreciation for the case itself. The processes of data analysis and the results are then presented and discussed. A review of the literature in relationship to the findings compares the new findings of this study to existing knowledge. A subsequent section discusses the utilization of the findings in practice, research, and education. The chapter ends with a brief summary.

OVERVIEW OF THE CASE STUDY METHOD

It is hoped that the utilization of the case study method of scientific inquiry will increase within the realm of nursing research. One could postulate that the increase will stem from a realization that the ontology of the method is philosophically and pragmatically congruent with the tenets of the discipline of nursing. As previously articulated, the case study method can be metamorphic; therefore, it is essential to acknowledge that this case study is an exemplar, not a dogma. The design of the case study method guiding this project has utility in the various domains of the nursing world, such as practice, research, and education. The substance of the case under study is not unfamiliar in contemporary nursing practice. It studies an essence of nursing, caring, in the context of a major health crisis, human immunodeficiency virus (HIV). This chapter will exemplify a variety of the processes presented in the preceding chapter.

Frequently, when completing a case study, an individual has a dual role, being both practitioner and researcher; such is the situation in this project. The case(s), the involved phenomenon, and the research question(s) in this type of study are not usually established a priori, as is the tradition with other research methods. In most situations where this type of study unfolds, these elements are identified as the case progresses. The practitioner entering into the situation of the case experiences the presence of an emerging phenomenon, a sense of uniqueness, that stirs the intuition and beckons to be examined. A change occurs when the practitioner begins to examine the case beyond the pragmatic bounds of usual or traditional practice, in search of answers to questions that describe and explain the unfolding situation at a theoretical, scientific level of discourse. The transition from the role of practitioner to the role of practitioner–researcher emerges at this point of theoretical, scientific query; this is when the case becomes a study. An example of the dual role of blending and synthesizing practice and research has been proposed by Newman (1990), who "advocates research as praxis and emphasizes process as content" (p. 37). Based on Newman's work, one can postulate that, in employing data-gathering processes of qualitative research, one is also simultaneously practicing; and, in practicing, one is also collecting data for research.

The case study method can also be utilized without the intent or context of practice. A researcher may develop and conduct a case study without initially being in a practice situation. The intent of the project can be stipulated in a research proposal, where the relationship of the researcher with the participants is for the purposes of scientific inquiry.

Introduction

The design of this case study utilizes some specific processes and procedures discussed in the previous chapter. This study has a single-case design; it is both descriptive and interpretative of a major life-event for an individual and his family. The elements of the study, as delineated in the previous chapter, are: context, the major life-event; boundaries, the experiences of the individual, family, and important others in context; time, the longevity of the case (nine days); intensity, a situational paradox of dissonance and harmony. What began as an assignment detailed as ordinary-with-an-element-of-discord was transformed into an extraordinary journey of harmony.

BACKGROUND OF THE CASE TO BE STUDIED

Jim Hall (henceforth, "Jim"), age 30, was discharged to his home from a medical center after extended treatment for HIV disease. His discharge plan from the medical center included a referral to a home health agency for total parental nutrition (TPN) via a central line ("to keep the family happy") and palliative nursing care. Jim's physician made a prognosis of one week of life post discharge. The physician was not in agreement with the discharge plan; it was his desire that Jim stay in the hospital until death. The patient and the family (his life-partner, mother, and father) insisted he be brought home. The physician also opposed the central line and TPN, but "gave in" to the patient's and family's wishes, which resulted in the need for a home health referral. Concern was expressed by the nursing staff at the medical center, the physician, and the supervisor of the home health agency that the life-partner and parents were a "negative influence" in that they frequently questioned and supported Jim's refusal of interventions. It was also noted that Jim had begun to refuse most of his medications, which was a concern for the "professional caregivers." During his stay at the medical center, Jim and his family frequently "demonstrated behaviors that were contradictory to the orders of the physician and requests of the nurses"; such transgressions included "eating foods that were not allowed on his diet" and "taking his own medications from home when they were not yet ordered or required a longer period of time to obtain than Mr. Hall could wait." Jim and his family were labeled as being "difficult and noncompliant." The essence of the initial plan of care from the home health agency was to provide skilled nursing service related to the TPN and central line, and to increase the compliance of Jim and his family regarding treatment.

As the practitioner, upon meeting Jim and his family and knowing the above history, I intuitively experienced the essence of intense caring in the situation, which at the time eluded words. The dissonance between what was reported and what was experienced spurred me toward a research approach in this practice situation; a case study was evolving.

This synopsis of the background of the case is necessary as a preamble to the case study report. The inclusion of a discussion of the background of the case as an introduction is left to the discretion of the researcher, and is usually determined based on the format chosen for the writing of the report. The organization of the content in the report utilizes the recommended sequencing by Lincoln and Guba (1985) as well as the standard style of research reports in nursing.

DESIGN OF THE CASE STUDY RESEARCH

Research Aim

The research aim that guided this case study was to understand how a dissonant situation evolved into one of harmony. To delineate the content and process of the research aim as it unfolded in the experience of the case, two research objectives underpinned the aim:

1. Understand the meaning evolving in the situation;
2. Describe the ways of being in the situation.

Explication of the Phenomenon

The rationale for choosing the case study method—and the purpose of the study—was to determine and examine the phenomenon that made this case a unique situation. The uniqueness lay in the individual's and family's ability to maintain their way of being in the midst of persistent forces in the health care system that were antithetical to the way they chose to be.

Conceptual Perspective

In case study research, as with other qualitative research designs, the term perspective is utilized because of the naturalistic approach to the research question. Researchers approach a phenomenon of interest, or a research question, with a particular view or conceptualization. Because the researcher in qualitative query is also the "instrument," collecting and analyzing data, it is essential that researchers make explicit their conceptualizations of the aim of the research at the onset of the study. The conceptual perspective makes clear the assumptions, preconceptions, and biases that the researcher holds. The conceptual perspective of the researcher is bracketed, or held in abeyance, as the research is conducted. The intent of this process is to decrease the influence of the assumptions, preconceptions, and biases in data collection and data analysis. Lincoln and Guba (1985) concurred with this practice by recommending that a section detailing the conceptualizations noted above be made explicit, in addition to the credentials of the researcher, to ensure the quality and integrity of the research.

The conceptualizations that I brought to this study are grounded in this personal philosophy of nursing as a discipline:

> *Nursing as a practice discipline is a human science. The operationalization of nursing is an art that is expressed in caring forms. The focal modes of the operationalization of nursing are practice and research. Practice and research are interrelated and interdependent. Human beings, health, and the environment are the core phenomenon of the discipline. The three are interrelated and simultaneous in nature and cannot be viewed as separate entities. Human beings are complex, irreducible beings that manifest their being through health. Being as health is conceived in the interrelationship of human beings and the environment. Nursing is the highest call to humanity. The practice of nursing is a process of bearing witness to and hosting the journey of humankind through the possibilities and paradoxes of choosing life.*

As the researcher, my beliefs and values are ontologically grounded in existential-phenomenological philosophy. My tradition of qualitative research has been peer-reviewed and deemed significant in nursing science.

Participants

The participants in this study were all the individuals involved in the case. The primary participants were Jim Hall; his life-partner of ten years, Bill; his mother, Susan; and his father, Steve. Primary participants are those individuals who are foundational to the case analysis. Other individuals who are peripheral to the unit of analysis are not excluded as participants; their involvement in the case may be transitory or contextual in nature. In the occurrence of a case study that emerges from a practice situation, the role of each participant in the study may not be clear until the study is

under way. It is also important to realize that the role of participants in an evolving study may transit as the case progresses. Participants in this study who were peripheral to the unit of analysis
were: Jim's older sister, Lucy, who lived in Europe; his next older
sister, Beth, who was in another part of the country at school;
other extended family members; the physician; the home health
agency's supervisor; and the practitioner-researcher. Both of
Jim's sisters were in contact with him and the other family members via mail and telephone on a regular basis. The researcher did
not have the opportunity for contact with them directly until after Jim's death.

Access to the participants or entré to the unit of analysis was
initially achieved for practice purposes. When a case study is initiated as a research project, the usual or traditional means of obtaining access to participants may be utilized.

Setting

The setting in which this case study transpired was the home of
Jim and Bill, specifically their bedroom, where Jim spent all of his
time during this study. Their home was in an elegantly designed
and decorated environment located directly on an Atlantic Ocean
beach. The style of the home was modern; its earth-tone color
scheme generated an aura of serenity, warmth, and softness. The
entire home always had a subdued floral aroma, emitted from esoteric live tropical flowers that were displayed throughout. The
sound of the waves hitting the shore of the beach in front of the
home provided a melodious background of tranquillity. The bedroom of the home had two walls of glass that opened onto a
wraparound balcony overlooking the sea. The "medical supplies,"
other than the obvious infusion pump, were stored out of sight,
which prevented the room from having a clinical appearance. It
was Jim's wish to utilize his home bed rather than a hospital bed
throughout this experience. The setting in this study was limited
because of Jim's physical limitations. (The setting in a case study
can be any environment or context in which the phenomenon of
the research exists.)

Protection of Human Rights

The protection of human rights is a critical element in any research study, including case study research. When a researcher wishes to conduct a case study, it is important to become familiar with the affiliated organization's or agency's policies and procedures for the protection of human rights, and the proper course to seek permission to conduct research.

In this case study, the agency involved had no institutional review board for the protection of human rights. Permission to conduct the study was obtained from the administration. More important, the participants—the family—granted their approval of the researcher's utilization of the case information for research purposes. Elements of the study that would be a threat to the anonymity or confidentiality of the participants in the report have been modified without diminishing the integrity of the data.

Data Gathering

Data for this case study were gathered utilizing the principles of data collection (Lincoln & Guba, 1985; Yin, 1989) discussed in the previous chapter. Data were achieved in a case journal as the study progressed. The case journal contained: copies of the nursing progress notes (standard agency procedure for the nurse), logging of telephone calls that included objective and subjective data, narrative entries chronicling participant-observer activities—conversations, observations, and intuitive experiences or impressions. As data were collected, the researcher compared and contrasted data sources: the impressions and perspectives of participants versus those of other participants; observational data versus reported data. The researcher also looked for consistencies and inconsistencies as the case progressed. During the process of the study, the researcher consulted with another qualitative researcher who acted as an external reviewer. The function of the external reviewer was to challenge what was unclear and confirm what was evident throughout the study. This process provided an adequate and reliable data base from which to conduct the study.

Presentation of the Data

Presentation of the data in a case study is a report or account of the case that is being studied. As discussed in the preceding chapter, a case study report can span from a book to sequential answers. Regardless of the form, the report should be engaging, objective, comprehensive yet salient, descriptive, and articulate. The format that is utilized in this study is a descriptive narrative. The descriptive narrative format was selected for logistical purposes, to provide an example of a case study report that was suitable for a chapter of a book. Because of this form's requirements, all of the data collected could not be presented. The synopsis of the case that follows provides the reader an opportunity to share the data and to see where in the case the outcomes emerged.

An introductory overview of the background of the case was presented before the case study method section. An overview of the case in the beginning of a report is necessary as a reference for the methodological discussion.

CASE REPORT

The Beginning of the Case

When I first went to Jim and Bill's home, I went with my usual plans, which were fairly traditional and prescribed for a first visit. I kept in mind, as I do every time I enter a person's home where I am providing care, that I was a guest, that it was their home, their life situation. Upon meeting the two men, I explained that my role was to be there for them in ways that would assist them with this life situation, as they saw fit. This approach seemed acceptable; I did not experience any of the "resistance" that had been reported. They shared the information that, prior to the onset of the case, Jim had experienced twelve hospitalizations related to HIV disease over the past three years. He first learned of his HIV status eight years earlier, and had been asymptomatic for five years. Two years into their relationship, Jim and Bill had made the decision to be tested for HIV, upon the advice of their physician. Both anticipated negative test results. Jim's test result was HIV positive. Bill's was HIV negative, and he continued to still test negative. Bill recalled how shocked and devastated they both had felt. He also shared experiences of guilt because he was negative and Jim was positive. Jim shared similar feelings of guilt, worrying that he was infectious to Bill. They both remembered the experience "like it was yesterday," of how people would ask each of them, "Who infected who?" Bill spoke of his feelings of isolation and stigma: "It was like we committed a crime. I felt like I was an appalling human being." With tears in his eyes, Jim recalled the hurt he had experienced: "I didn't do anything wrong! I didn't ask for this disease! I was looking for love, not sex, I only had sex with two other people before meeting Bill." We spent time talking about the blame that has been attached to this disease, and about how the idea of "guilty" or "innocent" victims of HIV stemmed from a lack of empathy and understanding. I remembered hearing people speak of the "innocent victims" of HIV and thought to myself, "Who are the 'guilty victims?' What must it be like not to be in the 'innocent' group?" Bill recalled similar experiences, as he gently rubbed the top of Jim's head: "Some people refused to believe that I had my first sexual experience with Jim, and that we have always been monogamous." Jim recounted: "There would always be someone that would imply that one of us must have been unfaithful to the other." Bill interjected: "In the beginning, and right through this whole ordeal, the only two people that have always been there and cared—I mean really cared; not curious, or placating—were Jim's parents." Jim agreed: "With my parents, it was never a question of being able to be myself, to just be whoever I was. I knew they always loved and cared about me." It seemed inhumane that someone who was about to die, and someone else who was about to lose the one he loved, had to deal with these situations. I recall thinking, "Why would I care about these things, how they got here?" What seemed important to me was the present: how they were and how I was with them. A trust between the two men and myself appeared evident by the end of the first visit, and was clearly present by the end of the second, as they shared more and more of themselves openly with me.

The Middle of the Case

Jim's father and mother, Steve and Susan, visited daily with Jim. Steve was a man who presented as solid, yet sensitive. He proclaimed, when we first met: "We love Jim, and we also love Bill. He's our son, and Bill is like a son." Susan acted in a maternal, nurturing way toward both Jim and Bill, and frequently would step out of the room with her husband to provide privacy for Jim and Bill with me. It was evident that both of Jim's parents respected his relationship with Bill as being not unlike that of a legal marriage. I always discussed things between Jim and Bill before including Jim's parents. To me, it was clearly the proper form to follow, as evidenced by the relationship the four shared. On two occasions, when reviewing my notes, my supervisor commented that I had recorded incidents of decision making in such a manner. She questioned my judgment because Steve and Susan were Jim's parents and Bill was "only a friend" with "no legal authority." I remember responding, "What is legal isn't always ethical." I assured her I wouldn't do anything illegal, nor would I do anything I thought was unethical. On one particular visit, Susan recalled when Jim started to become ill and required hospitalization: "I thought to myself, well this is it. I'm going to be focusing everything I have at the moment on him; physically, mentally, and spiritually, I'll be there in what ever way I'm needed." She always appeared to be a quiet, strong person. When I would ask her whether she needed anything, or whether I could do anything for her, she would always say, "Just a hug." We hugged frequently, from the first day to the last, and usually more than once during each visit. They weren't just hugs; they were embraces, holdings, that exuded warmth and love. One evening, as Steve and I sat on the balcony, he confided:

I remember staying all night, one of Jim's first nights in the hospital. I didn't know what to say or do. We spent the night discussing all the options or possibilities; discussing, not telling. I remember hearing doctors and nurses telling patients what they should do, and thought, who the hell are they? They're not living with this virus.

Jim, who had been listening from his bed as he faded in and out of sleep, muttered:

I got them realizing that this is my life and my situation. Nobody was going to tell me what to do.

Bill was lying by his side, embracing him. Jim sunk into Bill's arms as if they were a safety net, and slipped back into sleep. Just that morning, I had had a discussion with Jim's physician, who was displeased that Jim had refused the TPN and all of his medications. The physician wanted me to "convince him" to start taking both again. "He'll live longer" was his rationale. When Jim told me he wasn't taking either anymore, he said that the TPN felt terrible while it infused, and the meds made him vomit. He said he knew that he would dehydrate without the TPN and that he ran the risk of possible infection without the medications. He proclaimed: "I'd rather feel good than live longer." I told the physician that I wouldn't "convince him," that we had already discussed the possibilities of stopping both, and that Jim had made an informed decision, one that his family supported. The physician responded, as I recall: "I don't know why they bother with me; he never listens." I remember having two thoughts:

1. Do you ever listen to him?
2. They bother with you because they need to stay in the system; you're the gatekeeper.

It became clear that part of my role in this case was as a mediator between those being served and those providing the service. Jim and his family were in the position to make decisions regarding Jim's situation—not the physician, my supervisor, or myself.
Jim talked about his hospital stays:

When I was in the hospital I could always tell the people who really cared. I'd get that feeling—you must know the one—a feeling that another truly likes and enjoys what he or she is doing, I'd also get that opposite feeling too.

I thought to myself, "I know the feeling." I realized that what I had always thought was true was indeed true: people could tell whether nurses were really present to them. It also occurred to me how much I loved my work, how I felt honored to be part of people's lives at such critical moments, in such intimate ways. I began to think of nursing as an almost sacred calling.

Bill recalled times during the hospitalizations when he felt uncomfortable:

> *I could tell that there were people there that didn't approve of our life-style. I never wanted approval, just human respect. During those times, I found comfort when someone acted in a way that was, well, affirming my way of being, not judging or criticizing the way I am.*

I shared with them, on more than one occasion, how evident their love and regard were for one another, and what a special relationship they shared. Jim added, "It's so important when you're vulnerable to experience that you're being loved as another human, as a fellow human being, not some perverted freak that is only deserving of hate." I remember an in-depth discussion about the importance of acceptance versus tolerance. I thought how horrible it must feel to be tolerated like some type of nuisance, and pondered what it must be like to be in Jim's situation and experience these emotions. To me, these were two beautiful human beings, in a devastating situation, who were deserving of everything I had to offer them. I was privileged to share in their lives, as they lived this critical life situation.

The End of the Case

As nature would have it, this was the last day when Jim was awake and speaking. The next night, he would pass from life to death. His parting words to me that day were unforgettable. As I prepared to leave, he whispered softly:

> *Thank you for realizing that I am a sensitive, feeling person, and for not being rough with me, physically or emotionally.*

You never interfered in the way I wanted to be. You're very caring.

This was one of those moments when it was clear to me why I was in nursing, why I stay in nursing. I returned later that night, when Bill called to say he thought that Jim was passing rapidly. Jim passed quietly in his sleep, with Bill holding him, and his mother and father, along with myself, at his side. It was a beautiful experience. Later, the four of us spoke of what the last week had been like. Bill explained:

I am so happy that Jim was able to pass in the home we worked so hard to build together, not in some hospital. He left this world in a dignified manner, surrounded by the people who loved him, and who he loved.

He then added one of the most wonderful compliments I have ever received, "Even though we have only known you a short time, we love you. We couldn't have done this without you." Susan added, "I felt safe knowing I could always call you. I knew you were always there." I thanked them for allowing me to share in their lives. When I left, Steve walked me to my car. We embraced, and he said: "Thank you for being here, for being so sensitive and respectful to our son and to us."

My experience with this family seemed like a textbook example of the way things should be. I didn't know what I would find as I went back and analyzed the data of this case. As I left that last evening, however, I knew that something of importance for nursing existed in it. There was no dissonance in this family or situation, only harmony. The dissonance in this case was from outside the family, in the health care system.

PRESENTATION OF THE FINDINGS

Data Analysis

Data analysis in a case study begins during data collection, as stated in previous discussions. A phenomenological strategy of content analysis was utilized to produce the final outcomes of the study. The researcher read, and reread over and over, the data collected. Some qualitative researchers refer to this process as dwelling with the data (Parse, 1987). This researcher prefers the term "residing" with the data. Residing with the data reflects the continual conscious and unconscious processes of experiencing the data at various times, in various places, in various ways. These experiences occur not only during structured or scheduled periods of data analysis, but also in momentary flashes of thought that appear as the researcher is immersed in the process. In residing with the data, major themes surfaced. The themes that emerged utilizing this process were dignity, love, security, presence, respect, and sensitivity. The themes were then cross-referenced with descriptive statements from the participants to provide an example of empirical evidence for their existence as themes. Each theme that surfaced was then examined in relationship to each objective that underpinned the research aim. The researcher resided with the themes, pondering: What phenomenon do these themes underpin in the lived experience of the situation of this case? The phenomenon that emerged from the themes of this case study was caring. The lived experiences of this case were central to the phenomenon of caring. The themes were then formulated into a meaning statement that responded to the research aim, which was to understand how a dissonant situation evolved into one of harmony. The situation evolved through caring. The meaning statement that emerged from this case study was: Caring is a sensitive, respectful presence of one human being for the dignity and need for love and security of another. The data in the case were interpreted utilizing the phenomenological process of analysis depicted in Table 11-1. The reader of a case study report should be able to move through the levels of abstraction by following the analytical flow of discourse utilized by the researcher in the process of data analysis.

Review of the Literature

As with other methods of qualitative research, the review of the literature is not conducted until the data analysis is completed.

Table 11–1
The Phenomenological Process of Analysis

Research Aim	To understand how a dissonant situation evolved into one of harmony	
Research Objectives	To understand the meaning evolving in this situation	To describe the ways of being in this situation
Descriptive Participant Statements	"Being loved as another human, as a fellow human being"	"Focusing everything I have at the moment on him, physically, mentally, and spiritually"
	"Realizing that this is my life, my situation"	"Realizing that I am a sensitive, feeling person; not being rough physically or emotionally"
	"Being able to be myself, to just be"	"Affirming my way of being, not judging or criticizing the way I am"
	"Feeling that another truly likes and enjoys what he or she is doing"	"Discussing options or possibilities; discussing, not telling"
Themes	Dignity
Love
Security	Presence
Respect
Sensitivity
Phenomenon	Caring	
Meaning Statement	The meaning of caring in this situation was a sensitive, respectful presence of one human being for the dignity and need for love and security of another.	

The term caring has been utilized extensively in nursing. The literature reviewed in this study is philosophical and theoretical, intended to compare the findings with existing knowledge. The works of three scholars—Sartre, Heidegger, and Watson—are congruent and substantiate the structure developed.

The tenets of Sartre's philosophizing are evident in the findings of the study. Sartre (1966) postulated that human beings choose the way they are in situations. The choices faced by humankind are paradoxical, indicating that there is more than one way to be in any situation. Sartre stated that "to be conscious of another means to be conscious of what one is not" (Kaufmann, 1963, p. 259). This statement exemplifies the participant's statement that "realizing that is my life, my situation" as a dimension of the meaning of caring. Sartre's work further exemplified "discussing options or possibilities; discussing, not telling" as a way of caring, articulated by a participant. Nurses entering into caring situations bear witness to and participate in the revelation of different ways of being as they are chosen and lived.

The meaning of caring that was uncovered coincides with the beliefs of Heidegger regarding being. The basic theme of Heidegger's work was the quest for being, truth, and time. Heidegger credited himself as the first thinker in philosophy to have raised the question of being (Heidegger, 1972). Being is an attribute of being. Being assumes an active role in determining the fate of being (Spiegelberg, 1982). This statement is relevant in ways of caring. The participants' statements—"affirming my way of being, not judging or criticizing the way I am"; "realizing that I am a sensitive, feeling person; not being rough physically or emotionally"—provided an internal perspective of being, in the process of assuming an active role in determining the fate of being as described by Heidegger. The responsibility of caring in nursing is profound when viewed from this vantage. The participant's statement "being able to be myself, to just be" is in accord with Heidegger's beliefs of being. Being able to be true to self in being is essential in the meaning of caring for another, as well as one's own self, not only within nursing, but also within life.

The concept of caring in nursing can be nebulous at times, to the point that it is almost necessary to clarify the "type" or "brand" of caring one is referring to. In this study, caring is viewed as an expression of the art of nursing. The art of caring, whether it be practice or research, must be founded in a value system that holds humanity in the highest regard. Watson (1988) eloquently set forth the values that are critical in the caring forms of nursing:

> . . . *deep respect for the wonder and mysteries of life and the power of humans to change; a high regard and reverence for the spiritual-subjective center of the person with*

power to grow and change; a nonpaternalistic approach to helping a person gain more self-knowledge, self-control, and self-healing, regardless of the presenting health-illness condition. This value system is blended with carative factors such as humanistic-altruism, sensitivity to self and others, and a love for a trust of life and other humans. (p. 73)

The living of these values in the process of caring is the preservation of human dignity and restoration—indeed, of humanity itself. The themes of the meaning of caring that emerged in this study—dignity, love, and security—are reflected in Watson's work. Empirical referents of the meaning of caring in the study, in relation to Watson's work, are statements such as "being loved as another human, as a fellow human being" and "feeling that another truly likes and enjoys what he or she is doing." Similarly, the themes of presence, respect, and sensitivity in the study substantiate the value system that Watson declared was necessary for caring. The meaning of caring that emerged is conceptually consistent with and provides an empirical example of Watson's theoretical work. It became evident during data analysis that the values that Watson described were not evident during the dissonance in this case, but were evident during the harmony.

Discussion of the Findings

Research is not conducted merely for the sake of research. If the findings of nursing research are not shared and utilized in the domains of the discipline, the entire process can be futile. The three predominant contexts of nursing are practice, research, and education. A nurse researcher has a responsibility to provide implications for each of these contexts.

Theory should provide a guide or approach to practice in a scientific discipline. Meaning statements of lived experiences generated from research that has been theoretically based can be utilized to guide practice. This study generated a statement of meaning for the centrality of caring that is theoretically congruent with Watson's Theory of Human Care. The essence of the centrality of caring as a sensitive, respectful presence of one human being for the dignity and need for love and security of another can provide a guide for nursing practice. A nurse in practice would recognize the importance of dignity, love, and security as the content of caring, as presence, respect, and sensitivity unfolded during the process of caring. Consideration of the meaning of a lived experience that has been generated through research, as in this study, provides the nurse with an insight of the caring experience from the perspective of those who have lived it. Another implication for the utilization of these results in the practice setting is the examination of these findings by nurse managers and administrators as they seek to create an environment conducive to nursing that is caring. The centrality of caring is as essential to the nurse as it is to the individual being cared for. A caring environment for the nurse, an environment where the nurse experiences caring, would lend itself to caring nurses. It would be difficult to enliven the essences of caring that emerged in this study in an environment where they did not exist.

The meaning statement that emerged from this study can serve as the genesis for further studies. The phenomenon of caring that unfolded in this case study could also be studied utilizing other qualitative methods. The themes that emerged could be examined as phenomena in further research studies. This study could also be replicated utilizing the case study method or other methods, to provide further insights into experiences of caring.

The findings of this study have implications for curriculum development in nursing. Caring appears to be, and I believe should be, a universal concept in nursing curricula. If this is to be the case, then nursing students must have a philosophical understanding of the concept. It would also behoove educators to ponder the process and content of caring as they engage themselves with students and move among their colleagues.

SUMMARY

This chapter has provided a rudimentary example of an exploratory/descriptive case study, utilizing phenomenological methods of data analysis. As discussed in the previous chapter, clearly delineated methods for case studies are not prevalent in the same way that other research methods are. The clear and fundamental design of this case study was purposeful as a demonstration of the utility of the method in day-to-day nursing. The aesthetic quality of the case study method is its simplicity of design. It is critical to note that the simplicity does not decrease the rigor or scientific merit of the process or outcome; in fact, an opposite argument could be made. The reporting style utilized was traditional so that the method could be clearly understood and compared to other research methods.

In closing, the researcher shares this poem, which emerged from the experience of this case. The poem artistically expresses the meaning of caring as it unfolded:

The Centrality of Caring

Nurse, when you look at me what do you see?
Your brother, sister, mother, father,
Your spouse or partner, a Beloved friend,
yourself?

Please see me for who I am, a fellow human being,
No more important than you—no less
I am not a social deviant
I never intended for this to happen
I merely did the best I could
With the life situation that I found myself in

I never wanted to hurt anyone
I don't want to hurt you

All I ask, nurse, is that you recall
The journey that brought you to nursing
Please, look at my journey

Please be with me in the same caring way
As I move from earth
As that nurse who cared for my mother and I
As I came onto earth

Nurse, you are often the only one I have
You have been called to the highest order
To care for humanity
You are graced by the universe
Please see

Beauchamp, 1992

REFERENCES

Beauchamp, C. J. (1992). *The centrality of caring.* Unpublished poem.

Heidegger, M. (1972). *On time and being.* New York: Harper & Row.

Kaufmann, W. (1963). *Existentialism from Dostoevsky to Sartre.* New York: Meridian Books.

Lincoln, Y. S., & Guba, E. G. (1985). *Naturalistic inquiry.* Beverly Hills, CA: Sage.

Newman, M. A. (1990). Newman's theory of health as praxis. *Nursing Science Quarterly, 3*(1), 37–41.

Parse, R. R. (1987). *Nursing science: Major paradigms, theories, and critiques.* Philadelphia: Saunders.

Sartre, J. P. (1966). *Being and nothingness.* New York: Washington Square Press.

Spiegelberg, H. (1982). *The phenomenological movement; a historical introduction* (3rd ed.). Boston: Martinus Nijhoff.

Watson, M. J. (1988). *Nursing: Human science and human care.* New York: National League for Nursing.

Yin, R. K. (1989). *Case study research: Design and methods* (rev. ed.). Newbury Park, CA: Sage.

12

Historical Research: The Method

M. Louise Fitzpatrick

*T*he purpose of this chapter is to introduce nurse scholars to the field of historical research in nursing. Specifically, the recent developments in historical inquiry as a scholarly pursuit, the objectives of historical research, and, most importantly, the methods, approaches, and procedures associated with historical investigation, analysis, and interpretation will be explored. Historical inquiry, by its very nature, implies a degree of subjectivity in the interpretation and narration of past events. However, the rigor of the research process, corroboration of facts, and comprehensive examination of available data serve to provide the objective evidence on which analysis and interpretative historical exposition rely. The balanced combination of objectivity and subjectivity in the process of the research distinguishes history from the chronicling of events at one extreme and unsupported anecdotal narrative at the other. Like all scholarly investigations, historical research requires careful attention to method and procedure and adequate training of investigators in both the method and the contextual background of the subjects they select for study.

HISTORICAL INQUIRY IN NURSING

Historical inquiry in nursing, as a legitimate scholarly pursuit, received increased attention over the decades of the 1970s and 1980s. The renaissance of interest in the profession's heritage reflects the concern of a mature profession with its antecedents, not only as a means of informing itself, but to gain a backdrop for current and future directions. History serves a pragmatic purpose as well as a contextual one. It connects us with a heritage and confers on us an identity, personally and professionally. Simultaneous with this heightened interest in nursing's roots has come the expansion of opportunities for doctoral study in nursing. Logically, some individuals found historical research an exciting and productive path to take as part of their doctoral studies and, ultimately, their preferred research agendas.

Understandably, there was resistance to this movement in some sectors. In some universities, there were no nurse historians prepared to guide students. In others, history departments were reluctant to guide students who had not had previous education and experience in historical research methods. In the majority of situations, there was documentation by nurse faculty who, understanding the need for greater research productivity in the field, emphasized the need for clinical research over all else and did not place a value on history or on scholarly attempts to interpret the profession's past.

Scholtfeldt (1975), in her classic article, "Research in Nursing and Research Training for Nurses," encouraged history and the preparation of historiographers for nursing and commented on the dearth of prepared historiographers (p. 181). She contended that a reason might be the extent to which nursing history is presented to neophytes in ways that capture and nurture their interests, and the unavailability of educational opportunities designed to prepare nurses for historical inquiry.

Persistence, administrative support in certain universities, and maintenance of a high standard of performance and rigor in the preparation of nurse historians provided catalysts for the renaissance during the 1970s. Finally, a revised opinion has developed of history's value and worth as a scholarly research endeavor among nurses prepared for such investigations.

From a small cadre of individuals, a growing community of nurse historiographers has emerged. Funding for historical research in the field is possible to obtain, and centers for nursing history and research have developed in selected universities where doctoral study in nursing history is encouraged. Additionally, organizations such as the American Association for the History of Nursing have evolved, thereby providing a network for colleagues in the field and a focus for programs, research conferences, and related activities concerning historical research in nursing.

THE OBJECTIVES OF HISTORICAL RESEARCH

History, like philosophy, concerns itself with the thought side of human existence. As such, it has worth in and of itself. There is usually a tendency to justify historical research in professional fields like nursing from the standpoint of its helping to inform future decisions and to avoid repeating past mistakes. Such arguments have only slight merit because they serve a reductionist belief that historical facts can be distilled with a formula. History, although its goal is the establishment of fact that leads us to truth, cannot be reduced to statistical proof. The historian views events as unique. Therefore, it is impossible to ensure that any set of variables, acting in concert, will arithmetically result in some outcome. In human affairs, there are always intervening variables that make it impossible to control or precisely predict destiny. In addition, as Tholfsen posited, there is danger in demythologizing everything, and an understanding of the limits imposed by the past is what makes liberation and revolution possible (1977, p. 247).

Commager contended that the scientific historian studies the past because it is part of the evolutionary process and that this process is the key to solving problems (1966, p. 10). Allen Nevins believed that history is to be enjoyed, not endured, and attempted to popularize the results of scholarly research without corrupting it (Billington, 1975, p. xxi). In a practice discipline, the sharing of the results of historical inquiry in ways that are interesting and useful to the majority of the profession's members is probably an important consideration. Narration, presentation, and connection of solid historical interpretation with current trends, issues, and areas of professional interest are the keys to the utilization of such research findings by the contemporary professional and to the education of students about their corporate heritage.

If one of the reasons for pursuing historical research is to build up the body of knowledge in nursing, it is also essential that ways be found to make findings useful to other historians and to the public. The relation of nursing's contributions and activities to the history of women, women's work, and women's studies needs to be strengthened. Related to this is the public's perception and image of nursing. History, effectively used, can serve as the collective memory of nursing's accomplishments, not just its struggles; therefore, it can be a principal socializing agent for new members of the profession.

Increasingly, the products of historical research can be viewed in action-oriented dimensions. They can provide prototypes for the development of leaders, they can inform strategic plans of an organizational and political nature, and they can contribute to the development of clinical practice. The outcomes of the historical research process can provide useful analysis of the recent past, as well as an evaluation of events and circumstances that have been well-tempered by time. Without compromising the quality of scholarship, the products of historical research for public consumption can effectively shape the public's perception of nursing, by better informing others concerning the profession and its contributions.

Synthesizing the past and present through useful insights contributes to the work of those who are architects of the profession's future and brings historical research in nursing into an active and useful mode, while continuing to expand the knowledge and understanding of the profession's genesis and evolution for more esoteric reasons. Although the value of historical inquiry needs no justification as a scholarly pursuit when it is applied within professional disciplines, those within the disciplines of both history and the professional fields may still require reassurances concerning the preparation and ability of the investigator, the rigor of the research method, and the utilization of findings. For these reasons, among others, maintaining high quality in the research process and in the narrative exposition is extremely important.

Increasingly, nurse scholar-historians, like other career-minded researchers, are embarking on a line or program of related research activity that they pursue over the course of their careers. This has the net result of increasing their expertise, making a more sustained contribution to the field, and contributing in-depth substantive data to historical knowledge in the profession.

The development and evolution of nursing as an organized profession, a scholarly practice discipline, and a system of education provide a rich source of potential areas for study. Nursing's relationship to world events also provides endless opportunities for study and research. Although valuable and credible historical surveys that highlighted major benchmarks in the profession's development were written as texts from the 1920s to contemporary times, more in-depth scholarly investigations and historical analyses about specific events, institutions, individuals, and changes in clinical practice have emerged over the past twenty years. During this more recent period of scholarship, foundational work has given way to more conceptual areas of study such as feminist themes and their relationship to nursing's development.

THE NATURE OF HISTORICAL INQUIRY

Various schools of thought have influenced the field of historiography just as they have affected all disciplines and professions. The extent to which investigators subscribe to or are influenced by their philosophical approaches to history has critical effects on the research activity and influences the products of the studies. Historical inquiry, like all research, has the discovery of truth as its objective. It is systematic in its method, and objective evidence is determined and judged by using tools of validity and reliability (commonly referred to as methods of internal and external criteria) in historical research.

Today, the schools of thought that traditionally influenced historians are rarely in evidence in their extremes. Rather, an eclectic use of approaches from several schools is generally operational among contemporary scholars. One example of a school of thought that has had both negative and positive influences on the course of historical research was the Positivist or Neopositivist school. In this reductionist approach, the historical method attempts to parallel empirical methods in the natural sciences. There is an attempt to reduce history to universal laws. Discovery, verification, and categorization of data are used to provide objective evidences that in and of themselves serve as the interpretation of past events. There is an effort to quantify, to show cause–effect relationships, and to force interpretation of data through preexisting formulas, models, and generalizations. This school of thought concerns itself with conditions as predictors of outcomes rather than attempting to discern what specific conditions caused the known outcome. This school of thought employs the use of hypotheses liberally.

The use of constructs and frameworks has a place in historical explanation, but there should not be an attempt to force the development of universal axioms to explain a unique phenomenon—the historical event. It is possible, however, to use some survey methods and statistical analyses commonly employed in the social sciences to enhance presentation of objective evidence. This has been successfully accomplished in nursing by Kalisch (1981), in particular. These measures in and of themselves do not lend themselves to good historical interpretation but can support it.

Another school of thought that has had influence on contemporary history and interpretation is the Idealist school, which places procedure, intuition, and experience as ingredients for interpretation. This line of thinking posits that all events have an inside and outside view and that the historiographer must get inside the event and rethink the thought of the originator in the context of his or her time, place, and situation, to make adequate historical interpretations.

Today, historiography is influenced by elements of both schools. From the Positivist school have come attention to rigor in method, use of hypotheses, and instruments of statistical investigation and historical explanation. From the Idealist school have come the emphasis on making interpretations within an appropriate temporal and social context and the importance of viewing events as unique and diverse. From the Positivist school, we acknowledge the possibility of describing patterns that seem to exhibit themselves over time; this possibility is shared by the Idealists, who ascribe what is exhibited to unique and interrelated circumstances. Interconnectedness, or a relationship of the parts of the whole, is necessary if coherent and meaningful historical explanation is to result from the research. Although the use of hypotheses is not common among inexperienced investigators, hypotheses can be used effectively in historical inquiry. The danger in their use is a tendency for the investigator to be attracted to and therefore collect only data that will assist in upholding a hypothesis, while inadvertently ignoring other data. This potential bias in data collection can influence the analysis and interpretation of a historical study and is therefore discouraged for novice investigators.

The use of theoretical frameworks, models, or approaches in the conduct of historical studies and their interpretation requires familiarity with the framework and sophistication in the analysis and interpretation of history. The more common or popular frameworks and approaches used by historians include:

1. *Great Person.* This approach focuses attention on individuals and their personal power within a social context. It is particularly useful when the objective of the research is a biographical study or there is a desire to provide emphasis on people who make changes, rather than the changes themselves.

2. *Deterministic.* This approach minimizes the importance and power of individuals in shaping history and relies primarily on predetermined moral/ethical or religious codes for making judgments and explaining historical phenomena.

3. *Sociological.* This approach emphasizes the primacy of social forces and their influence on people and groups as determinants of historical events. Using such a framework, historical phenomena are explained using social trends and

cultural events as instruments for interpretation of specific occurrences.

4. *Political/Economic.* This approach may employ the use of an ideology as a framework for interpretation of historical events and is frequently used in combination with the Great Person approach. The use of Marxism or other ideologies as a framework for explaining historical events is one example of this approach.

5. *Psychological.* This approach requires a solid grasp of psychology as well as facility in the historical method of research. It attempts to explain the thinking, motivations, and behaviors of individuals in a historical sense, using psychological theories as instruments for analysis and explanation. Erikson's biography, *Young Man Luther* (1962), is an example of such an approach. Both historians and psychologists have frequently raised valid concerns about the adequacy of either group when it takes on such complex interpretation.

THE PROCESS OF HISTORICAL RESEARCH

The initial stages of development in a historical study are critical to the process and the successful production of the product. Selection of a topic should be considered carefully and in light of its value as a contribution to the field. Frequently, seminal work in an area can provide the foundation for a logical extension and expansion of research on a specific topic. The degree of preparation of the investigator in historical research method, as well as the investigator's knowledge, history of the period under study, and background in nursing history, can considerably influence the ease of application of the research process and the confidence that can be placed on the result of the investigation. Frequently, the exposition of true interpretative history, as opposed to the development of chronicle, turns on these variables.

When a topic has been selected for study, the framing of the title becomes critical: the title takes on the same significance as the research question in other kinds of studies. Each word in the title is critical to communicating the thesis of the study and the relative emphasis that will be given to specific dimensions named in the title. Frequently, a time period will be specified, and words in the title will become devices to delimit the topic and determine the study's scope.

Early in the process, a thorough investigation and location of sources should ensue. It is possible that the most fascinating topics will become impossible research challenges unless, at the outset, the investigator can ensure the existence of sufficient data to study and research. Location of potential sources such as archives, libraries, and personal collections of individuals can be of great value in determining one's ability to execute the research and to further justify the study. In many instances, embarking on a historical study is like becoming a detective who leaves no stone unturned. Written sources and individuals can be of significant assistance in locating data and ensuring its adequacy for the investigation. Location of sources logically leads to an initial inventory of items that become helpful in shaping the process of the study and collecting data later.

The importance of taking sufficient time to craft the study design systematically, to consider the appropriateness of using or not using hypotheses or specific constructs, and to develop a plan and system that facilitate data collection and analysis cannot be minimized. Although data collection in such research tends to be time-consuming, additional time spent in preliminary steps will ensure more ease of analysis, interpretation, and exposition when the study develops beyond the data collection phase. Developing topical and chronological classification systems can be extremely helpful for filing collected data in ways that make it possible to retrieve them and to read notes in a variety of configurations preliminary to analysis and interpretation.

Sources of Evidence

Contemporary scholars generally agree that a variety of relevant sources, both primary and secondary, are valuable in providing data for historical investigations. Primary sources, either written or in the form of individual verbal responses, provide a firsthand account of an event from one who was present. Examples of primary sources include official documentary material such as verbatim minutes and proceedings, and interviews with individuals who were present at an event. Although recollection can be faulty and some documents may reflect the subjectivity of the recorder, in general, these are considered to provide strength to the discovery of truth and establishment of fact.

Secondary sources can also provide rich data. These are accounts of events at least once removed. They are not hearsay; they are data that can be accepted with confidence despite the fact that they are interpretative reports of events. Some of these may include articles written about an event, notes taken at a meeting or summaries of meetings, or narrative descriptions of events by individuals who were not present at the occurrence. Reliability of sources is not related to a particular category. Frequently, a secondary source may be more reliable than a primary one, such as an interview, which may be colored by egocentrism, hyperbole, and selective memory. A guiding and important principle in selecting and collecting available data is: (1) take measures to ensure balance when sources disagree, and (2) include sufficient amounts of available data in order to establish reliability.

The data collection stage, the longest stage of the historical research process, can be tedious and isolating. In order to guide data collection, it is helpful to develop a research outline that raises pertinent questions under each topic or time period. This serves to guide the investigator and maps the area of exploration that needs to be addressed through the process of data collection. The outline, while usually broad, should help to focus the investigator and sharpen the parameters of the study as related to the thesis contained in the title. Ideally, it leads to the articulation of specific questions to be asked of the data.

Establishing Fact from Objective Evidence

Two important elements in the research process involve measures of validity and reliability that form the basis for establishing fact. In historical inquiry, validity takes on the form of external criticism of the data. Questions may be raised about authenticity, origin, and originality of documents. Techniques to verify the authenticity of an author's handwriting, and composition of paper at various time periods, may also be expressed in more elaborate studies. Reliability is the primary means by which fact is established. The strength of the data leading to conclusions that result in the determination of fact depends on tests of reliability. When absolute fact cannot be established, probability and possibility become alternatives. Corroboration of data becomes the critical element in the process. As contrasted with validity, reliability is related to the internal criticism of data. Therefore, correct understanding of language, which itself evolves and changes over the decades, is important. Because parlance changes over time, accurate interpretation of the meaning of words in their particular social and temporal milieu becomes essential. Related to this is the adequacy of understanding the customs of a time period, which may be reflected through the language. Placing both words and events within an appropriate context is a basic ingredient for good analogies and interpretation.

Although there is resistance today to the use of formulas for the determination of historical fact, the following guidelines may be helpful to the investigator when setting out the requirements for establishing fact. Two independent primary sources that corroborate one another establish fact, as does one primary source corroborated by an independent secondary source that contains no substantial contrary evidences. When this is not possible, probability can be the goal. This requires data from one primary source with no substantial contradictory evidence, or from two or more primary sources that disagree only in some minor aspects. If neither fact nor probability can be established or when corroboration can occur only from secondary sources, possibility can be established using data from a primary source that cannot be critically evaluated. In short, reliability in historical research is an attempt to establish truth. Validity and reliability become critical elements in the conduct of the research and in the critique of the quality of a completed study. Historical evidence and proof are cited in references and footnotes. Frequently, multiple references are used to reflect the process of corroboration. Content footnotes that further explain information in the text are also useful devices for the historiographer.

Interviews, whether they are primary or secondary source materials, are usually best conducted after data collection from documents has taken place. This provides the opportunity for further clarification and corroboration of written material. Frequently, anecdotal material provided in interviews helps to connect disparate pieces of already collected data and assists the historiographer in interpreting the evolution and pattern of events.

When all known data have been reviewed and collected, the investigator usually becomes aware of a repetition that emerges in further data collection and is able to complete the process, confident that essential information has been gathered.

Development of Interpretative Report

The next phase of the study, sometimes taking weeks, involves careful review, reading, and analysis of the collected data. Simultaneous with this process is the construction of a highly specific writing outline. The more detailed the outline, the easier it becomes to engage in the interpretative and narrative phase of the investigation. A good writing outline helps to form the gestalt. The particular and unique are viewed in relation to the whole without losing their integrity. In addition, careful reading of the data provides understanding of the interconnectedness among events and moves the process from analysis to synthesis and, finally, to interpretation. Perhaps synthesis is the most difficult of the processes, development of the narrative the most creative, and giving meaning to facts through interpretation the most critical. Historical explanation expressed through the use of a unifying construct or framework, or narration based on the predetermined topical or chronological outline emerges through expository writing. At this point, subjectivity plays an essential part in bringing the research process to its logical conclusion. Subjectivity in the interpretation of objective evidence is central to the historical research process and distinguishes history from chronicle; researcher bias in the collection and selection of data must be carefully avoided. In the search for truth, objective evidence and facts provide the foundation for understanding the past; but interpretation by the individual investigator provides the perspectives and views that fill out our understanding of the past and raise new questions for study.

SUMMARY

The use of the historical research process in nursing is a valuable approach to expanding nursing's understanding of itself, and for interpreting the field and its contributions to others. It provides a scholarly means of connecting the field to the whole of human experience. Its liberating and liberalizing quality assists the profession further to define its identity through understanding of its heritage and to provide direction for its future. As a research method, it links nurse scholars with their colleagues in the humanities. As a scholarly pursuit within the professional field, historical inquiry, properly executed, has become essential to the refinement of nursing's understanding of itself.

REFERENCES

Billington, R. (Ed.). (1975). *Allan Nevins on history.* New York: Scribner's.

Commager, H. S. (1966). *The study of history.* Columbus, Ohio: Merrill.

Erikson, E. (1962). *Young man Luther: A study in psychoanalysis and history.* New York: Norton.

Kalisch, P. (1981). Communicating clinical nursing issues through the newspaper. *Nursing Research, 30*(3), 132–138.

Scholtfeldt, R. (1975). Research in nursing and research training for nurses: Retrospect and prospect. *Nursing Research, 24*(3), 177–183.

Tholfsen, T. (1977). The ambitious virtues of the study of history. *Teachers College Record, 79*(2), 245–257.

13

The Development of Organized Nursing and the Pan-American Exposition at Buffalo in 1901: Doing Historical Research

Nettie Birnbach

INTRODUCTION

The Pan-American Exposition held in Buffalo, New York, from May 1 to November 1, 1901, was conceived by James G. Blaine, former U.S. Secretary of State under President Benjamin Harrison. The exposition's purposes were to highlight examples of nineteenth-century development in the western hemisphere as well as demonstrate the positive relationships among countries of the Americas

(Pan-American Exposition, 1901, pp. 8-17). Besides featuring entertainment, cultural programs, lavish exhibits, and scientific displays, the exposition gave nursing public exposure by providing an opportunity for nurses and nursing organizations from the United States and abroad to meet to discuss common concerns and interests (Committee on Publication, 1901, pp. 21-22).

METHODOLOGY

The decision to investigate this particular event and its place in the history of nursing stems from prior knowledge of the era in which the event occurred and familiarity with the written testimony of participants who confirmed the impact of the event on nursing's progress. The title infers a relationship between nursing's organizational growth and the activities at the exposition. The purposes of this investigation, therefore, are to determine the specific nature of that relationship; analyze the effects of organizational activities on the development of nursing; identify key nursing figures and evaluate their contributions; and assess the socioeconomic and political climate affecting nursing at that time. The study combines the sociological, political/economic, and great-man approaches to historiography as defined in the chapter on historical method.

The use of primary data sources—original catalogs, programs, minutes, official proceedings, and reports prepared by the principals involved—fosters more accurate historical interpretation by permitting the researcher to interact with the past. Secondary sources—newspaper and journal articles, monographs in nursing history, and historical works of general interest—provides supportive information that facilitates corroboration. Placing events and people in their logical historical context reduces the likelihood of isolating nursing from the mainstream and contributes a broader perspective to the narrative.

The search for historical resources germane to the study led to Buffalo, site of the Pan-American Exposition. Several local historical societies and the historical collection at the Buffalo Public Library provided data relevant to the participation of Buffalo nurses in planning the activities of the nursing organizations that met during the exposition. The archives of the Smithsonian Institutions in Washington, DC, provided original programs, catalogs, and ancillary materials related to the exposition itself, and the official proceedings of the major nursing associations were rich sources of data on the topics discussed, issues debated, and other business transacted during the meetings.

FACTORS INFLUENCING NURSING

Increasing nursing's visibility by including a meeting of nurses in an event of international importance was not a new phenomenon. The precedent was established in 1893 when a nursing congress was convened at the World's Columbian Exposition in Chicago. The thrust of nursing's deliberations in Chicago was organization, and the outcome in the United States was the founding of the American Society of Superintendents of Training Schools for Nurses (Superintendents' Society) (Roberts, 1959, p. 25). At that time, organization was viewed as the means for advancing appropriate educational standards for nurses and initiating strategies to curb the sudden proliferation of unsound nurse training programs.

Although the need for trained nurses was first recognized during the Civil War, when great numbers of sick and wounded required nursing care, it was not until 1873 that systematic nurse training began in this country.[1] The development of nursing schools coincided with postwar changes that had a profound effect on the social, political, and economic structure of American life.

Women were becoming increasingly visible as wage earners, largely due to economic instability precipitated by the high cost of the war. The economic depression of 1873 generated financial problems for many families, and an increasing number of women were forced to seek work. By the late 1870s, teaching and nursing

---

[1] It is generally acknowledged that, in 1873, Bellevue Hospital in New York, the New Haven Hospital in Connecticut, and the Massachusetts General Hospital in Boston initiated the earliest systematic training of nurses.

were viewed by society as acceptable occupations for women. Nursing was particularly favored because it presented little threat to the male-dominated world of work (Jacobi, 1883, pp. 773–787; Warrington, 1879, pp. 490–503). As the number of women entering training schools increased, additional schools were needed.

Paralleling these events was the growing agitation for women's rights. The movement initiated by Elizabeth Cady Stanton, Lucretia Mott, and others at Seneca Falls, New York, in 1848 gathered momentum after the war. Joined by women like Julia Ward Howe, Lucy Stone, and Susan B. Anthony, the movement grew in scope and national prominence. The Women's Congress held in New York in October, 1873, focused on the need to improve educational and occupational opportunities for women as well as their political status (Browne, 1873). By the 1880s, the number of employed women exceeded 2.5 million, and education was available to more women than ever before (Merriam, 1920, p. 16).

Concurrently, there was marked population expansion in many urban centers. The rapid growth of industry, aided by an extensive rail transportation network, drew people from quiet rural areas to the bustling cities. The shift from an agricultural to an industrial society created problems, including those related to health. As cities grew in size, overcrowding resulted in substandard living conditions, an increase in crime, and serious fire hazards. An influx of immigrants in the years following the Civil War added to the already burgeoning urban population. In 1873, for example, approximately 400,000 people entered the United States from abroad (Curti, 1951, p. 491). Immigration continued unabated, and, in 1892, Ellis Island opened to receive immigrants for examination and processing. The lack of labor laws, rampant political corruption, and nonenforcement of sanitation codes compounded existing problems. Although upper-class families began to amass great wealth during this period, the laboring class continued to endure poverty and deprivation.

Humanitarian activities directed at ameliorating the suffering of the underprivileged and improving the general welfare of the public were gradually introduced by a variety of official and voluntary groups. Progressive reform was the overriding goal of select political and social groups. Dedication to social justice characterized

the work of individuals like Jane Addams at the Hull House Settlement in Chicago and Lillian Wald at the Henry Street Settlement in
New York. As public recognition grew, these efforts became more
organized and more widely supported. Nursing's contributions
were primary: direct services were provided to individuals and
families through home nursing programs. Fitzpatrick has provided
a description of specific reforms and the role of nursing during
this period (1975, pp. 4–8).

Scientific discoveries also contributed to the need for trained
nurses. The isolation of disease-causing organisms and the subsequent development of vaccines and treatment, improved surgical
and obstetrical techniques, and technological advances reduced
previously inherent risks in hospitalization.

Nurse training schools developed slowly at first; by 1880, fif-
teen schools were in operation in the United States. Hospital authorities gradually recognized the advantages to be gained from a
ready supply of inexpensive labor. As new hospitals emerged,
training schools were incorporated into many of these facilities
and nursing students became their work force. By 1890, the number of training schools had grown to thirty-five, and notable inconsistencies were evident from school to school. Few standards
existed with respect to length of program, admission requirements, and curriculum. Yet training schools continued to prolifer-
ate and no mechanism existed to control this expansion.

Recognizing the need for organization in order to effect reform,
the Superintendents' Society established at the 1893 Chicago Exposition undertook the task of developing uniform educational
standards for nurses. Lavinia Dock later wrote that the proceedings
of the Nursing Congress in Chicago contained the "seedlings of almost all the later lines of growth in the nursing profession . . . ."
(1912, p. 141).

THE TWENTIETH CENTURY

The years leading to the turn of the century were turbulent and
dynamic. Identified as the "Fateful Decade" by a nurse historian

(Christy, 1975, pp. 1163–1165), the period was characterized by a number of significant events. The financial panic of 1893, resulting from a sudden drop in the price of gold, led to massive unemployment and an economic depression. In 1894, Jacob S. Coxey led an "army" of the unemployed from Ohio to Washington, DC, to ask Congress to enact emergency legislation to create jobs. In 1896, the *Plessy v. Ferguson* decision created the "separate but equal" doctrine. In the same year, William McKinley was elected 25th president of the United States. In 1897, the discovery of gold in the Yukon Territory generated a gold rush second only to that of the 1840s.

Advancement continued in science, medicine, technology, and education. Although higher education was more readily available to women and labor unions focused on the female worker to a greater extent, male domination prevailed in every facet of life—the arts, literature, humanities, sciences, politics, and religion. By the end of the nineteenth century, the number of women wage earners had markedly increased; however, most worked in factories or business offices. Women in Wyoming, Colorado, Idaho, Utah, and Montana were permitted to vote, but universal suffrage was still unattainable and the prevailing male attitude continued to view women's place as the home.

A strong social reform movement led by journalists, educators, sociologists, and health care professionals was emerging during this period. Writers like Lincoln Steffans, Ida Tarbell, Ray Stannard Baker, and Upton Sinclair were beginning to develop the literature of exposure, which addressed corruption and the exploitation of the public by various big business enterprises. Theodore Roosevelt would later refer to this group of reformers as the "muckrakers."

For nursing at this time, protection of the public's health and the welfare of the individual nurse were matters of vital concern. Recognizing the progress made in medical education as a consequence of the activities of medicine's national organization, the Superintendents' Society moved toward establishment of a national organization for nurses as one of its priorities. In 1896, the first steps were taken to organize nursing on a national scale and on February 12, 1897, the Associated Alumnae of Trained Nurses of the United States and Canada was officially established (Associated Alumnae).[2]

According to the 12th Census, the total population of the United States in 1900 was 75,995,000. Life expectancy was 48 for males and 51 for females, and people looked forward to the new century with optimism and a continuously expanding spirit of reform.

With respect to nursing, the issue of standards for nursing education was a matter of great urgency by 1900. The number of nursing schools increased to 432, and nursing's leadership group was alarmed by the disparities in the quality of the nursing programs among schools. Similar problems were acknowledged by nurses in Great Britain, Ireland, France, and other countries. The movement toward a national legal credentialing mechanism for nursing practice was already in progress in Great Britain under the leadership of Ethel Gordon Fenwick. In the United States, however, the regulation of professions was the right of the individual states. Thus, the movement to credential and register American nurses would require separate legislation state-by-state. The Associated Alumnae initiated strategies to establish state nurses' associations—"the last link in the chain of organization" (Robb, 1900, p. 101).

Like nursing, medicine was contending with the issue of overcrowding in the profession, and stronger controls were needed if fraudulent practice was to be eliminated. Between 1890 and 1904, organized medicine demonstrated impressive strength and unity in seeking revision of the laws affecting practice. Standards for state licensure established by the American Medical Association contributed to the upgrading of medical education (Shryock, 1967, p. 111). The legal profession also was struggling with the issue of acceptable standards for practice but the existence of varying legal codes among the states created impediments to reform. Consequently, it was not until 1921 that law established its licensing procedures.

---

[2] In the process of incorporating, Canadian nurses were excluded from membership because of a conflict with state regulations. In 1911, the Associated Alumnae of Trained Nurses of the United States became the American Nurses Association.

The movement of the professions toward legislative reform reflected the trend toward progressive change in this country. The awakening of the nation's social consciousness by the "muckrakers" through the exposure of abuses in health-related industries like food and medicine production eventually resulted in the enactment of legislative constraints that mandated compliance with elevated standards. Formerly held doctrines opposing governmental intervention in private enterprise were replaced by positions supportive of official restraints. The middle class particularly clamored for state and municipal enforcement of regulatory mechanisms (Schlesinger, 1933, pp. 395–396). The increased awareness of the need to protect the public, as reflected in the implementation of numerous statutes during the closing years of the nineteenth century, more than likely provided an external stimulus to nursing's leaders as they consolidated their efforts in the pursuit of legal regulation for nursing and control of the profession. By 1901, state nurses' associations were established in New York, Virginia, and Illinois.

THE EXPOSITION

Economic conditions in the United States improved during the early years of the twentieth century. Income levels for American workers rose and many families enjoyed a higher standard of living. The introduction of new labor-saving devices for the home decreased the time needed for household chores. Conveniences like the automobile improved transportation; the telephone increased communication capability; and electricity facilitated the use of new machinery and other inventions. The popularity of President McKinley was confirmed in 1900 when he was reelected to serve a second term.

The prospect of an international exposition in Buffalo in 1901 was greeted with enthusiasm. The previous World's Columbian Exposition in Chicago had been highly successful in attracting the public and was of particular importance to women through its international focus on women's work. The Pan-American theme of the 1901 exposition and the repeated attention given to women would prove to be equally attractive to Americans and visitors from foreign countries who traveled to Buffalo.

An outstanding feature of the exposition was the harmonious color scheme carried out on the facades and in the interiors of its buildings. The attractiveness of the arrangement gave rise to the term "Rainbow City" (Waldron, 1901, p. 1).[3]

Occupying 350 acres and built at a cost of $10 million, the exposition displayed up-to-date sanitary procedures and equipment (e.g., modern plumbing and garbage disposal; Arnold, 1901, p. 2) and focused attention on electrical advancements like various types of lighting, incubators, electrically operated elevators, and other machines and appliances. Many of the electrical exhibits were illuminated at night. One in particular, the Great Electric Tower, stood prominently in the center of the exhibition grounds (*Official Catalogue and Guide Book to the Pan-American Exposition,* 1901, pp. 26–27).

Besides beautiful sculpture, flower gardens, a women's building, and exhibits devoted to ethnology and the graphic arts, there was a mile of streets called "The Midway" with as many as forty different attractions. The most sensational and most popular was the "Trip to the Moon." People boarded an "air-ship" that simulated travel away from earth to the planets (Waldron, 1901, p. 15).

BOARD OF WOMEN MANAGERS

A Board of Women Managers, organized in 1900, had responsibility for the women's building and its utilization. The board arranged exhibits of women's work and sent invitations to women's groups to meet during the exposition. One of the members of the board was Annie Damer, a prominent nurse in the Buffalo area who was also President of the local Buffalo Nurses Association (Board of Women Managers of the Pan-American Exposition, 1901–1902). Damer wrote to Ethel Fenwick, President of the International Council of Nurses, to invite the Council to meet in Buffalo

[3] Select photographs of the buildings and sculpture are in the September, 1901, issue of the *American Journal of Nursing.*

in 1901. Arrangements had already been made for the Associated Alumnae and the Superintendents' Society to hold their conventions at the same time. Damer suggested that an international congress of nurses be held to coincide with the many planned nursing meetings (Breay & Fenwick, 1931, p. 14).

Other groups meeting at the exposition included the New York State Federation of Women's Clubs, the National Council of Women, and the Spanish-American War Nurses. The Board of Women Managers had successfully executed their plan to promote the visibility of women in general and nursing organizations in particular.

INTERNATIONAL STATUS OF ORGANIZED NURSING

In the United States, the Superintendents' Society was comprised of superintendents of nurse training schools. In Great Britain, a similar configuration applied to the Matron's Council of Great Britain and Ireland. Founded in 1894, the Council focused on issues of concern to nurses and initiated reforms relative to nursing education and credentialing. In June, 1899, the Council addressed nursing topics at the International Congress of Women. At that meeting, Ethel Gordon Fenwick, former matron of St. Bartholomew's Hospital in London, proposed to establish an International Council of Nursing (Dock, 1900, p. 114). Besides the United States and Great Britain, nursing organizations were operational in Denmark, Holland, and France, among other countries. According to Fenwick, an International Council of Nursing would "provide a means of communication between nurses of all nations . . . . to confer upon questions relating to the welfare of their patients and their profession" (1900b, p. 789).

Ethel Gordon Manson Fenwick was born in Scotland on January 26, 1857. When she was a young child, her father died, her mother remarried, and the family moved to England. When she was in her early twenties, Ethel Manson completed her nurse's training at the Royal Infirmary in Manchester and in 1881 was appointed Matron at St. Bartholomew's Hospital in London, a position she maintained for six years. Following her marriage to Dr. Bedford

Fenwick in 1887, she resigned her position and began her crusade for nurse registration in Great Britain. It was Fenwick's conviction that registration for qualified nurses was in the best interests of both the public and nursing (*American Journal of Nursing*, 1901c, pp. 861–867).

In 1888, Fenwick organized the British Nurses Association; its objective was registration. In 1893, she acquired the *Nursing Record* and used its pages to publicize the causes to which she was committed. Although the British Nurses Association suffered multiple defeats in its struggle to achieve legal recognition for nurses, Fenwick persevered and became an international spokesperson for organization and registration. She had a central role in planning the British women's exhibit at the Columbian Exposition in Chicago and orchestrated the International Nursing Congress held there (Hector, 1973, pp. 42–45).

After founding the International Council of Nurses (ICN), in 1899, Fenwick was named its first president and devoted her energy to strengthening nursing's international ties. At a meeting of the ICN in London in July, 1900, Agnes Snively of Canada and Lavinia Dock of the United States (who was secretary of the ICN) were charged with establishing a nursing committee to plan for an International Congress of Nurses to be held September 18, 19, and 20, at the Pan-American Exposition at Buffalo in 1901 (*American Journal of Nursing*, 1900, p. 62). Isabel Hampton Robb, Linda Richards, Isabel McIsaac, and several others joined with Snively and Dock to form the nursing committee. Working in conjunction with the local Board of Women Managers, the nursing committee developed strategies to promote the attendance of nurses at the congress. Letters requesting foreign and domestic nursing associations to send delegates were sent to Great Britain, Scotland, Sweden, Holland, Italy, Australia, and other nations (*American Journal of Nursing*, 1901a, p. 373).

Plans were already under way for the Superintendents' Society, the Associated Alumnae, and the ICN to hold business meetings and/or conventions prior to the Congress. All three organizations were scheduled to meet on September 16, at different times, in the Women's Educational and Industrial Union Building on Niagara Square. September 17 was reserved for additional meetings, should there be a need for more time (*American Journal of Nursing*, 1901b, pp. 747–748).

The International Congress was scheduled to meet in the Women's Educational and Industrial Union Building from September 18th through the 20th. Although the building was not on the exposition grounds, it did provide the space needed for the various associations and for a large group of nurses to congregate. The final nurses' meeting was held in the Temple of Music at the exposition on September 21 (Bennitt, 1901; Breay & Fenwick, 1931, pp. 17–19; *Proceedings of the Eighth Annual Convention of the American Society of Superintendents of Training Schools for Nurses,* 1902, p. 3). It was customary for the exposition managers to designate specific dates for the recognition of select groups. September 21 was Nurses Associated Alumnae Day, a day for honoring nurses.

THE INTERNATIONAL CONGRESS OF NURSES

The Congress convened on Wednesday, September 18, and began its proceedings on a sad note. President William McKinley had been shot while attending a reception at the exposition on September 6. For several days, it seemed that the president might recover, but the onset of infection led to his death on September 14. That same day, Vice-President Theodore Roosevelt was quietly sworn in as the 26th President of the United States at the home of Dr. Wilcox, a well known Buffalo physician and friend of Roosevelt (Archives of the Theodore Roosevelt Inaugural National Historic Site).

Irrespective of the atmosphere of mourning prevailing in Buffalo, the nurses were welcomed to the city by various officials, and the opening ceremonies included a resolution to extend condolences to Mrs. McKinley. In her address to the congress, Isabel McIsaac, Presiding Officer, called attention to the many problems confronting nursing. She cited "the uniform requirements for admission to our schools, the uniform curriculum, what shall constitute a trained nurse, state registration, local and national organization . . ." among others (Committee on Publication, 1901, p. 19).

American nurses attending the congress came from all sections of the United States, and foreign representation included Canada, Great Britain, Scotland, Cuba, India, Australia, South Africa, and many more. Reports on nursing education and organization had been sent to the congress from nurses throughout the world, and the papers presented covered topics such as hospital administration, nurses' societies, preparatory instruction of student nurses, women on hospital boards, army nursing in the United States and India, district nursing, and inspection of tenement housing (Committee on Publication, 1901, pp. 27-271).

THE ROLE OF MRS. FENWICK

Fenwick delivered two eloquent addresses at the Buffalo proceedings. The first, "The Organization and Registration of Nurses," was presented on September 20 and advocated membership in nursing societies through alumnae associations. She proposed that each country establish a national council of nurses which in turn would be eligible for membership in the International Council of Nurses. Fenwick further recommended that nursing take control of its own regulation and advancement through a system of registration that would guarantee that trained nurses were appropriately qualified (Committee on Publication, pp. 335-343).

Her second address, delivered at the Temple of Music on September 21, was "A Plea for the Higher Education of Trained Nurses," which noted the additional educational requirements imposed on nursing by scientific progress. Among the immediate goals to be attained she identified "preliminary education . . . post-graduate teaching . . . [and] special instruction as teachers." She praised the nurses of the United States for taking the lead in inaugurating the postgraduate Hospital Economics course at Teachers College, Columbia University (begun in 1899), and encouraged the audience to undertake similar programs in other institutions of higher learning. She emphasized that "the time has come when nurses need their educational centers, their endowed colleges, their chairs of nursing, their university degrees, and State registration" (Committee on Publication, pp. 363-368).

The transactions of the congress centered on nursing's control of education and practice through legally authorized strategies. A resolution unanimously adopted stated:

It is the duty of the nursing profession of every country to work for suitable legislative enactments regulating the education of nurses, and protecting the interests of the public, by securing State examinations and public registration, with the proper penalties for enforcing same (Committee on Publication, p. 351).

Another resolution adopted by the assembly strongly protested the custom of sending student nurses on private duty assignments in patients' homes during their period of training (Palmer, 1901a, p. 147).

The action taken by those assembled confirmed that the autonomous regulation of nursing had become organized nursing's primary objective.

THE ROLE OF SYLVEEN V. NYE

Sylveen V. Nye, first president of the New York State Nurses Association (NYSNA), was a native New Yorker and member of a distinguished family. Nye graduated in 1890 from the Indianapolis City Hospital Training School for Nurses at the age of 30. In 1894, she settled in Buffalo, New York, where she remained until her retirement in 1926. Her professional experience comprised employment as head nurse, private duty nurse, and administrator, but the position that occupied the major part of her career was with the Women's Department of the New York Life Insurance Company (*American Journal of Nursing,* 1936, p. 1173; *Quarterly News,* 1937, p. 19).

Nye's significant leadership skills became apparent in 1895 when she orchestrated the establishment of the Buffalo Nurses Association (BNA). Founded for the purpose of bringing nurses together to share common concerns, the association's objectives focused first on local needs and later on statewide issues.

Recognizing that the growing demand for qualified nurses presented an opportunity for nursing to advance, Nye advocated the organization of a state association for nurses in New York. She believed that through a state organization nursing could achieve the legislation required to implement uniform standards for training schools, legal recognition of the title "Nurse," and other measures that would protect the public from the untrained. Early in 1900, Nye met informally with a group of equally committed nurse leaders to examine the feasibility of founding a state association. A committee was formed with Nye as chairman, and planning was initiated for a statewide meeting to be held in the spring of 1901. Fifty-six nurses assembled in Albany on April 16 and 17, 1901. There, NYSNA became the first state nurses' association in the country and Nye was elected its first president (Nye, 1900, pp. 397–400).

Nye also participated in the proceedings of the International Congress of Nurses by delivering an address on the organization and registration of nurses immediately following Fenwick's discussion of the same topics. Nye agreed with the idea of organization and registration but differed from Fenwick with respect to the methods of achieving those goals. She espoused membership of individual nurses in state societies rather than through alumnae associations. She favored the inclusion of all nurses who graduated from recognized schools and viewed that mechanism as the most equitable way to achieve the broadest representation. In devising strategies to achieve legislation, Nye proposed acquiring the support of medicine and hospital authorities, stating that it would be a mistake to ignore their advice (Nye, 1901, pp. 343–347).

Opposing viewpoints regarding the implementation of strategies were not uncommon as organized nursing progressed through its formative years. The international forum provided by the exposition permitted nursing to address commonalities and differences from country to country and to develop a mutually acceptable agenda for the future. Recognizing their commitment to the public welfare, the nurses assembled in Buffalo unanimously agreed to work toward local, national, and international organization for the purpose of upgrading nursing education and practice.

The inclusion of a nursing congress in each of two early international expositions reflected strategic planning designed to publicize nursing issues. In reviewing the outcomes of the Buffalo Congress, Sophia Palmer, first editor-in-chief of the *American Journal of Nursing,* predicted that the results of the 1901 meeting would surpass those of 1893 (1901b, pp. 941–942). Her prophecy was verified by the events that followed. The transactions sparked the determination of both American and foreign nurses and many embarked on campaigns to advance nursing on an international level.

OUTCOMES

Following the exposition, efforts to establish more national associations abroad were successful. Nurses organized in Germany, Ireland, and China, and regulation of the educational preparation of nurses was their priority (Dock & Stewart, 1920, pp. 252–298).

The organization of state associations for the purpose of improving nursing education and achieving credentialing for qualified nurses was overwhelmingly supported in the United States. However, differences emerged with respect to implementation and titling. Some states opted to retain the two-year nurse training program; others moved to a three-year model. Curriculum content reflected broad variations and the question of an appropriate title for the credentialed nurse generated suggestions like Trained Nurse, Graduate Nurse, and Registered Nurse, among others. Registered Nurse was ultimately selected and became the focus of proposed legislation (Birnbach, 1982, pp. 72–73).

Despite divergent viewpoints on some issues, there existed a unique spirit of common purpose among American nurses as they moved forward to attain their goals. In 1903, four states enacted registration laws;[4] by 1909, state nurses' associations were formed in thirty-three states. Twenty-two years after the 1901 exposition, legislation regulating nursing was in effect in forty-eight states, Hawaii, and the District of Columbia (Birnbach, 1982, pp. 110–111).

In a prevailing climate of progressivism that focused attention on the needs of society, nursing seized the moment to initiate

[4] North Carolina, New Jersey, New York, and Virginia, respectively, enacted legislation.

strategies to reform nursing education and practice and to establish the RN credential for those nurses who met the required standards.

CONCLUSION

Resolutions that were adopted and discussions that took place at the nursing congress in Buffalo helped shape the purpose from which organized nursing could proceed. Educational reform and the enactment of regulatory mechanisms became vehicles for distinguishing between competent and incompetent nurses and, over time, produced desirable results.

Unquestionably, the women's movement, in conjunction with other external forces already delineated, influenced nursing's decision to expedite the drive for reform. Fenwick confirmed the relationship when she said that "the evolution of the trained nurse . . . depends upon the evolution of the woman" (Fenwick, 1900a, pp. 56-57). Although stereotypical notions surrounding gender differences were obstacles facing nursing and the absence of universal suffrage was an additional barrier, organized nursing was able to effectively promote and obtain official endorsement of its proposals.

The worldwide growth of national nursing organizations provided the means for international connectedness and collaboration in the exchange of ideas and exploration of shared areas of concern. The five hundred nurses who entered their names in the register at the Buffalo congress began a tradition that strengthened the International Council of Nurses and made its survival a reality to this day.

REFERENCES

American Journal of Nursing (1900). Announcements. *American Journal of Nursing, 1*(1), 62.

American Journal of Nursing (1901a). Official Reports of Societies. *American Journal of Nursing, 1*(5), 373-375.

American Journal of Nursing (1901b). Official Reports of Societies. *American Journal of Nursing, 1*(10), 747-748.

American Journal of Nursing (1901c). Foreign delegates and organizations: Ethel Gordon Fenwick. *American Journal of Nursing, 1*(12), 861-867.

American Journal of Nursing (1936). Obituaries. *American Journal of Nursing, 36*(11), 1172-1173.

Archives of the Theodore Roosevelt Inaugural National Historic Site. Buffalo, NY: Wilcox Mansion.

Arnold, C. (1901). *Glimpses of the Pan-American Exposition.* Buffalo: The Courier Co.

Bennitt, M. (1901). *Bennitt illustrated souvenir guide, Pan-American Exposition.* Buffalo, NY: Goff Publishing.

Birnbach, N. (1982). *The genesis of the nurse registration movement in the United States, 1893-1903.* Unpublished doctoral dissertation, Teachers College, Columbia University.

Board of Women Managers of the Pan-American Exposition. (1901-1902). *Handwritten minutes of the Board of Women Managers.* Buffalo, NY: Board of Women Managers.

Breay, M., & Fenwick, E. (1931). *History of the International Council of Nurses, 1899-1925.* Geneva, Switzerland: The International Council of Nurses.

Browne, C. (1873). The woman's congress. *Chicago Journal,* November 26, 1873. In the Scrapbooks of Julia Ward Howe, Schlesinger Library, Radcliffe College.

Christy, T. (1975). Nurses in American history: The fateful decade, 1890-1900. *American Journal of Nursing, 75*(7), pp. 1163-1165.

Committee on Publication. (1901). *Third International Congress of Nurses.* Cleveland, OH: J.B. Savage.

Curti, M. (1951). *The growth of American thought,* 2nd ed. New York: Harper & Row.

Dock, L. (1900). The International Council of Nurses. *American Journal of Nursing, 1*(2), pp. 114-118.

Dock, L. (1912). *A history of nursing: Vol. III.* New York: Putnam.

Dock, L., & Stewart, I. (1920). *A short history of nursing.* New York: Putnam.

Fenwick, Mrs. B. (1900a). The evolution of the trained nurse. *The Outlook, 64*(1), 56-57.

Fenwick, E. (1900b). The International Council of Nurses. *American Journal of Nursing, 1*(11), pp. 785-790.

Fitzpatrick, M. L. (1975). *The national organization for public health nursing, 1912-1952: Development of a practice field.* New York: National League for Nursing.

Hector, W. (1973). *The work of Mrs. Bedford Fenwick and the rise of professional nursing.* London: Royal College of Nursing.

Jacobi, A. (1883). The historical development of modern nursing. *Popular Science Monthly, 23*(10), 773-787.

Merriam, C. (1920). *American political ideas 1865-1917.* New York: Macmillan Co.

Nye, S. (1900). The proposed New York State Nurses Association. *Trained Nurse and Hospital Review, 25*(6), 397-400.

Nye, S. (1901). Organization and registration. In Committee on Publication (Ed.), *Third International Congress of Nurses* (pp. 343-347). Cleveland, OH: J.B. Savage.

Official catalogue and guide book to the Pan-American Exposition (1901). Buffalo, NY: Arhart Publishing.

Palmer, S. (1901a). Editor's miscellany. *American Journal of Nursing, 2*(2), 147.

Palmer, S. (1901b). The editor. *American Journal of Nursing, 1*(12), 941-942.

Pan-American Exposition. (1901). *Art handbook: Official handbook of architecture and sculpture and art catalogue to the Pan-American Exposition.* Buffalo, NY: David Gray.

Proceedings of the eighth annual convention of the American Society of Superintendents of Training Schools for Nurses (1902). Harrisburg: Harrisburg Publishing.

Quarterly News (1937). Sylveen V. Nye. *Quarterly News, 9*(1), 19.

Robb, I. (1900). Address of the president. *American Journal of Nursing, 1*(2), pp. 97-104.

Roberts, M. (1959). *American nursing: history and interpretation.* New York: Macmillan.

Schlesinger, A. (1933). *The rise of the city: 1878-1898.* New York: Macmillan.

Shryock, R. (1967). *Medical licensing in america, 1650-1965.* Baltimore: Johns Hopkins Press.

Waldron, H. (1901). *With pen and camera at the Pan-American Exposition.* Portland, ME: Chisholm Brothers.

Warrington, H. (1879). Hospital nurses and ladies. *Contemporary Review, 34*(2), 490-503.

Part Three

Other Considerations in Qualitative Research

The following chapters address a variety of questions and concerns frequently expressed not only by students of nursing science but also by teachers, consultants, and reviewers of qualitative research. The content represents our best thinking at this time in response to those questions and concerns. An effort has been made to acknowledge and describe controversy, in part to communicate the openness of our responses. We have modified our views over the years and expect to continue to do so. The references for each chapter potentially expand the content through study of other sources.

Chapter 14 discusses ethical considerations in the context of qualitative research process and in accord with the spirit of the qualitative paradigm. Specific guidelines are offered as either complementary or supplementary to those discussed in some of the methods chapters. In Chapter 15, the challenges of the review processes for study proposals are discussed, with special attention to funding concerns; in Chapter 16, specific guidelines are presented for developing proposals and presenting research reports. Chapter 17 addresses the issue of combining qualitative and quantitative approaches, placing it in the context of divergent views of these two paradigms and inviting readers to arrive at their own positions on this controversy. Lastly, Chapter 18 reviews various approaches to the evaluation of qualitative research and, with reference to a study of proposal reviews, offers specific suggestions for gaining a positive evaluation of proposed research.

14

Ethical Considerations in Qualitative Research*

Patricia L. Munhall

A s members of the scientific community, nurse researchers have become adept at identifying and applying criteria for evaluating the various aspects of quantitative research. We may even have surpassed our colleagues in other disciplines in the level of rigor applied when evaluating the design, method, and protection of human subjects of a study.

With regard to the protection of human subjects, I like to think that rigor is founded on a profound reverence for human beings and their experiences. As nurse researchers, we have become increasingly sophisticated in our qualitative research endeavors and

* Reprinted with permission of *Western Journal of Nursing Research*, *10*(2), 150–162, 1988.

have begun to identify distinct considerations and criteria for viewing the ethical dimensions of qualitative research.

Naturalistic, direct involvement and participation with people necessitates acknowledging the subjective nature and activity of the researcher as the main "tool" of research. Qualitatively oriented nurse researchers prize this direct involvement, yet contextually are faced by the canonization of objectivity detachment of prevailing convention. In contrast, qualitative nurse researchers face the "nitty gritty," the serendipitous, the passions, the complexity of subjectivity, and attachment to people and their vicissitudes.

The purpose of this chapter is to provide one of the stepping stones needed to differentiate criteria that are essential and appropriate for qualitative research methods in nursing. This discussion will focus on selected ethical considerations with the following themes interwoven throughout: ethical means and ends, collaborators as means, conflict methodology, models of fieldwork, and process consent. Potential for role conflict within the investigator is discussed from the perspective of the therapeutic imperative and the research imperative.

UNDERLYING ASSUMPTIONS AND DILEMMAS

In the tradition of qualitative research methods, I would like to state, or bracket out here, my own beliefs and values and their implications for ethical considerations when doing qualitative nursing research:

1. The therapeutic imperative of nursing (advocacy) takes precedence over the research imperative (advancing knowledge) if conflict develops.
2. Nursing reflects a deontological ethical system (people are not to be treated as means). However, if individuals consent to be part of our research, they have, in essence, joined the research enterprise. Instead of being called subjects or objects, they are now collaborators (Punch, 1986).
3. Informed consent is a static, past-tense concept. Qualitative research is an ongoing, dynamic, changing process. Because

of unforeseeable events and consequences, a past-tense consent is not appropriate. We need to facilitate negotiation and renegotiation to protect our collaborators' human rights. Therefore, a verblike consent seems necessary and the concept of process consenting reflects the ongoing dynamic nature of qualitative research.

ETHICAL MEANS AND ENDS

Bellah (1981) sets our stage for ethical dialogue with the premise that all inquiry has normative commitments. Arguing that all social inquiry is linked to ethical reflection, he uses the term "moral sciences" interchangeably with "social sciences." He states: "Social science must consider ends as well as means as objects of rational reflection" (p. 2).

Laudan (1977) focuses also on the consequence side of science when he states: "Science is essentially a problem-solving activity" (p. 66). Wilson and Fitzpatrick (1984) state that the purpose of nursing science is "to render reality intelligible as it relates to human health and development" (p. 41).

The question to be asked from an ethical perspective then is: Toward what goal and for what end? For our purposes here, let us suggest that for the most part, nurse researchers are very much interested in "problem solving" or "problem-preventing" research and that our motives are to produce an end that is in some way considered "good." In this way, research assumes a normative commitment, something that "ought" to be. The most apparent example of this is that many of our research endeavors focus on facilitating "health." The search for a means to produce a desired health outcome requires critical ethical reflection.

Other aims we have in addition or in conjunction to the attainment of health are assisting people to reach their potential, to self-actualize, and to reach their maximum well-being. Actually, many of these ends are equivalent to or similes of the concept of health.

Acknowledgment that our aims have normative commitments is critical because we then move on to ways (means) to achieve our decided good. In essence, our aims become prescriptive. An example may serve to illustrate this point.

Ethical Aims

One of our normative commitments is to help individuals achieve their maximum potential. In this pursuit we do a qualitative study of a group of "underachievers" who are not attaining full intellectual potential or physical health potential. The ethical questions that arise include whether the ethical aim is to assist those subjects we study or future generations. What do the underachievers, whom we study, have to gain from our studying them? Further, is it a given that our mission is to help people reach their maximum potential if unrequested?

Although our society has accepted and promoted some goods, we need to reflect upon them. Some may actually be in opposition to others. For example, a "steady state" or some form of "equilibrium" may indeed *be in opposition* to an achievement ethic. In qualitative research, knowledge of our collaborators' aims and normative commitments are an intrinsic component of the research process. We need to reflect on our own, and perhaps more important, their normative commitments.

Ethical Means

In *The Prince,* Machiavelli proclaimed his aim of a free, independent Italy, free from outside governance as an end that was readily proclaimed as good. However, his means to that end illustrated moral vacuity. Machiavelli believed that corruption is natural to man. However, by generalizing a behavior to *all* "men," he justifies his means in order to obtain an end. Human experimentation is based on the "ends justifying the means" principle.

Changing people's behaviors, often an aim in the helping professions, contrasts sharply with understanding different behaviors and accepting and supporting those differences. Perhaps not all people need or want to reach their maximum potential. Some philosophers such as Kant believe humans have a moral obligation to reach their maximum potential. The question then becomes, Do nurses have a moral obligation to help others attain a moral obligation? This is an example of an ethical consideration which needs in-depth exploration from nurse researchers.

Aims Versus Means

Ethical consideration in qualitative research (and quantitative as well, though it is not spelled out) entails knowing explicitly and implicitly what our ethical means and aims are. Entering and participating with our collaborators seems a precious experience that calls upon us to reflect, know, and bracket what our ethical means and ends are. A negotiated view requires such reflection.

Perhaps the most critical ethical obligation that qualitative nurse researchers have is to describe the experiences of others in the most faithful way possible. This ethical obligation is to describe and report in the most authentic manner possible the experience that unfolds even if contrary to your aims. Perhaps it might appear wonderful not to strive to maximum achievement of one's potential! Not having to achieve a level of significance to accomplish your aim may be the highest degree of freedom possible when doing research.

THERAPEUTIC VERSUS RESEARCH IMPERATIVE

Ethics is a tangled web of principles where one can usually see the position of the opposition as having some legitimacy. That is why ethical dilemmas are thorny, at best. In the instance of the therapeutic imperative and the research imperative, the ethical systems of deontology and utilitarianism potentially conflict. The nurse who is doing research needs to acknowledge what her therapeutic imperative is. Is it deontological, where the individual is not a means to an end but an end as such? Is it advocacy for human beings? Is it based on justice, beneficence, and respect for patients' rights? The researcher also needs to reflect on the research imperative. Is it utilitarian, where people are used as means to further knowledge? Is the researcher posing possibly uncomfortable conditions for her participants? Is the researcher working under a utilitarian posture where the ends may justify the means? In qualitative research, some conflicts that present dilemmas for researchers are as follows:

Means	Ends
Entry	Departure
Confidence	Disappointment
Elation	Despondency
Commitment	Perceived betrayal
Friendship	Desertion

From a utilitarian perspective, those results listed at the right may seem unavoidable in fieldwork. From the deontological perspective, they are ethically problematic.

Role conflict evolves from behavioral expectations that may differ in the nurse's therapeutic imperative and in the researcher's imperative. Given the potential for harm in fieldwork, consideration must be given to these dilemmas so as to minimize or prevent them from occurring. Communication is a vital process, as is a team or joint approach to research. Perhaps even the term *participant-observer* could be abandoned, simply titling all those involved as *participants* or, as mentioned, *collaborators*. It may be helpful to understand, from a human perspective, that if there is to be a departure, that all involved are prepared and that the researcher, too, often does feel sad. In essence, there is a real "joining" of feelings and understandings.

IS BEING A COLLABORATOR A MEANS TO AN END?

Suppose a nurse-anthropologist-researcher asked you to participate in her study titled, "Contemporary Women's Hassles: An Exploratory Study," and she asked whether she could visit you in your home at various times when you were available to "sort of" observe and interview you. Also, she asks, would it be all right to visit you in your office? Rock (1979) states: "No sociologist I know would himself agree to become a subject of observational research" (p. 261).

Well, what is at stake here? When I think of this, very much is at stake, and we need to walk in our collaborators' shoes. Sure, there are hassles for the contemporary woman, but having this researcher come into my home seems not only another hassle, but perhaps a crisis! One needs to be concerned about the usual ethical considerations of fieldwork: privacy, confidentiality, achieving accurate portrayal, and inclusion and exclusion of information. In this instance, however, as in many others, the psychological burden and threat that an outsider might pose need serious consideration. Regardless of all of our efforts to act in the collaborators' best interest, some invasion, as it were, occurs to the person or people involved. The end that we hope to accomplish may be laudable, but we are cajoling ourselves, I think, if we are not aware that there is some inconvenience or discomfort in the process of being observed. The unknown consequences of the observation, it seems, could contribute to pervasive anxiety state for the participants, whether consciously or unconsciously. Rather than the casual "within two to three weeks the person or persons seemed comfortable with my presence" or "I was virtually unnoticed after two or three weeks," we need, as advocates, to attend to other possibilities that occur with observations. We can ask ourselves, "Would we be comfortable until the results were in?" Empathizing with and attending to the process of being an observee must be ongoing on the researcher's part. We may feel blended into a culture, but that does not mean the observees are experientially where we are.

As was mentioned, nursing seems to espouse the deontological principles, that human beings are to be treated as ends and not means. In contrast to that system is utilitarianism, which argues that the ends justify the means. From that perspective, one can use another person for the good of others and to advance further knowledge. Technically, the research enterprise turns people into means, and though one could argue that this occurs far less with qualitative research, the potential still remains. We have come to some peace with this issue through the process of informed consent, where, in effect, the individual joins the research enterprise. Joining the effort accords individuals the opportunities of contributing to society, of being of service and perhaps advancing a cause of their own. We may not have thought of informed consent from that perspective, but ethically it helps to resolve the means–end dilemma and also makes the term collaborator much more accurate.

INFORMED CONSENT IN QUALITATIVE RESEARCH

Fieldwork that is existential and authentic involves the negotiation of trust between the researcher and the participants. Entering into fields in the various roles of participant-observer is a privilege. We are "allowed" into someone else's world with its customs, practices, and events, which we promise to describe faithfully and without bias. While we are negotiating entry into this world, we invite the participants to become part of the research enterprise and validate that agreement with an informed consent.

Informed consent has been defined as:

knowing consent of an individual or his legally authorized representative, so situated as to be able to exercise free power of choice without undue inducement or any element of force, fraud, deceit, duress, or other forms of constraint or coercion. (Annas, Glantz, & Katz, 1977, p. 291)

Typically, informed consents include the title, purpose, and explanation of the research and the procedures to be followed. Risks and benefits are to be clearly spelled out. A statement that the participant has had the opportunity to ask questions and that the participant is free to withdraw at any time is also included (Field & Morse, 1985). This model of informed consent evolved out of experimental research; some of it is applicable to qualitative research, but to resolve some of the aforementioned dilemmas more seems needed.

PROCESS CONSENT

Because qualitative research is conducted in an ever-changing field, informed consent should be an ongoing process. Over time, consent needs to be renegotiated as unexpected events or consequences occur. I may, in a weak moment, sign a consent for our previously mentioned researcher to observe me in my home, but without the full realization of what the consequences might be. To be ethical in this situation, the researcher needs to assess the effects of involvement in the field and continually acquire new permissions. Maybe children will react negatively to an outsider in their home, and perhaps the contemporary woman will find keeping some semblance of cleanliness of her home on a daily basis is just the hassle that will take her over the edge.

Common sense plays a large part in renegotiating informed consent. If our focus should change, we need to ask participants for permission to change the first agreement. This is important from the perspective of sensitivity to our collaborators as well. They may wonder why you "lost" interest in a particular part of the field and chose something that you obviously have found "special." Continually informing and asking permission establishes the needed trust to go on further in an ethical manner.

Secrets

Another area that needs ethical consideration in fieldwork is confidentiality of the exchanges between the researcher and the participants. Both informed and process consent should carefully delineate the data to be included in the study. Role conflict can be generated when the participant wants to tell you a secret or an off-the-record remark. The "nurse" listens to this, and in fact, knows that a bond has been established that is valuable. However, the "nurse researcher" and participants will probably be better off if the researcher gently reminds the participant of the purpose of the study and that all communication is supposed to be part of the study (Field & Morse, 1985). If it is possible, as may be the case in a health care facility, the participant can be referred to an appropriate person with any information not relevant to the study. The idea here is to discourage participants from telling secrets unless these secrets can be part of the study. This, of course, needs to be done with the utmost care, for secrets are treasures, *but more important, imply promises to keep them.* Most often these problems can be discussed quite openly with collaborators.

Witnessing unethical or illegal conduct can pose another ethical dilemma. If we are nurses, and as such, the client's advocates, we cannot place the research imperative above the therapeutic imperative. Some (Estroff & Churchill, 1984) suggest that clear procedures be established prior to the start of the study that spell out the channels the researcher will go through if unethical or illegal practices are witnessed. Researchers are morally obliged from the therapeutic imperative to report such violations. The ethical dilemma of whistle-blowing helps us to understand this particular problem.

Findings and Publication

Anonymity of subjects individually or as a group is often a requisite of qualitative research. However, sometimes individuals and cultures allow themselves to be identified. An understanding about anonymity, of course, is part of the informed and process consent. What is often not mentioned or planned for is publication and dissemination of findings. With all research, what the researcher intends to do with the findings needs to be a part of the consent. A longitudinal view from point of entry to publication needs to be agreed upon with our collaborators. Being observed can have quite different consequences than reading a description of yourself or of your culture or hearing from someone who has such information. To prevent misunderstandings, all involved need to agree upon the various stages and activities of the entire project. What will happen to the descriptions? Will they be presented at conference? Will they be published, and where, and for what purpose? Our collaborators need to agree to dissemination of findings, from an ethical perspective of deontology, because they are part of the entire project. Because we may not foresee the consequences of publication, it is wise in this litigious society to protect not only our collaborators but also ourselves.

CONFLICT METHODOLOGY

Conflict methodology in fieldwork is built on the interactionist and ethnomethodological perspective, adding the belief that ordinary social life is characterized by deceit and impression management (Douglas, 1979). Opponents of this method maintain that the researcher is justified in using similar techniques, because it is the explicit purpose of research to expose the powerful and that deception is "legitimate" (Punch, 1986, p. 32).

The argument is based on an end that may in itself be highly moral (recall Machiavelli); yet the means are acknowledgedly unethical, but within the conflict methodological view, justified. There are ethical arguments advanced for conflict methodology, but if civilization hangs on to the Kantian principle, certainly this is a most dangerous practice.

The counter argument to justifying deceit is nicely summed up by Warwick (1982):

Social scientists have not only a right but an obligation to study controversial and politically sensitive subjects . . . but this obligation does not carry with it the right to deceive, exploit or manipulate people. My concern with backlash centers primarily on the alienation of ordinary individuals by research methods which leave them feeling that they have been cheated, deceived, or used. (p. 55)

In nursing research, deception, exploitation, or manipulation of people would be ethically antithetical to all we philosophically stand for professionally. Our concept of client advocacy precludes the use of conflict methodology. In addition we need to be alert to *nuances* in our research that could cause individuals to feel "cheated, deceived, or used." I have often heard collaborators comment that they were supposed to receive a copy of the research report but never did. Thus they feel cheated. In some of our methods and consents, the collaborators actually see the report or description before finalization for their response and agreement to the portrayal. This may also assist invalidation and an accurate portrayal. From an ethical perspective, we need to determine which models of fieldwork seem consistent with our belief system.

MODELS OF FIELDWORK

The extent to which invasion into a social setting is ethical or not is often a matter of common sense. The researcher needs to be aware of what is not being told, as well as what is being said. Also, the extent to which the research is a covert or overt operation is open to ethical evaluation. Here, again, the ethical aim needs to be clear. There is a fine line between doing anthropological research and an "investigation" in the journalistic or "FBI" sense.

Punch (1986) conceives of three models of fieldwork and relates them to ethical features of trust and deceit:

1. The hypothetical "problemless" project, when for instance, a graduate student gains entry into a commune, shares daily life, is accepted, departs to write a description, and allows the culture involved to read and validate what has been written. There is no high trauma, drama, or problems, and as Punch (1986) points out, this type of study is like the classical ethnography when the investigator could be sure that the Ashanti and Nuer would not be scouring the anthropological journals with their lawyers for negative references to tribal life. Today I am not sure we can even say that!

2. The "knotty" project, when the institution erects barriers against outsiders and gaining access becomes difficult. An example of this might be a state mental institution where those associated with certain practices fear publication in the interest of preserving the institution's and their own reputation.

3. The "ripping and running" project, when there is deliberate concealment, which in addition to being ethically indefensible, is illegal. This model depends upon an unrevealed person posing as a member of the group. This practice has the connotations of spying and undercover investigating and certainly violates civil liberties.

Many of us doing fieldwork like to believe that, as moral agents, we may come to identify problems and abuses within cultures or institutions. Because of that ethical aim, we may be tempted to justify unethical means, such as bending the truth, to gain entry in order to obtain an accurate portrayal. Such practices again constitute conflict methodology and have serious consequences for collaborators and researchers in the field.

The second and third models of fieldwork hold the potential for moral, social, and political change. However, in the long run, using these two models will have the effect of "closed doors" in the field due to loss of trust, credibility, and confidence in nurse researchers. The last model of fieldwork violates the very foundation of our nursing practice. Whistle-blowing again is the topic that needs to be addressed and certainly is not limited to practices witnessed by researchers. For instance, in any type of health care facility where unethical practices exist, the moral obligation of reporting such practices belongs to all involved. However, as was mentioned under process consent, preplanning for such events, should they occur, is one way of ensuring that your course of action is known and has been agreed upon prior to the commencement of the study.

SUMMARY REMARKS

There is much more to be discussed within the topic of ethical consideration of qualitative research. There is much still to be discussed about qualitative research methods in nursing. So these remarks are not concluding but contribute to the dialogue centered on the developing interest in these methods. One facet is clear, though: One cannot transpose criteria for quantitative research and apply them to qualitative research.

The static, past tense of informed consent does not adequately protect human subjects in qualitative studies. For that matter, it may not always for quantitative methods.

The most glaring difference, however, springs from the dynamic, process-oriented qualities of qualitative research. Qualitative research could be thought of as a verb, a process, with the ethical components constantly being scrutinized. "Process consenting" might be a way to remind ourselves of the ongoing nature of discussing with our collaborators the means and the aims of our study.

In addition, our therapeutic imperative and research imperative need to be as clear as possible. From an ethical perspective, the therapeutic imperative provides the research imperative, so that efforts to avoid any difficulties or disadvantages to the collaborator need our constant vigilance if the research is to proceed ethically.

Because we, as nurses, have the ethical theme of deontology threaded throughout our philosophies, I think we are humanistically ahead of many other disciplines in considering the ethics of our research enterprise. Our egos are not split. We are patient-client advocates, where trust, compassion, and empathy encompass all our nursing endeavors, including research.

REFERENCES

Annas, D. J., Glantz, L. H., & Katz, B. J. (1977). *Informed consent to human experimentation: The subject's dilemma.* Boston: Ballinger.

Bellah, R. (1981). The ethical aims of social inquiry. *Teachers College Record, 83*(1), 1–18.

Douglas, J. D. (1979). Living morality versus bureaucratic fist. In C. B. Klockars & F. W. O'Connor (Eds.), *Deviance and decency.* Beverly Hills, CA: Sage.

Estroff, S. E., & Churchill, L. R. (1984). Comment (Ethical dilemmas). *Anthropology Newsletter, 25*(7).

Field, P., & Morse, J. (1985). *Nursing research: The application of qualitative approaches.* Rockville, MD: Aspen.

Laudan, L. (1977). *Progress and its problems: Towards a theory of scientific growth.* Berkeley: University of California Press.

Punch, M. (1986). *The politics and ethics of fieldwork.* Beverly Hills, CA: Sage.

Rock, P. (1979). *The making of symbolic interactionism.* London: Macmillan.

Warwick, D. P. (1982). Tearsome trade: Means and ends in social research. In M. Bulmer (Ed.), *Social research ethics.* London: Macmillan.

Wilson, L., & Fitzpatrick, J. (1984). Dialectic thinking as a means of understanding systems in development: Relevance to Roger's principles. *Advances in Nursing Service, 6*(2), 41.

15

Institutional Review of Qualitative Research Proposals: A Task of No Small Consequence*

Patricia L. Munhall

PLACING THE TASK IN CONTEXT

A colleague of mine sent her research proposal to a large university hospital where the sample for her study was to be derived. She followed the format precisely and was somewhat surprised when she was asked to appear before the Institutional Review Board (IRB) of the hospital. When she arrived she was astonished to find

* Reprinted with permission from Sage Publications; Qualitative Nursing Research: A Contemporary Dialogue, J. Morse (Ed.), 1989, 1991, pp. 258–271.

26 members of the Board present. They discussed the project with her for two hours, and engaged in what appeared to be an internal struggle over the design and conceptual framework of the study, before granting her permission to conduct the study.

My colleague's study was a traditional quantitative research project. Ironically, the study was not to be conducted within the institution itself; rather, the nurse-researcher wanted to do a follow-up mailing to all patients who had had hip-replacement surgery. My purpose in this chapter is to place the review of qualitative research proposals in a perspective where this context can be understood. According to Noble (1985), IRBs often pose problems for researchers, *regardless* of their research method: "A frequent solution . . . is to engage in minimally clinical projects, such as research involving healthy, intelligent, middle-class clients . . ." (p. 293).

Using this solution, many researchers have looked for subjects outside of institutions. That is one alternative, but since many nurse-researchers are committed to research within institutions, the aim of this chapter will be to facilitate the IRB process, specifically with qualitative research proposals.

The Setting

In this chapter, the presentation of qualitative research methods to IRBs in institutional settings will be addressed. Similarities of IRB requirements for qualitative and quantitative research designs will be discussed. Departures and additions specific to qualitative research methods will be analyzed, with emphasis on the educational aspect of research proposals. Also, the idea of process consent will be examined, and the appearance of qualitative researchers before IRBs with research proposals will be discussed.

Institutional Review Boards are the conscience of an institution. They are deeply concerned with human rights and human dignity. The principles of patient autonomy and rights of privacy, confidentiality, anonymity, self-determination, and safety are critical components of the philosophical statements of IRBs.

The most important aspect of any research proposal is the education of our colleagues about qualitative methods and the assurance that we share the same concerns for the dignity and rights of our human subjects. A psychological principle pervades this need for education as most people are generally invested in the status quo, that is, the familiar. Individuals on IRBs are, for the most part, accustomed to the traditional quantitative research design and thus feel a certain amount of confidence when reviewing these proposals. Qualitative research designs within the traditional medical science setting present problems for these individuals and raise questions simply because the reviewers are unfamiliar with the more unstructured qualitative research methods. This leaves the qualitative nurse-researcher with a task of no small consequence.

The Challenges

Qualitative research in institutional settings presents different challenges from those of more traditional research methods. The three main challenges in receiving permission to conduct qualitative research in institutions are:

1. The IRB's unfamiliarity with the methods, language, and legitimacy of qualitative research;
2. The structural-functionalist perspective that pervades most institutions;
3. The conscious or unconscious perception of the similarity of qualitative research methods with investigative type journalism.

Although these challenges are interrelated, each one will be addressed separately.

The Unfamiliarity with Qualitative Research Methods

Most IRBs (and in fact, most grant review panels) have members who are unfamiliar with the aims and outcomes of qualitative research. Presently, many IRBs are developing guidelines and are uncertain about the role they play in the institution. Their task is complex—so complex that a request for the release of names to do a follow-up mailing to individuals who are no longer patients (as previously described) resulted in a major meeting of the IRB. The receipt of a proposal with a method called "phenomenology" may also result in an invitation to provide further information.

Phenomenological studies aim at understanding a phenomenon by studying the essences of a life experience with thoughtful attention, and they search for what it means to be human in the attempt to discover plausible insight. Many members of IRBs are not familiar with such language in a research proposal. They will ask, "What is phenomenology?" or "What is grounded theory?" Though these questions do not spell disaster for proposed qualitative research projects, they do complicate matters because these important questions are asked from the structural-functional perspective of institutions.

The Structural-Functional Approach of Institutions

The structural-functional perspective is often viewed as the sacrosanct way of organizing a bureaucratic institution. Roles are prescribed, functions are distributed, behavior and outcomes are predictable, and all should go well according to fixed rules and procedures. The values in our health care institutions seem removed from or, at best, unrelated to qualitative research aims. For the most part, without our health care institutions, pragmatic goals prevail. There should be an action, an intervention, and a concrete observable task with a measurable outcome. Pragmatism in research is narrowly perceived, for example, the idea of testing something to solve some problem. The idea that understanding preceding experience or any lived experience has pragmatic value is not self-evident from the highly structured functional perspective. From this perspective, the search for "meaning" appears irrelevant. It is this search for meaning that creates confusion in some minds about the difference between qualitative research and investigative journalism.

Similarity of Qualitative Methods with Investigative Journalism

All research methods are essentially investigations, but perhaps, they are more threatening to individuals when unstructured interviews and the possibility of threatening participant observation technique are part of the research design. Quantitative research designs are by nature more specific, the variables are already known, and the researcher searches for relationships between variables. On the other hand, discovery, the finding out about something otherwise not fully understood, is often the aim of qualitative research designs.

Within institutions, such studies may be perceived as threatening. Interviewing patients may cause staff to worry about negative information the patient may give, for example, complaints, reporting incidents, and so forth. If there is to be observation, who does not experience some anxiety about the idea of being observed? Fear, then, is an important feeling to consider, and one that cannot be summarily dismissed, for what if you do "discover" some "negative" findings that do not reflect well on the institution or staff?

These challenges must be addressed in any proposal that goes before an Institutional Review Board. The strategies for meeting these challenges include education and translation, establishing compatible values, and generating trust.

MEETING THE CHALLENGES

Education and Translation

Becoming sympathetic to the concerns and psychological dynamics of the individuals on Institutional Review Boards is the best place to start. In many cases, qualitative research proposals may not be understood by these individuals, may be contrary to the way they think, and may be threatening to them. In addressing these challenges, one should realize that the normal human response to change is resistance. Many qualitative nurse-researchers in institutions have reported that "resistance" was the only response to their research proposal and that they have had to change their proposal or move out of the institution. Although this is unfortunate, this situation can be avoided if qualitative nurse-researchers will educate their colleagues who sit on IRBs about the nature and philosophy of qualitative methods.

Most board members are thoroughly familiar with the methods associated with the Western Mind-Set of objectivity, control, prediction, and so forth. No one needs to explain "ex post facto," correlation, experimental designs, or statistical test, but phenomenology, grounded theory, ethnography, or whatever qualitative research method is going to be used must be explained. Not only must it be explained, but it must be presented in language that can be understood by individuals familiar with deductive, pragmatic, numerical ideologies.

There is a need to explain in concrete terms the primacy of perception, embodiment, and the philosophical concepts. All these ideas should be clearly stated in language that the reader will understand. For example, in submitting a proposal for a qualitative research project that will examine the needs of patients who have had a mastectomy so that appropriate nursing interventions can be developed, language such as "the lived experience" of having a mastectomy, consciousness, and essences may be used but need to be explained. Is this a capitulation, a compromising of our principles? On the contrary, it is the recognition that it can take years to understand these concepts and that, in a proposal, there is a limited amount of time and space for explanation. So instead of a capitulation, it is actually a pragmatic action for a pragmatic setting. If the institution reflects a structural-functionalist approach, it is unrealistic to think that this perspective will not also be reflected in the process of an IRB review.

Compatible Values

In structural-functional bureaucracies, the reality is that the search for meaning, apprehending essential relationships among essences, thematic analysis of cultures, perceiving another's world, and discovering core variables are at odds with the predominant problem-task orientation. Helping patients find meaning does not rank high among institutional objectives. So this objective must be stated in the proposal in pragmatic terms, such as, this study will result in improved nursing care or act as the basis for developing nursing intervention. Also, the qualitative method must appear structured, even if there are fluidity and some flexibility in the design. As far as possible, research aims should be compatible with the aims of the institution. The members of the IRB must not think they are making an exception by accepting a qualitative research proposal, because it appears different from their value orientation. It is best, from any point of view, to *demonstrate the convergence of values* between the institution and the qualitative study by stating how the study's *quest for discovery is laying the groundwork for nursing intervention.*

Generating Trust

Developing trust and alleviating fear and/or anxiety within the institution is critical to a successful qualitative research proposal, and it is also one of the more awkward challenges. This difficulty arises from the perplexing situation in which the staff worry about the researcher having access to potentially damaging information or observing poor nursing care. They wonder what the researcher is going to do with possible "negative" findings.

This difficulty can be dealt with by pointing out that quantitative researchers in institutions may also witness and be part of the same environmental activities as qualitative researchers, and that the staff themselves are probably aware of whatever problems exist. Ideally, ethics committees or quality assurance programs address these problems, yet there is always the possibility that qualitative research may uncover some problems, and consequently, the staff may feel threatened.

The first step in dealing with this problem is to include a category for "unanticipated findings" in the proposal and to carefully spell out what channels the nurse-researcher will use to share such findings. If the members of the IRB understand that *findings that indicate problems are important to discover* so that they can then be solved, members and staff might be more assured. Again, education is important for achieving this perceptual shift. Traditionally, IRBs are familiar with research that attempts to *solve problems.* The value of research that may *identify problems* so that they too may be addressed needs to be stressed, and stressed, and stressed. Indeed, it is critical to identify the right problem *before* testing solutions.

Sometimes this is difficult to do, such as when patients complain during interviews about poor nursing care. A good qualitative researcher looks at the larger context (before reporting such a result, ethics demands that the lens of the study must be widened) and finds that there is inadequate staffing. Although the administration may not be happy with that finding, the nurses on the unit will be glad to have such an important need substantiated. At other times the issue is thornier. Perhaps the poor nursing care is the result of an incompetent nurse. Although the nurse-researcher cannot be the only one to know of this, he or she is ethically obligated to report these findings through the channels that are established prior to starting the project (see the example in Field & Morse, 1985, pp. 48-49). While this is essentially "whistle-blowing," with its attendant consequences, sometimes good, sometimes bad, this action embodies the belief that "the therapeutic imperative of nursing (advocacy) takes precedence over the research imperative (advancing knowledge) if conflict develops" (Chapter 14, this volume).

These problems have fewer ramifications for researchers not researching in their home institution, and if possible, it may be wise not to conduct research in one's home institution. Also, IRBs have members who wish to protect their institution and/or their own reputation. This is a difficult problem that should be addressed in qualitative research proposals in positive, helpful terms and fully discussed with staff. They too need to be fully informed about the research project.

Similarities Between Qualitative and Quantitative Proposals

There are many similar areas in qualitative and quantitative proposals that are of concern to Institutional Review Boards. More than likely, both type of methods will be using the same form, and the researcher will be asked to address the following areas:

1. Objective of study
2. Research methodology

3. Characteristics of group(s) involved
4. Special groups (children of compromised adults)
5. Type of content
6. Confidentiality of data
7. Possible risk involved
8. Nonbeneficial research

Although there may be other variables, ensuring that individual rights and human dignity are protected needs to be demonstrated and documented. Often, Institutional Review Boards have more elaborate requests than those listed above, and qualitative research proposals are often evaluated on adherence to traditional scientific method. Scientific legitimacy, then, is being evaluated rather than human subjects' protection. This may not be a problem 10 years from now, but today, proposals come back from IRBs with questions that indicate reluctance to approve the proposal because the Board does not understand the method and its concomitant language. As was previously suggested, educating members of IRBs about the scientific legitimacy of qualitative studies is an additional task for qualitative nurse-researchers. What follows are some distinguishing characteristics of qualitative research that need to be addressed in IRB proposals.

Departure and Additions for Qualitative Research Proposals

Depending on the institution, a brief overview of the aim and purpose of qualitative research methodology may precede the proposal or, perhaps, be the introductory paragraph. This does not have to be a highly sophisticated discourse about worldviews and paradigms, with quotes from Husserl, Erasmus, or Speigelberg; rather, a simple paragraph explaining how qualitative research methodology seeks to discover new knowledge, uses narrative descriptions in the findings, involves interviews with individuals, and so forth, is all that is necessary. Stating that these aspects of the methodology can be used to build upon one another may be important. Nurse-researchers often get into difficulty by discussing intersubjectively, going "to the things themselves," living the question, and so on. Understandable language is critical.

Objective of the Study. As was previously discussed, the objective of the study should ultimately be stated in pragmatic language. Often the aim of qualitative research is stated in existential terms. Remember the setting and take the existential purpose one step further by showing how the study might, for example, (a) improve staff performance or (b) assist the patient in recovery.

This approach is appropriate because it is the qualitative research baseline that enables quantitative researchers to develop hypotheses for nursing intervention, staff performance, and assisting patients in their recovery. Stress the importance of the study in pragmatic terms.

Research Method. This is perhaps the most important part of the proposal and it offers the best opportunity for educating members of IRBs. Introduce the method, the rationale for choosing the method, and the outcome of this method. Take the reader through a step-by-step narrative in language that is familiar. This may mean taking the proposal that was written for nursing colleagues of a similar bent and translating it for individuals who may be puzzled over the use of the word "phenomenon." For example, instead of saying "lived experience," just say "experience." In fact, someone once asked me what other kind of experience there is! Perhaps replacing the phrase "ontological commitment" with "it is my belief that" will also be helpful.

Although it may be human to want to impress one's colleagues with a high level of abstraction, it will probably be counterproductive. In any case, it seems paradoxical when qualitative research is actually very interested in the concrete. No one wants to feel inadequate, and it seems unwise to send out proposals loaded with unfamiliar language. Again, in order to achieve IRB approval, *members must be able to read* qualitative research proposals *without a dictionary.*

So qualitative researchers need to be clear and emphatic about their research methods. They need to teach about the method and its pragmatic usefulness to nursing sciences in language that will not distract the readers but keep them focused on the substance.

Consequence.   There is a debate in the literature as to whether informed consent is necessary when observations and discourse occur during nurses' routine work (Noble, 1985; Oberst, 1985). Interviews have often been exempt from formal informed consent procedures if verbal consent by an individual is given. However, I fear we will be on a slippery slope if too many of these exceptions to the written consent process are allowed. Common sense needs to prevail.

Within institutions, qualitative researchers need to anticipate a request for informed consent. If more than one interview or observation is going to take place, the idea of a process consent seems to exemplify a negotiated view of not only the "phenomenon" but also the study itself (Chapter 14). All consents need to take into consideration the individual's capacity, full disclosure of the research activity, and voluntariness to enter and, of course, to withdraw freely. An inclusive consent can be found in Field and Morse (1985).

A proposal for process consent is suggested because an informed consent represents a past-tense concept. Qualitative research is often an ongoing, dynamic, changing process. A process consent offers the opportunity to actualize a negotiated view and to change arrangements if necessary. A process consent encourages mutual participation and, perhaps, mutual affirmation for the participants and the researcher.

A process consent for qualitative nursing research should be developed with the research participants' input, ideas, and suggestions and reviewed at specific times if necessary. This approach is appropriate if the researcher is going to be doing observations or participant observations over a period of time. In addition to the informed consent, a process consent should address some of the processes listed in Table 15-1.

It is probably wise to have information about self-disclosed secrets in the process consent. It should be stated that all data obtained will be part of the study. In other words, secrets should be discouraged if they cannot be included in the study. It is best to explain to the participants that some secrets pose a dilemma for researchers who are also concerned about the patient's well-being. The question of secrets and patients' confidentiality needs to be

Table 15–1
Process Consent

Researcher and Participant as Collaborators come to agree upon
  how you will enter the field
  how often, for how long
  how you will leave the field
  how you will prepare to leave
  how you will share the information
  how you will keep the information anonymous and confidential
  how you will assure an accurate portrayal
  what you will do if focus changes
  what you will do with "unanticipated findings"
  what you will do with secrets and confidential material
  what you will do with inclusion and exclusion of information
  where are the findings to go

Comments by participant

Comments by researcher

Dates reviewed and changes made

Signatures

Note: Each study would require a specific process consent depending on the substance of the study. This is in addition to the usual components of informed consent.

planned, and ethical dilemmas need to be considered before the proposal is written (see Chapter 14).

Confidentiality and Anonymity.   The same guarantee of confidentiality of data and anonymity of participants that quantitative researchers give must be made a general principle of qualitative research. This is only a general principle because some institutions allow their identity to be known, especially if the study is going to reflect positively on them. Also, some individuals enjoy being identified in certain kinds of interviews or studies. However, the general principle is to maintain confidentiality and anonymity.

In qualitative research, can we promise confidentiality when we include precise quotations from the transcripts in our publications? The answer is "no," but we can provide anonymity by protecting the identity of the participant. Consequently, individuals and institutions will want assurances that only the researcher(s) will have access to the data and that there will be no identifying evidence, such as names on cassettes, names on computer print-outs, and so forth. They will also want information about how and where the data will be stored.

In this section of the proposal, it might be helpful to identify the lines of communication that have been established for reporting findings. Also, information concerning the plans for disseminating the findings (i.e., publication, presentation, and who will receive final reports) should be included and mutually agreed upon.

Possible Risks.   Qualitative research is considered noninvasive, but in a sense, that is a limited perception of the word. While it is true that qualitative researchers do not physically alter the participants with an intervention, there is an invasion of their space and psyche. However, while this is often therapeutic, it can pose possible risks if certain precautions are not taken.

It is well substantiated that talking has therapeutic benefits. Patients in institutions, or staff for that matter, often find relief just "getting it out of their system" or "off their chest." Nursing intervention often speaks to the provision of opportunities for patients to ventilate their feelings, and interviews provide such an opportunity. Also, attention is usually viewed as a positive experience, and being important enough to study can be viewed positively. That someone's experience is worth studying can have a validating effect.

Are there risks in qualitative research? One reviewer from an IRB asked about "triggering" an emotional response within the informant. This cannot be lightly dismissed if the experiences under study are highly charged. Because of their training, nurse-researchers are usually able to intervene appropriately and make good assessments about how a patient is responding. It may be normal if a patient becomes upset during an interview, and the nurse-researcher must be supportive and manage the interview with good clinical judgment. Arrangements also should be made with the patient's primary caretaker to support the patient after leaving the field. Aamodt (1986) writes:

In the Human Subject Consent Forms we had said there were no psychological or social risks. Because communication in response to client feelings is an expected nursing intervention, to ignore such a need could be classified as irresponsible. We planned that interviewers would not be the primary caretaker of the child, and when the situation demanded it, the child and parent were referred to the primary caretaker. (p. 167)

An inaccurate portrayal of participants or situations can also cause harm. A statement of how you intend to ensure accurate description of participants and situations should also be included in this section of the proposal. Validation by the participants is respectful and necessary for authentic representation. The harm/benefit question is succinctly placed in context by Morse (1988) when she states:

Are the risks to the participant any greater than the everyday risk from confiding in a friend? And the "friend" in this context is a registered nurse who is accustomed to handling confidential information, counseling the dying and the distressed, observing and listening. Yet, suddenly, because the information is obtained under the auspices of "research" (rather than practice), the activities of the nurse may be considered by the IRB as potentially harmful. We must learn to trust our colleagues. (p. 214)

Nonbeneficial Research

This section of the proposal addresses research that is devoid of therapeutic purpose for the participant. Again, the opportunity to verbalize and be appreciated for sharing often does have therapeutic effects. This section should not be problematic, particularly in light of what has previously been discussed.

Presenting to the IRB

When presenting to an IRB panel, anticipate as many questions as possible. Consider this a wonderful opportunity to discuss your study. However, educating IRB members about your research methods and translating them into clear, concrete, pragmatic terms should also be done in the verbal presentation. Know who the board members are and avoid answering questions in a philosophical or existential style. If there is a member of the clergy on the board, he or she might understand your answer, but the lawyer, the physician, the two laypeople, the banker, and the accountant might not, so keep your discussion clear and precise. Remember, the intentions of the IRB are the same as yours: to protect the patient.

In summary, writing clearly, especially philosophical translation, suggesting compatible values between the institution's goals and the research goals, developing trust, and establishing clear lines of communication are important areas to consider when submitting a qualitative research proposal to an Institutional Review Board.

REFERENCES

Aamodt, A. (1986). Discovering the child's view of alopecia: Doing ethnography. In P. Munhall & C. Oiler (Eds.), *Nursing research: A qualitative perspective* (pp. 163–171). Norwalk, CT: Appleton-Century-Crofts.

Field, P., & Morse, J. (1985). *Nursing research: The application of qualitative approaches.* London: Croom Helm.

Morse, J. (1988). Commentaries on special issue. *Western Journal of Nursing Research,* 10(2), 213–216.

Munhall, P. (1988). Ethical considerations in qualitative research. *Western Journal of Nursing Research,* 10(2), 150–162.

Munhall, P., & Oiler, C. (1986). *Nursing Research: A qualitative perspective.* Norwalk, CT: Appleton-Century-Crofts.

Noble, M. (1985). Written informed consent: Closing the door to clinical research. *Nursing Outlook,* 33(6), 292–293.

Oberst, M. (1985). Another look at informed consent. *Nursing Outlook,* 33(6), 294–295.

16

Qualitative Research Proposals and Reports

Carolyn Oiler Boyd
Patricia L. Munhall

*L*ofland and Lofland (1984) emphasized that a qualitative research project begins with the investigator's personal concerns
and involves determining what he or she cares about independent
of social science. Personal concerns are thus primary and may or
may not coincide with those judged to be of significance in a given
discipline. These authors stated:

> *"Starting where you are" provides the necessary meaningful
> linkages between the personal and the emotional, on the
> one hand, and the stringent intellectual operations to come,
> on the other hand. Without a foundation in personal senti-
> ment all the rest easily becomes so much ritualistic, hollow
> cant. (p. 10)*

Although personal interest and investment are not unique features of qualitative research, attention to personal concerns and use of that involvement are uniquely important in the qualitative research tradition. This stands in marked contrast to the common practice of delineating a research agenda based on priorities set by funding agencies, or some other sanctioning authority. The influence of conventional sanctions on research poses a dilemma for researchers who are dependent on external approval of their work, and may be managed at times by casting the proposal in terms that will convince readers of the significance of the proposed research for science. In this chapter, the problem of sanctions is addressed along with other influences on not only what we study, but how. An effort is made to accommodate the legitimate concerns of qualitative researchers who seek approval from funding agencies and/or from dissertation committees that are relatively unfamiliar with the qualitative paradigm or that interpret and judge qualitative proposals with a positivist orientation. At the same time, however, we intend to protect the nexus of qualitative research philosophy with its methodology and thereby preserve the congruency of substance and form in qualitative research.

In Marshall and Rossman's text, *Designing Qualitative Research* (1989), the bent toward a positivist interpretation of qualitative research is revealed in an emphasis on a thorough review of the literature and formulation of guiding hypotheses. Although these authors repeatedly stress the importance of flexibility in design to accommodate the unknown and what may emerge in the conduct of the inquiry, their position appears to be one of compromise with the requirements of the positivist paradigm. Qualitative research from such a position is characterized more by its salient strategies and techniques (that is, by the generation of word data with an effort to maintain the sociocultural context of people's verbal expressions) than by its philosophical premises and broader implications. Nevertheless, this chapter will reflect some of the same advice as that given by Marshall and Rossman because, regardless of one's philosophical orientation, when a proposal must be approved by the guardians of the dominant paradigm in our world, the positivist frame must be addressed. We suggest therefore, that qualitative proposals provide readers with:

1. Education and description about the method from its aim to its outcome. Such detail also enhances confirmability by leaving a decision trail.
2. Justification for using the method through a logically developed explanation of why the researcher chose it.
3. Translation of language unique to the method in terms that are likely to be understood by readers.

In time, with greater acceptance of qualitative research on its own terms, compromises and translations may no longer be necessary except for those who practice qualitative research as a hybrid model in the positivist tradition.

GETTING STARTED

On some level, most researchers settle on a research topic because of some personal reason. Even for the opportunistic researcher with an eye on funding priorities, personal interest is usually aroused with ties to the researcher as person. For the qualitative researcher, this is a strategic tool in the research project; it provides the energy and the motivation to persevere with the challenges and tedium inherent in any scholarly work. More importantly, however, personal interest can position the researcher to attend to the phenomenon under study in a certain way; it establishes figure and ground for the research endeavor in what can be highly personalized ways that make the research a passion, a preoccupation, an intimate companion. All this is enabling for the qualitative researcher, making it possible for him or her to be in a state of what Schutz (1970) referred to as wide-awakeness (pp. 68–69). The personal sentiment of which Lofland and Lofland spoke is more than an idle curiosity, more than a mere research interest or agenda. It merges with aspects of one's life that encompass the professional but goes beyond it. As a colleague remarked, "I find that I am increasingly interested in geriatrics as I grow closer to being elderly myself." Similarly, some of the authors of this text have had occasion to share notes on the menopausal experience as we search for meaning in this time of our lives. And, as required in phenomenological research, Lauterbach has acknowledged her personal investment in meanings associated with the loss of a pregnancy in her research presentation in Chapter 5. Rather than biases to confess and then to eliminate, such personal investment in the research topic can be exploited to enhance the research process. The first step in developing a proposal is thus to identify a phenomenon about which one has a vested interest. This step is, of course, private and largely invisible. There are, no doubt, multiple instances, if not an established convention, of glossing over this consideration in deference to more practical issues in proposal development.

If the researcher is a "purist," he or she has taken up a position philosophically that establishes a particular way of regarding the nature of being human and of reality and truth, usually in connection with a way of regarding the nature of nursing. For such a qualitative researcher, all questions and problems in the domain (nursing) will be qualitative questions, circumventing the need to dwell on whether to use a qualitative approach in the research at hand. This point bears some elaboration. As a point of departure, the qualitative researcher acknowledges the following premises for his or her work, although these may be stated in various ways:

1. Human realities are constituted in human involvement with a world of people, objects, events, circumstances.
2. There are multiple points of view that may be taken up in this intending toward a world. The facts of the world alone do not equate with human realities.
3. Reality is constituted in a complex interaction of one's historicity, which includes the common stock of knowledge passed on through the culture in which one resides, and a chosen perspective in the world.
4. Although an objective world may be focused for attention in research, human reality is chosen for attention in nursing research, thus necessitating attention to the complex context in which those realities emerge for humans.

Thus, to understand people is to comprehend them in their contexts, mindful of the concrete world in which they are enmeshed, and attentive to the variety of ways in which it is possible for them to be in that world. The qualitative paradigm thus determines the kind of question posed for research; all questions are qualitative in nature.

On the other hand, for the researcher who reconciles the qualitative and quantitative paradigms, these premises may or may not be considered important or addressed. Because the philosophy and ideology of the qualitative paradigm are not consciously and explicitly adopted as a point of departure, the research idea does not alone determine how the research will be carried through. Rather, a more conventional approach is adopted in which a research question/problem is posed, and after ascertaining its significance to the domain, a decision-making process is used to determine whether qualitative methods are best suited to the question/problem. Regardless of whether a philosophy drives the question, the adoption of a qualitative design must be defended, however, and discussion of the premises listed above can serve later in proposal development to achieve this.

One can start from the perspective of the qualitative paradigm or be led to it by the nature of the phenomenon under study and the state-of-the-art concerning knowledge about it. At the very least, however, getting started requires reflection on one's own position in the world. In a discussion of getting started in phenomenological inquiry, Van Manen (1990) talked of orienting to the phenomenon:

> *It is important, therefore, for the researcher to focus carefully on the question of what possible human experience is to be made topical for phenomenological investigation. . . . This starting point of phenomenological research is largely a matter of identifying what it is that deeply interests you. . . . [T]o orient oneself to a phenomenon always implies a particular interest, station or vantage point in life. (p. 40)*

For nurse researchers, this advice means that we orient to life as nurse or perhaps as nurse educator or nurse administrator. It is primarily this orientation that should characterize selection of a phenomenon for study, if the study is to qualify as a *nursing* study. Parenthetically, what it means to orient to life as nurse is itself an interesting question that, despite a long history of contemplation, still eludes us as a discipline. This question is further confounded by some nurse researchers' orientation as nurse researchers or as social scientists rather than as nurses as such. There are yet other orientations to life; for example, as a mother or middle-aged woman or as a person with a chronic illness or as an artist, any of which may also enter into a nurse researcher's selection of a research focus. These latter orientations have the potential to enhance the intensity and passion with which one begins a study as well as the data to which one has access during the study. It is also true that such involvement through one's given orientations presents challenges to the researcher in managing preconceived conceptualizations during the study—the price of gaining the high ground of insight.

FORMULATING THE RESEARCH QUESTION

Qualitative research questions are characterized by their focus on what is often cited as "lived experience." They are also characteristically stated broadly through language that allows for the flexibility required in the research process while communicating a starting position of openness about the phenomenon under study. If a position of humility is not warranted by the state-of-the-art concerning the phenomenon, research is not indicated. Both features figure prominently in the process of formulating the research question.

As in all research proposals, the question undergoes revision as the proposal is developed and decisions about the study plan are made, however tentative this plan may be. For a qualitative study, the question is born by focusing one's attention on a selected interest. Some qualitative researchers specify the utility of selecting an interest about which one knows little, at least in a formal way, in order to augment the researcher's openness in the conduct of the inquiry. Others, quite naturally, orient to interests that have been central to their careers in nursing. Still others select interests that have been piqued by personal experience that is tied to their professional lives. A psychiatric nurse, for example, might become interested in how people live through infertility and infertility technology if she has herself been diagnosed as infertile.

All qualitative research questions are psychosocial in nature in the sense that they are concerned with living through various health-related circumstances. The focus is on awarenesses, meanings, and the various ways in which these awarenesses and meanings are given expression as well as their consequences for health and the quality of people's lives. In the earlier example, the researcher's lack of professional knowledge about infertility could be used to advantage in that she would be less likely to be encumbered by ready-made, scientific conceptualizations that might obscure her fresh vision of the human experience involved. Like the substance of fiction, the selected interest carries with it an angst of some sort that will figure into defending the significance of the study. This may be a matter of discontent with measurement of variables, sensibilities about patient experience, or adequacy of nursing interventions in certain situations. The angst, however, regardless of its source, provides fuel for the research endeavor.

The overriding consideration in formulating qualitative research questions, and in refining them as the proposal is shaped, is whether they focus on some aspect of human experience *in its context*. Context refers to "the world" in which people live out their lives, the world in which human meanings are constituted. Each qualitative method brings a particular orientation to the research question, but all concern themselves broadly with the task of understanding something about the human condition and why and how it comes to be that way. All recognize that human choices, manipulations, interpretations, and "sense making" figure prominently in the way things are.

The selection of a research focus establishes that phenomenon as important. In so many aspects of women's lives, the phenomenon may profit from being carefully attended to and the research question may focus on providing a rich description of it. A qualitative researcher who cites increased sensitivity to the phenomenon as an aim or purpose of the study is suggesting that this phenomenon is an important one for us to pay attention to and to understand. In so doing, a statement is made about the boundaries and mission of the discipline, and there is an implicit intention to alter the discipline's sensibilities about the objects of its concerns as well as the adopted perspectives on those objects. In other cases, the aim is to go beyond description of what it is to description that sheds light on how and why it is. The point of understanding how and why of any given human condition is, for nursing, threefold:

1. Such understandings enter into the sense making of which we are capable, and these, of course, influence our actions in patients' health circumstances;
2. They constitute impetus and rationale for our actions;
3. When qualitative research is conducted in tandem with quantitative studies, such understanding contributes to identification of relevant variables, conceptualizations of such variables, and possible relationships among variables.

The particular focus of qualitative studies, then, is on human experiencing in the contexts in which such experiencing is studied. The constantly changing landscape of our contexts as well as the variety of contexts in which human behavior can be observed provide an infinite call for qualitative research activity. Presumably, the nursing discipline's concern with health and with doing something constructive about people's health provides the overriding context for all nursing research endeavors regardless of various views on how direct the connection of the research with nursing practice should be. Beyond this overriding context, the qualitative researcher specifies that he or she is interested in the various ways in which people construct their ideas about health matters and how these ideas are played out in their lives, given the worlds to which they are tied. The research question may isolate any of these aspects of this interest and, for example, specify an inquiry into what people perceive in a given situation, or how they interpret the meaning of that situation, or what can be discerned about the connection between their meanings and their actions in the situation. Some qualitative research questions indicate the intention to investigate the entire domain of the qualitative interest for a select group or for a select situation. These distinctions in the scope of the research question have numerous implications for the type of qualitative research approach best suited to the study and the attending decisions concerning research design or method.

In all cases, the emphasis in qualitative research is on the perspective wielded by those who are in the situation. Research results, then, contribute to insights about why and how human conditions come to be. Such insights are, of course, explanatory, dispelling the idea that qualitative research produces description alone. Research that produces description of human perspective itself, if a rich description, simultaneously produces insight about why that perspective is chosen and how it figures into the way things are. The power of description needs to be reconceptualized in order to better acknowledge its role in a much needed revision of the explanation of phases and processes in theory development.

SIGNIFICANCE OF THE STUDY

It goes without saying that any research study must be important for the development of knowledge in the discipline, or for social science generally. Passable theories may become outdated as the contexts in which people live out their lives change (inevitable in health care because of the ongoing changes in health care technology and delivery). Theories may be revealed as biased, or relevant to only a portion of those to whom they are applied, or in some other way inadequate as a framework for nursing practice. The phenomena with which they are concerned may be recognized as being infinitely more complex than their accounts of reality, particularly when they have been developed in the absence of adequate attention to lived experiences or with exclusive attention to objective reality in a conception of reality as dualistic. Any of these judgments concerning the adequacy of formal knowledge in the discipline might serve to defend the significance of a qualitative research study.

Significance of a study, then, arises from a judgment that what we know collectively as a discipline is not enough, and is grounded in a sufficient review of the literature to document that the proposed study will contribute to knowledge in some way. Perhaps one of the most common pitfalls in developing a proposal is benighted ambition, a well-meaning intention to fill in a knowledge gap completely. Not only is this impractical within a single research project, but also, it is impossible from the point of view that knowledge changes and must be recreated anew forever.

The review of the literature to establish the significance of a study varies from the review in quantitative research in this vital respect: what is already known is recognized as partial and tentative and possesses the quality of data rather than a conceptual framework that guides, leads, and filters the researcher's observations and analyses. For the researcher who is studying a phenomenon within the parameters of a specialty in which he or she has been involved in the course of his or her career, the literature review serves a second important purpose that is unique to qualitative research; that is, acknowledging what is already known enables the researcher to bracket this knowledge so that fresh insights may emerge in the course of the study. Particular attention to conventional or customary ways of understanding the phenomenon under study is needed, rather than a comprehensive review that accounts for every point of view. A regard for what is already known as *data* rather than as fixed reference points also serves this purpose when presented critically by raising questions about this knowledge. These questions will also serve in the refinement of the research question and may be introduced as guiding questions for the research, thus satisfying some researchers' need for more detailed structure in the research question.

SELECTION OF A QUALITATIVE RESEARCH APPROACH

One of the most common questions of doctoral students who have studied the qualitative paradigm concerns which of the many methodologies reported in the literature should be selected to study a given research question. The research question itself is often silent on the matter, an outcome of the precision of the paradigm in directing researchers to the types of questions that are qualitative in nature, or perhaps, the power of the paradigm to generate universally (in that paradigm) relevant questions. Selection of a specific approach, then, becomes a function of other considerations. Any of the following considerations might apply:

1. Those orientations identified in the phase of "getting started" constitute a conceptual orientation that is subsumed within the qualitative research paradigm. If one is particularly interested in intrapsychic processes, for example, phenomenology or case study methods would be compatible and lend direction to design decisions. Alternatively, an orientation to interpersonal processes might lead one to grounded theory, and an interest in the cultural contexts of human behavior might lead one to ethnography or historical research.

2. Contemplation of the options in qualitative methodology might lead the researcher to select one over others because of its anchor in a disciplinary perspective that is believed to have potential in the investigation of nursing phenomena. Hutchinson, for example, (see Chapter 6) although learned in the various qualitative methodologies, preferred the grounded theory approach and its anchor in the sociological theory of symbolic interactionism. Each qualitative method carries with it a grounding in the works of particular philosophers and theorists, any one of which might hold particular appeal to a researcher.

3. At times, the researcher may be quite committed to a particular way of stating his or her research question, which in turn points to one method over the others. The research questions listed below are all concerned generally with families and chronic health problems. The way in which each is stated, however, illustrates the implications for selection of method.

   a. What are the challenges for these families and how do they address them? (grounded theory)

   b. What is the nature of human relationships in a cystic fibrosis clinic? (ethnography)

   c. What are the meanings of health for these families? (phenomenology)

   d. How does Family X perceive and manage health care and day-to-day living? (case study)

   e. What is our sociocultural-political legacy in concepts, values, and attitudes about chronic health problems? (historical research)

A research question that asks broadly "What is the lived experience of families in which there are members with chronic health problems?" does not provide sufficient direction in the selection of qualitative method or in the many decisions that must be made about design; without the support of subquestions, it is simply too broad to be useful beyond the "getting started" stage.

4. Some research questions that fail to give a clue to the most useful and/or appropriate method are compounded by the researcher's lack of commitment to any particular perspective offered by the various methods. In this case (and as sometimes practiced by researchers), the method may be synthesized from the particulars of the options. Although there are legitimate questions about this practice, it may represent researchers' interest in developing creative applications of borrowed methods within the discipline of nursing. Such creative and experimental work in methodology is laudable, particularly when it reflects more than a simple cut-and-paste approach.

5. Lastly, a researcher may simply wish to learn a selected method well, and will use that method to refine the research question as well as to direct the plan for the research.

In our experience, dissertation committees are usually most comfortable with selection of a design from the literature and faithful adherence to the methods included in that design. Although it is a common practice in published qualitative research reports to cite the use of a particular method for data analysis (for example, Colaizzi's method of data analysis [1978] or the constant comparative method from grounded theory), it is not unusual to find little else in the report that identifies it as, for example, phenomenological or as grounded theory. Rather, such studies are generically qualitative; using the constant comparative method does make a study grounded theory, for example. There are models for us in the education literature for such an eclectic approach to qualitative research design. However, readers should be aware of what may be thin ice in this approach in nursing. We believe that nursing will profit from experimentation with qualitative methods and that social scientists who have developed qualitative designs are no more legitimate sources for designs than methodologists who have emerged or who may emerge in our own discipline. There is, however, a lingering malignant doubt about ideas in nursing that can't be traced directly and clearly to other disciplines.

To summarize, refinement of the research question is accomplished in tandem with selection of the qualitative approach. It should reflect the particular orientation or perspective that the selected qualitative approach lends to the study. When an eclectic approach is to be used, the researcher will need to explain how his or her choices in the design reflect his or her nursing perspective (or other orientations). In keeping with the idea of researcher-as-instrument in qualitative research, careful attention to the researcher's orientations and perspectives in an explicit way is expected throughout the research process. In the proposal phase, identifying and explicating those orientations and perspectives are part of bracketing (in phenomenological terms) or controlling and monitoring researcher bias (in positivist terms).

INTRODUCTION TO THE STUDY

The first section of the qualitative proposal is usually titled "Introduction" and includes the research question, the aim of the study, the researcher's explanation of its significance for nursing, and identification of the qualitative approach that will be used to conduct the inquiry. As explicated in the preceding sections of this chapter, the way in which these components of the introduction are communicated and explained is critical for a positive review of the proposal.

The overall purpose of the introduction is to orient the reader to the phenomenon under study and to the general design of the study. It demonstrates how the aim of the study has implications and relevance for nursing, and clearly focuses on the substance of the study. What the researcher needs to convey is his or her perceived justification for studying the selected phenomenon.

Because of the openness of qualitative research to fresh insights, in general, the language used to state the research question will contain phrases such as:

"What is it like to [be in this circumstance]?"

"What is [this phenomenon]?"

"What is going on [in this situation]?"

"What is the nature of [this experience]?"

Identification of a context in which the phenomenon occurs provides further definition of the research question and may be discussed narratively rather than through precision in the research question as such.

The aim of the study should be stated explicitly and related to the strengths of qualitative methodology. Knafl and Howard (1984, 1986) described four purposes for qualitative studies that may assist with this articulation: instrumentation, illustration, sensitization, and conceptualization. Most qualitative studies aim to enhance conceptualization through description of lived experiences that have eluded our theories. From this point of view, discovery is an apt way to refer to the aim of such studies. It is obvious that reference to the literature is necessary to document the relevance of any of these four aims and to support the researcher's claims of the significance of the study for nursing. A brief overview of the particular qualitative method selected for the study should be included and should flow logically from the presentation of the research question.

REVIEW OF THE LITERATURE/EVOLUTION OF THE STUDY

The literature review conducted to document relevance and significance also serves the purpose of establishing the historical, experiential, and scientific contexts of the study for the researcher. As stated earlier, this acknowledgment is an aid to the researcher in bracketing assumptions and preconceptions. It is entirely appro-

priate for the researcher to speak of personal experience to illuminate his or her orientation(s) and process of getting started in this
research project. Inclusion of such information contributes to the
reader's understanding of the full context of the study's origins.

The critical guideline for the researcher in his or her review of
the literature is to recognize this phase of proposal development
as instrumental in opening up the inquiry rather than narrowing it
down to a selected conceptual framework. Regarding the review
of contexts as initial data collection is a helpful attitude to assume,
and may be expressed through a critical questioning of one's experiences and of the adequacy of established theory to explain those
experiences. Upon reading this section of the proposal, the logic
of using qualitative methodology to achieve the research aim
should be clear.

THE RESEARCH DESIGN

Proposal readers frequently need to be educated about the selected
qualitative approach or design; for this reason, we suggest that the
selected design be presented and explained in a separate section.
Some repetition of information is inevitable in this approach, but
we have found that this is useful to readers unfamiliar with the various qualitative designs available to the qualitative researcher.

Design includes the philosophical/theoretical premises for research within that design as well as the kinds of questions that can
be addressed and a host of particulars concerning methods to answer those questions. In grounded theory, for example, symbolic
interactionism is a critical framework for research and thus must
be understood and used in the research. In phenomenology, several interpretations of method are reported in the literature; each
has implications for the design of studies, from formulation of the
question to the substance and form of the research product. In order to make the researcher's decisions sensible and plans comprehensible, the selected design must be presented and explained in
considerable detail. Because integrating this presentation and explanation into other sections of the proposal is not usually satisfactory for the reader, we suggest that it be addressed in a clearly
identified, separate section (preceding the section titled "Research

Method") in which many of the particulars of the design are applied in the study. The following guidelines emphasize the importance of definition, translation, description, explanation, documentation, and illustration in this section of the proposal:

1. Reiterate the philosophical/theoretical premises of the design.
2. Use primary sources to document the description of the design. In a grounded theory study, for example, Glaser and Strauss's (1967) work is indispensable.
3. Translate or paraphrase language that has meanings unique to the design. The term "lived experience," for example, is particularly puzzling to many.
4. Reiterate the rationale for selecting the design, emphasizing how it will help to answer the research question and why this is important to the nursing discipline. For example, if the identification of basic social psychological processes shared by people in common circumstances will contribute to the development of nursing interventions in their shared social psychological problem, this should be highlighted. Citations of studies that used the design can be especially effective in substantiating the claims that are made.
5. Describe the design's methods for generating and analyzing data. Examples from other studies may be useful in clarifying steps of analysis in particular.
6. Predictable questions about reliability and validity should be addressed through a description of the design's provisions for rigor. Kirk and Miller (1986) provided a handy reference on reliability and validity in qualitative research by reframing and responding to the questions in terms appropriate to the qualitative paradigm.

THE RESEARCH METHOD

The research method—that is, the plan to collect and analyze data that will answer the research question—is one element of the design. In qualitative proposals, method is tentative to allow for ongoing decision making through interaction with research participants and discovery of the unforeseen. Some of the same methodological questions addressed in quantitative proposals are equally germane to qualitative proposals. The relevance of each question varies with the research question and the overall nature of the method.

In this section of the proposal, it is helpful to repeat the aim of the study and to relate the methodological particulars to that aim. The language of the design can be used freely, having been defined and explained in the preceding section, and the researcher can now focus on how the design will be carried out within the specific parameters of his or her study.

Sample, Setting, Unit of Analysis (What Will the Sources of Data Be?)

A research question may delineate that research participants' perceptions are the source of data, and the method will reflect this by describing methods to solicit those perceptions. Often, the source is participants' responses to the researcher's questioning through interview. If the occasion for the interview is directly tied to the research project, it is possible and desirable to indicate how the interview will be initiated and sustained. In this case, an interview guide is purposeful and should be included in the proposal. This holds true also for the broad, open question such as "What is it like for you to take care of your mother in her old age?" that constitutes the only prompt from the researcher. More often, however, qualitative interviews are conducted in a conversational manner, and an interview guide merely indicates, rather than prescribes, how the researcher will direct attention to the research question in that conversation. Like social conversations, the course of the qualitative interview cannot be predicted with any precision, nor would this be desirable.

A recurring question concerning sources of data is the matter of sample size. As in quantitative research, the answer is ambiguous—that is, "It depends." In studies that use a single source of data such as a one-time interview or a written response to the research question, one would expect to see larger numbers of participants included in the design. In studies that use repeated interviews that extend over long periods of time, fewer participants might be acceptable. One of the considerations in this decision concerns the amount of data that is likely to be produced by the selected data-generating method, particularly in the context of the overall time frame for the research project. When multiple methods of data generation are included in the study, the "sample" would include not only people who have agreed to provide data but also the documents examined or the journals recorded or the researcher's own field notes, for example. In our study of nurses' values, the sample consisted of 121 nurses' poems and photographs numbering in excess of 700 individual entries.

Although there are no formulas to apply in determining sample size, a common rule of thumb is that data are collected until redundancy in the data occurs or the researcher finds that no new data are emerging. Experienced qualitative researchers, particularly ethnographers and grounded theorists, recommend that field research should be planned for several months to a year. Some methodologists (van Kaam, 1969, for example) specify large samples, but most are mute on the matter, leaving the number question open in deference to the more significant issue of adequacy of the data base for the research question. Unlike quantitative research, in which statistical procedures determine the necessary sample size, qualitative research leaves the question open to judgment. This holds true even in the case study design; here, the case is the sample of one, but what the researcher identifies as sources of data about this one case is parallel to the concern with sample size in quantitative research.

In most qualitative designs, the sample is selected in accord with pre-established criteria or guidelines. These should be described and, when possible, a plan to collect demographic data descriptive of research participants will enable the researcher to provide an account of this dimension of the context for the study.

Data Collection Procedures, Ethics
(How Will Data Be Solicited from These Sources?)

Once the researcher has decided what form(s) of expression will constitute the data for the project, the next question concerns how, when, and where to solicit those expressions. Our study of nurses' values is illustrative of this aspect of the plan. In this study, the aim was "to enhance understanding about nursing perspective: the human values, value conflicts, and value questions expressed by nurses in their poems and photographs" (Munhall & Oiler, 1987). Multiple possibilities presented themselves for data generation concerning nursing perspective. From among them, we selected nurses' expressions in poetry and photography, in the recognition that these expressions might provide a more direct path to values than interview or questionnaire, for example. The idea of using nurses' aesthetic expressions seemed particularly congruent with our phenomenological orientation as well as our appreciation for the preverbal nature of nursing perspective for most nurses. Still, decisions needed to be made concerning how to solicit these aesthetic expressions. A call for nurses' poems and photographs became the method for solicitation and was distributed as widely as our resources allowed. The call was published as a classified ad in *The American Nurse,* and fliers were distributed to 300 hospitals randomly selected from a national listing of JCAH accredited hospitals, all Sigma Theta Tau Chapters, and all newsletter editors of state nurses associations. Alternatively, nurses might have been asked to write poems or to take photographs for this research project, or they might have been asked to respond to selected works of art, or they might have been interviewed about their nursing practices.

Questions and problems of gaining access to data include obtaining informed consent and plans for negotiating ground rules in an ongoing way. (Readers are referred to Chapter 14 for further detail concerning the ethics of qualitative studies and to the methods chapters for additional considerations for data collection procedures.) For studies that are conducted over a period of time, a time frame for data collection points should be tentatively planned.

Data Management (How Will Data Be Managed During the Data Collection Process?)

A variety of strategies for managing qualitative data are described in this text as well as in the many references cited for expanded readings on qualitative methods. Typically, interview data are transcribed to facilitate the researcher's contemplation of the data during analysis. Field notes are often formatted to enable the researcher to record observations and to facilitate his or her reflections on the research process and the simultaneous data analysis process.

Data Analysis (How Will Data Be Analyzed?)

Data analysis procedures in qualitative research have drawn criticism because of their ambiguous nature. Despite the development of a variety of strategies to make the process of analysis explicit and reproducible, there remains a fundamental ambiguity that is inherent in the creativity of the process. Many methodologists have listed analytic steps that may be adopted to the satisfaction of all concerned. The use of expert judges to validate the researcher's analysis is commonplace, as is the practice of validating findings with research participants. Ironically, these strategies, which were developed largely to quell the concerns about bias in the research, sometimes have the effect of limiting the researcher's interpretations.

The importance of data analysis as a creative process cannot be overemphasized. It remains, regardless of the strategies employed to systematize it, a unique rendering of the meaning(s) of the phenomenon under study. The term researcher-as-instrument in its widest sense refers not only to the researcher's influence (through his or her orientations) on what is studied and how it is studied, but also to the possibilities and limits of his or her sense making in data analysis. Like other creative acts, data analysis is a matter of composing an order and does claim to be the only possible order that could be brought to bear. Despite the difficulty of articulating in any precise way exactly how insights and orders are achieved, we offer the guidelines for data analysis listed below as having been useful for others. We suggest that strategies be planned that will help to:

1. Ponder the meaning of data in parts and as a whole and on repeated occasions.

2. Search for repeated instances that support each interpretation.

3. Reach for complex interpretations to account for variations in the data; contradictions in the data sometimes call attention to "real" contradictions in people's lives.

4. Use all the data available, including field notes, the literature, and any other sources of inspiration. Do not be limited to transcribed interview data merely because they seem more scientific.

5. Identify the technical aspects of data analysis. If data analysis procedures from one of the qualitative methods is useful, adopt it in the design. Recognize that what you are doing is adopting a procedure rather than an entire design (unless, of course, you are).

6. Relate the findings to preexisting knowledge, keeping in mind that although the project may be an end in itself in some ways, to qualify as science, it must be entered into a dialogue with one's colleagues. In the proposal phase, merely indicating a plan to do this may be sufficient. Some concepts, theories, and research may be identified in the proposal as a function of reviewing the literature for the purposes cited earlier; other relevant literature may be a part of the discovery in the research process, and this may need to be explained as part of the flexibility required in qualitative studies.

Reliability and Validity (How Will Reliability and Validity Be Assured?)

Although questions of rigor may be adequately addressed in other sections of the proposal, they are sufficiently troublesome for many readers to warrant repetition in the method section. Here, the particular strategies that the researcher will use to ensure reliability and validity should be described in whatever language was used to explain the meaning of rigor in the selected design earlier. The strengths of the selected design and its application in the study should be emphasized, but limitations should also be acknowledged. The usual reference to sample size and generalizability should not be listed as limitations because they do not hold the same meaning for qualitative research and would serve to obfuscate the proposal by mixing paradigms (unless, of course, mixed paradigms are part of the study).

IMPLICATIONS AND THE FORM OF THE RESEARCH REPORT

All qualitative studies produce description that is intended to be full and rich with detail. Standard forms for communicating research findings are generally concerned with efficiency and thus are in opposition to the primary purpose of qualitative research and present troublesome challenges to qualitative researchers. There are, however, multiple options for the form of such descriptions, some of which aid the researcher in meeting the challenges; others call for new forms of communication in the discipline.

Expository writing is generally the form selected, with some variation based on the qualitative design selected. In a grounded theory study, for example, figures and models often complement the presentation of the theory. Colaizzi's (1978) phenomenology produces what he refers to as an exhaustive description of essences, which encapsulates recurring themes in interview data. Presentation of qualitative themes in tabled lists is a common format. Miles and Huberman (1984) described a variety of quantitatively inspired approaches to the presentation of findings that hold appeal for some. Other possibilities include vignettes and short stories or case study formats even though case study design may not have been used. Selections from the data themselves may present options. For example, an exhibit of photographs might be arranged as the primary report format or as complementary to it.

The form of presentation will often be determined by the intended audience and/or the vehicle. Journal articles and dissertations, for example, will limit options dramatically. In many instances, findings may be presented in different ways for different audiences, serendipitously calling on the researcher to rewrite findings, which can be an occasion for continued refinement of the analysis. We now have a 10-year accumulation of nursing literature on qualitative methodologies and on the debate about whether qualitative research is a legitimate tool of nursing science. In view of this, the attention given to the rationale for selection of a qualitative method and to elaborate explanations of the method itself may be attenuated in the interest of focusing more on the findings and their implications. In our view, the significance of findings for the discipline tend to be short-changed in many reports, a failing that is often attributed to the brevity required in journals and conference presentations. This is a practice that can be changed now that there is greater sophistication in the discipline about qualitative approaches to knowledge development; the practice needs to change in order to bridge qualitative research findings to nursing practices and subsequent nursing research.

In any case, the proposal should indicate tentative plans for discussion of the meaning of the findings and for disseminating findings. The discussion should bring the inquiry together as a whole, including scholarly reflection on the historical, scientific, and experiential contexts acknowledged in earlier sections of the proposal. In the course of data gathering, other aspects of these contexts and new contexts may have emerged, and these too should be related to the findings in order to enter them into the discipline's discourse about the phenomenon under study. One cannot predict the nature of the synthesis that is performed in the discussion, but the intention to perform a synthesis can be planned.

APPENDICES AND REFERENCES

As in any research proposal, communications relevant to the study, consent forms, and other supporting documents (such as an interview guide, if one is used) are appended to the proposal. References should reflect the researcher's mastery of relevant literature concerning the selected design as well as the phenomenon under study, particularly as it is understood and discussed in the nursing discipline.

THE FINAL RESEARCH REPORT

In view of the interest in qualitative methodology and the discipline's relatively novice status in the use of qualitative designs, the final research report will be of interest not only for the research product but also for the research process. This observation does not distinguish qualitative research reports from those that spring from the dominant positivist paradigm, but it does suggest that the labor of explaining and defending the qualitative choice is meaningful.

Table 16-1 provides an outline for a formal research proposal. Overall, the first three sections of the proposal (Introduction, Review of the Literature/Evolution of the Study, Research Design) remain the same for a formal research report that is consistent with common dissertation requirements (see Table 16-2). Converting the future tense to the past tense would be the only revision. The section on research method, however, requires considerable expansion, in accord with what actually happened in the research process. Specific illustrations of various features of the research process should be included to substantiate generalities. For example, in Haase's (1987) study of courage in hospitalized adolescents, the analytic steps of identifying significant statements in transcribed interview data, formulating restatements, and articulating formulated meanings are illustrated through the reporting of selected data. Alternatively, such illustrations might be intro-

Table 16–1
Outline for Qualitative Research Proposals

Proposal Section	Section Substance	Comments
Introduction	1. Phenomenon of interest. 2. Identification of research question. 3. Aim of study. 4. Justification for design and significance of study. 5. Overview of design.	Acknowledges the researcher's orientation/ perspective.

Table 16–1 (Continued)

Proposal Section	Section Substance	Comments
Review of the Literature/Evolution of the Study	1. Historical, experiential, and scientific contexts of the study.	Details researcher's orientation/perspective and strengthens arguments for design and significance.
Research Design	1. Philosophical/theoretical premises. 2. Methodological techniques and strategies for data gathering and analysis. 3. Relation to research question and aim of study. 4. Reliability and validity provisions.	Educates the reader.
Research Method	1. Sample, setting, unit of analysis. 2. Data collection procedures. 3. Ethics. 4. Data management strategies. 5. Data analysis procedures. 6. Reliability and validity provisions. 7. Timetable.	Specifies application of design in this study.
Plan for Discussion and Dissemination	1. Plan for scientific literature review. 2. Plan for report format.	Registers research project as scientific and strengthens argument for significance.
Appendices	1. Correspondence, consent forms, interview guides, and other supporting documents.	
References	1. Methodological references. 2. Scientific literature about the phenomenon under study.	

Table 16–2
Outline for Qualitative Research Reports

Report Section	Section Substance	Comments
Introduction	Same as proposal. Outline of remaining report.	Convert proposal's future tense to past tense.
Review of Literature/Evolution of the Study	Same as proposal.	Expand in breadth and depth as indicated by research process.
Research Design	Same as proposal.	
Research Method	Same as proposal, except for modifications as indicated by actual research process.	Illustrate use of method with actual data and examples from research process.
Findings	Description in a selected form(s) and in accord with design.	Substantiate narrative amply with "raw" data.
Discussion	Meanings and understandings. Implications.	Relate to scientific literature and to contexts described in Section #2.
Appendices	Update as indicated by research process.	
References	Update as indicated by research process.	

duced in the presentation and explanation of the design, an option that did not exist in the proposal phase.

Literature that was reviewed in data gathering should be cited in the Research Method section, and its use in the research process should be described. In those studies that postpone a formal review of scientific literature for the Discussion section, the literature review should be placed in that section. The Findings and Discussion sections are usually reported separately, although we have observed successful exceptions to this sequence. The form of the Findings section is usually narrative, peppered with supportive "raw" data that might include quotes from participants, poems, or field note entries, for example. The aim of meaningful qualitative description should guide the researcher's choices among data reporting forms, and might include graphics as complementary to the narrative. In the Discussion section, as noted earlier, the study's claims to significance for the discipline are realized when the report is effective and complete. Here, the relation of the study to what is believed, known, thought, or understood is explicated in a contemplative review of relevant scientific literature. Appendices and references are modified as indicated by what actually transpired in the conduct of the research project.

THE ABSTRACT

Abstracts are commonly required for dissertations, journals, and research conference planners. Traditional formats are again troublesome for the qualitative researcher. Rather than sacrifice substance to form, we suggest that formats be modified to accommodate the nature of the qualitative paradigm. Table 16-3 presents an alternative that is consistent with the outlines for proposals and reports.

Table 16–3
Outline for Qualitative Research Abstracts

Abstract Section	Section Substance
Research Question and Aim	Identification of phenomenon studied. Significance of the study for nursing.
Evolution of the Study	Historical, experiential, and scientific contexts for the study. Rationale for qualitative approach.
Design	Overview of selected design. Overview of its application in this study.
Findings	Synopsis of major findings.
Discussion	Reflections on the findings. Synopsis of meanings, understandings, implications.

SUMMARY

In essence, a well-developed qualitative proposal provides:

1. A clear statement that specifies the phenomenon to be studied;
2. Documentation of a need for study, with specification of the significance of the study for nursing (or social science in general);
3. Acknowledgment of the researcher's a priori orientation(s) and perspective(s) with articulated questions about the attendant presuppositions;
4. Identification of the qualitative approach with a rationale for its selection;
5. Specification of the design with attention to:
   a. what data are sought,
   b. how and when those data will be solicited,
   c. how relationships with research participants will be initiated, maintained, and terminated,
   d. how data will be managed,
   e. how data will be analyzed and related to preexisting knowledge,
   f. how findings will be reported.

Table 16-1 provides an outline for qualitative research proposals in accord with this chapter's discussion of the proposal as a process as well as a concrete product. Variation in the outline is not only possible (without transgressing the tenets of the qualitative paradigm), but also may be necessary or desired as determined by particular interpretations of the various qualitative designs and/or by the researcher's needs in a given situation.

As long as qualitative research approaches have the status of being an oddity, qualitative methodology will require careful attention and explication. In our state of heightened consciousness about methods, however, it is helpful to recall Schutz's (1970) advice on the matter:

> *Methodology is not the preceptor or the tutor of the scientist.*
> *It is always his pupil, and there is no greater master in his*
> *scientific field who could not teach the methodologists how*
> *to proceed. But the really great teacher always has to learn*
> *from his pupils. . . . In this role, the methodologist has to*
> *ask intelligent questions about the technique of his teacher.*
> *And if those questions help others to think over what they*
> *really do, and perhaps to eliminate certain intrinsic diffi-*
> *culties hidden in the foundation of the scientific edifice*
> *where the scientists never set foot, methodology has per-*
> *formed its task (p. 315).*

With this in mind, every qualitative study stands to teach us something about methodology. To the extent that qualitative studies
bring us closer to the lived realities of health care recipients and
their nurses in shared circumstances, qualitative methodology will
also learn from the teacher of nursing practice. As we move ahead
in insisting on a place for qualitative research in nursing science,
we hope that there will be methodological progress that requires
rewriting this chapter and text to accommodate what we learn
from one another along the way.

REFERENCES

Colaizzi, P. (1978). Psychological research as the phenomenologist
    views it. In Valle and King (Eds.), *Existential phenomenological al-*
    ternatives for psychology. New York: Oxford University Press.

Glaser, B. & Strauss, A. (1967). *The discovery of grounded theory.*
    Chicago: Aldine.

Haase, J. (1987). Components of courage in chronically ill adoles-
    cents: A phenomenological study. *Advances in Nursing Science, 9,*
    64–80.

Kirk, J., & Miller, M. (1986). *Reliability and validity in qualitative re-*
    search. Newbury Park, CA: Sage.

Knafl, K., & Howard, M. (1984). Interpreting, reporting, and evaluat-
    ing qualitative research. *Research in Nursing and Health,* 7(1), 17–
    24.

Knafl, K., & Howard, M. (1986). Interpreting, reporting, and evaluating qualitative research. In P. Munhall & C. Oiler (Eds.), *Nursing research: A qualitative perspective.* Norwalk, CT: Appleton-Century-Crofts.

Lofland, J., & Lofland, L. (1984). *Analyzing social settings: A guide to qualitative observation and analysis.* Belmont, CA: Wadsworth.

Marshall, C., & Rossman, G. (1989). *Designing qualitative research.* Newbury Park, CA: Sage.

Miles, M., & Huberman, A. (1984). *Qualitative data analysis: A sourcebook of new methods.* Newbury Park, CA: Sage.

Munhall, P., & Oiler, C. (1987). Human values in nursing: Esthetic expressions. Poster presentation at the American Nurses Association, Council of Nurse Researchers International Nursing Research Conference, Washington, DC.

Schutz, A. (1970). *On phenomenology and social relations.* Chicago: University of Chicago Press.

van Kaam, A. (1969). *Existential foundations of psychology.* New York: Doubleday.

Van Manen, M. (1990). *Researching lived experience: Human science for an action-sensitive pedagogy.* New York: SUNY Press.

ADDITIONAL REFERENCES

Bogdan, R., & Biklen, S. (1982). *Qualitative research for education: An introduction to theory and methods.* Boston: Allyn & Bacon.

Cobb, A., & Hagemaster, J. (1987). Ten criteria for evaluating qualitative research proposals. *Journal of Nursing Education, 26*(4), 138–142.

Lincoln, Y., & Guba, E. (1985). *Naturalistic inquiry.* Newbury Park, CA: Sage.

17

Combining Qualitative and Quantitative Approaches

Carolyn Oiler Boyd

*C*ombining research methods in a study, or research triangulation, is an issue in the nursing discipline as it has been for many years in psychology and sociology, and it is one of the manifestations of the division between the qualitative and quantitative traditions in research. Fielding and Fielding (1986, p. 10) noted that this issue, in psychology, is apparent in the tension between clinical and experimental methods; in sociology, it is apparent in the separation between fieldwork and statistical work. Further, they traced the differences in points of view to the hypothetico-deductive approach in quantitative research and the analytic-inductive approach in qualitative research. A third point of view posits the advisability of using both approaches to arrive at a superior research product; it is this view that draws protests from some camps, and that will serve as the primary focus of attention in this chapter.

Knafl and Breitmayer (1989) reported that, originally, the term "research triangulation" was "a technical term used in surveying and navigation to describe a technique whereby two known or visible points are used to plot the location of a third point" (p. 210). They explained that its first appearance in the social sciences occurred in the 1950s as a metaphor to refer to the use of multiple methods to measure a single construct. The earliest references to triangulation in the research methodology literature, then, were concerned with enhancing the validity of quantitative findings through confirmation, or convergence, of findings from two or more instruments and/or data collection procedures and techniques. Today, amid controversy, research triangulation is a term that refers broadly to the research practice of combining methods within a single tradition (quantitative or qualitative) or across those traditions. The overriding purposes of triangulation are to increase the reliability and validity of a study and/or to increase the comprehensiveness of a study, including those studies that are carried out in phases over a protracted period of time.

In this chapter, the purposes of triangulation, types of triangulation, and applications in nursing studies are discussed, serving, in part, to enable the reader to engage in or to observe the controversy with a clear sense of the broad and particular meanings of triangulation and how it has been, and could be, used in nursing research. The controversy over combining qualitative and quantitative approaches in a single study is presented with an effort to transcend a simplistic view of the differences between the qualitative and quantitative traditions in research in the arguments either for or against this practice.

PURPOSES OF TRIANGULATION

As stated above, there are two overriding purposes for combining methods in research. The first of these is to increase the reliability and validity of a study, otherwise known as convergence or confirmation. In essentially quantitative studies, when there is measurement of discrete variables, the researcher may perceive a need to provide confirmation of findings from measurement. This could be accomplished by triangulating in another measure of the same variables. Qualitative strategies such as interviews might be conceived as such a measure just as the addition of another instrument is so conceived. For the quantitative researcher, all the traditional rules of quantitative research continue to apply, and the integrity of the research remains essentially quantitative. Findings from this other measure or measures would be expected to converge with, or confirm, those obtained through initial or primary measurement if that instrument is reliable and valid. Convergence might be the purpose of administering a scale measuring a construct of caregiver burden in an essentially qualitative study as well. However, one sees fewer examples of this in the literature. It is becoming increasingly common nevertheless—a function perhaps of qualitative researchers needing to document in statistical form that their qualitative findings are valid from the positivist point of view. This problem with the concept of truth in research continues to vex qualitative researchers despite excellent explanations of how reliability and validity are interpreted and protected in qualitative approaches.

The second primary purpose of triangulation is to increase the comprehensiveness of a study. The idea here is that one method provides at best a partial picture of a complex phenomenon with many perspectives or aspects that need to be understood. Two or more methods are thus selected within one or the other of the research traditions or across those traditions. Some common ways to express this purpose are:

- *To provide qualitatively derived richness or detail in description and/or explanation of a phenomenon.* In quantitative inquiry, this is usually viewed as complementary to the quantitative findings. In a qualitative inquiry, this purpose is generally at the heart of the research, and often is expressed in the research design through the inclusion of multiple methods selected from within the qualitative tradition.

- *To achieve a more complete understanding of the phenomenon under study, especially when the phenomenon has multiple aspects or perspectives to consider.* For the quantitative researcher, the option that meets the purpose of comprehensiveness might be conceived in terms of two types of measurement as, for example, the use of a broadly designed survey of adult women in a selected geographical area to ascertain usage patterns of mammography services, and a more detailed questionnaire administered to a random sample to obtain detail concerning such questions as how subjects determine a need for such services. Or researchers might regard some aspects of the phenomenon under study as measurable and others as needing to be explored qualitatively, leading to triangulation across research traditions. Such triangulation might, for example, include solicitation of data from nurses about caring as an aim and activity, from nursing management about their views, from patients about being cared for, and from nonparticipant observers of the interpersonal exchange in nursing care delivery. Or, comprehensiveness might be considered temporally and data might be generated at multiple points in time, producing multiple perspectives on, for example, the experiences of a child during and after the divorce of his or her parents.

- *To compensate for the weakness of one method via the strengths of the other; that is, to maximize validity of a quantitative study or to achieve a holistic understanding in a qualitative study.* In a quantitative study of loneliness in institutionalized elderly, for example, the measurement process may be recognized as posing a threat to validity. Qualitative method might be triangulated into such a study by collecting observational data descriptive of the manifestations of loneliness, and thereby the threat is counteracted. In a qualitative study of the same phenomenon, the addition of a measure of loneliness administered to elderly residents might be included in the study's design to compensate for possible reactivity to the research process.

It bears mentioning that there is often a relative emphasis in triangulated studies as essentially quantitative or qualitative. Methodological options are viewed by some as a menu of data generation strategies or techniques and are used accordingly, with a sense of full freedom to select strategies that best serve identified purposes. There may, however, be important differences in the application of those strategies and in the gestalt of the design and analysis, based on the researcher's allegiance to one research tradition over the other.

Both purposes of triangulation—to enhance reliability and validity and to increase comprehensiveness—are accommodated by routine features of many qualitative inquiries. The incorporation of multiple data sources provides a check on the reliability of researcher-as-instrument and increases the credibility of findings. The conduct of an inquiry over a protracted period of time and the validation of findings with informants or the inclusion of judges in analysis of data accomplish this as well. In this sense, most qualitative studies are triangulated by nature. The issue, then, is clearly concerned with triangulation across qualitative and quantitative methods. In this narrower sense of the meaning of triangulation, the purposes discussed above emerge from and relate to the quantitative paradigm in nursing research. Researchers who choose this approach in their studies thus reveal a positive regard for the coexistence of both research traditions if not an explicit allegiance to the quantitative paradigm.

TYPES OF TRIANGULATION

There are four types of triangulation distinguished in the literature: theoretical, data, investigator, and methodological triangulation (Denzin, 1978). Each of these will be explained briefly, with an emphasis on methodological triangulation, which serves to focus the argument about combining qualitative and quantitative methods.

Theoretical Triangulation

Theoretical triangulation is the use of several different frames of reference in analysis of data. This type of triangulation is commonplace in qualitative research once data are analyzed in the discussion of findings and how they relate to the existing theory, research findings, and clinical practices. However, theoretical triangulation usually refers to the effort to test two or more theories with the same data base by using each theory, in turn, to analyze the data. For example, in Campbell's (1989) study of women's responses to battering, she compared two theoretical models, grief and learned helplessness, for their relative explanatory applicability for these responses.

Data Triangulation

Data triangulation refers to the use of a variety of sampling strategies or multiple data sources. This too is characteristic of qualitative studies, particularly those using grounded theory and ethnographic approaches (and, properly, those adhering to phenomenological criteria). It is geared toward enhancing the internal validity of findings. Informant guardedness, for example, would be revealed during the prolonged period of fieldwork in which one "samples" that informant repeatedly. Researcher bias, as another example, is less likely to be maintained in the avalanche of data that contradicts him or her. In quantitative studies, this type of triangulation is seen when researchers use different measures of the same variable—for example, different measures of pain. It also refers to such strategies as data collection from the same subjects over time and sampling from more than one group and more than one situation. For example, measuring professional values of graduating seniors, recent graduates, and RN students might aim at revealing the effect of the curriculum on socialization into the profession.

Investigator Triangulation

Investigator triangulation refers to the use of multiple observers in a single study, as seen in studies conducted by research teams. This type of triangulation usually introduces theoretical triangulation by virtue of the various theoretical perspectives introduced by the team members. It also serves as a check on researcher bias and thereby contributes to internal validity in a qualitative study.

Methodological Triangulation

Methodological triangulation is simply the use of multiple methods in a single study, and as such this type of triangulation is the focus of attention in the controversy over combining qualitative and quantitative approaches. There are two subtypes of methodological triangulation: within method and between or across method triangulation. Within method triangulation is illustrated when one method, such as survey, is selected and several different data collection strategies are used within that method, as, for example, the use of several measures of social support. This subtype is employed for the purpose of establishing convergent validity of confirmation of findings on one measure by the findings on the other. The second subtype, between or across method triangulation, is an approach that combines qualitative and quantitative approaches. It serves the purpose of establishing convergent validity as in the within method subtype or the purpose of disclosing paradox and contradiction in the findings.

APPLICATIONS

Comprehensiveness in a quantitative study can be achieved through the use of case study to illustrate the full meaning of quantitative findings. Qualitative data obtained from interview are not uncommonly used to clarify and amplify responses to questionnaires and scales. Alternatively, in qualitative studies, responses to questionnaires or scales can be used to give direction to the fieldwork, giving the researcher some beginning orientation to people's concerns or their beliefs, for example.

To achieve convergence, researchers may validate empirical constructs through interview or observational data. They may verify quantitative findings with qualitative findings, or vice versa. In either case, the findings from one type of data generation are compared and contrasted with those from another type of data generation. If findings converge, they point in the same direction, to the same conclusions. In some cases, there may be "left-over" findings that require explanation. They don't fit in with the bulk of findings, but they don't contradict them either. Flaws may be located in the instrumentation or in data collection procedures or in statistical analysis procedures; that is, there may be a failure in comprehensiveness. The deviant findings in such a case may give direction to future instrument development, for example. In other cases, the qualitative and quantitative findings may "fight" each other, offering up contradiction. Again, the researcher may search for flaws in the study. Finding none, one might turn again to the purpose of comprehensiveness as a possible explanation for contradiction. In qualitative research in particular, contradiction may simply point to a need for expansion in concepts so that the range of human variety is adequately accounted for in the data. Here, the quantitative researcher's concerns with means and medians are at odds philosophically with the qualitative researcher's concerns with the range of human possibilities. The odd case, the one that doesn't fit in with the others, is critical to disclosing those possibilities. The search for possible ways to be human in any given context is of particular interest to the phenomenological researcher, and of general interest for all qualitative researchers. Nonetheless, the tension between the particular and the universal is experienced not only between the quantitative and qualitative orientations; it is also a tension within the qualitative tradition. The purpose of comprehensiveness is for some qualitative researchers interpreted to mean that a research interest in coping or in using the health care delivery system, for example, is necessarily concerned with an accounting for the variety that we believe exists.

Two studies using multiple triangulation, and recently reported in the literature, will be reviewed to illustrate ways in which triangulation might be used. The first is an essentially qualitative study, according to the authors' designation; the second is an essentially quantitative study.

Knafl and Breitmayer (1989) reported on their use of multiple triangulation to achieve comprehensiveness in a qualitative study in-process of how families define and manage a child's chronic illness. In Table 17–1, these authors' framework for evaluating the comprehensiveness of their study is indicated by citing each type of triangulation and the approach and purpose/goal for that type.

Table 17–1
Framework for Evaluating the Completeness of a Qualitative Study Using Multiple Triangulation

Type of Triangulation	Approach	Purpose/Goal
Investigator	Four member team	Substantive, theoretical, and methodological diversity.
Data Source	Person Time Situation	Represent individual perspectives over time and across a variety of situations. Theoretical sample.
Method	Intensive interviews Child Behavior Checklist (CBCL) Family Environment Scale (FES) Harter Perception Profile (HPP)	Identify individual definitions and management behaviors. Explore outcomes of definitions and behaviors.
Unit of Analysis	Individual Family	Conceptualize individual and family unit response.
Theory	Development Application	Conceptualize family management style. Interpret individual and family unit response patterns.

Note: From "Triangulation in Qualitative Research: Issues of Conceptual Clarity and Purpose" by K. Knafl and B. Breitmayer, 1989. In *Qualitative Nursing Research: A Contemporary Dialogue* (pp. 213–214), Ed. by J. Morse. Newbury Park, CA: Sage Publishers, Inc. Reprinted by permission.

For investigator triangulation, four team members were assembled who had a general interest in how families respond to a member's chronic illness. The team members were diverse, however, in terms of their particular expertise with parents, children, or siblings; knowledge about differing aspects of the relevant literature; theoretical backgrounds; and research training. This diversity produced in the research team a complementarity that contributed to the purpose of comprehensiveness in the research.

Data triangulation was used across the three dimensions of person, time, and situation by collecting data from: (1) chronically ill children, their parents, and their siblings (person); (2) families in which a child had been recently diagnosed and families in which a child had been diagnosed for some time (situation); and (3) two data collection sessions, spaced twelve months apart (time). Two levels of data analysis, the individual and the family unit, were featured in this study, to emphasize the person dimension of the data triangulation. Methodological triangulation was used through combining qualitative and quantitative data generation strategies: structured instruments, observations, and intensive interviews. Theoretical triangulation in this theory-generating (as opposed to theory-testing) study was to be used in two ways: first, existing theories were to be used to interpret the data; and second, at the conclusion of the research process, findings were to be discussed in relation to other theories of family response to chronic illness (Knafl & Breitmayer, 1989, pp. 214-218).

All four types of triangulation were also illustrated in Murphy's (1989) report of a study that aimed to assess the relationships between disaster-related stress and mental and physical health outcomes after the Mt. St. Helens volcanic eruption in 1980. Both purposes of convergence and comprehensiveness were served by triangulation in this study. The mediating effects of self-efficacy and social support on the stress–health relationship were examined, and the effects of mass media coverage on recovery were explored. Table 17-2 summarizes the main features of multiple triangulation in this study.

Data triangulation involved collecting data from 5 mutually exclusive types of study participants as listed in Table 17-2. Study instruments, arranged in 3 random orders, were mailed 1 year and 3 years postdisaster. This enabled the researchers to compare data across the study groups and longitudinally, from 1 year to 3 years postdisaster. Follow-up interviews were conducted with subsamples from each of the 5 study groups in order to obtain in-depth information regarding perceived disaster stress, coping strategies used, and perceived recovery. Investigator triangulation was achieved through the involvement of multiple researchers in this 8-year research project, and included multiple interviewers and initial and secondary analyses of data. Data analysis involved various theoretical and methodological approaches by the research team members. Theoretical triangulation was used to test the

Table 17–2
Multiple Triangulation: Application in a Study of the
Relationship Between Disaster-Related Stress and
Health Outcomes (Murphy, 1989)

Type of Triangulation	Approach Features
Data	Study groups:
	1. Bereaved group without property loss
	2. Bereaved group with property loss
	3. Permanent property loss
	4. Vacation home loss
	5. No disaster loss
	Instruments randomly arranged, mailed at 1 year and 3 years postdisaster
	Follow-up interviews with subsample from each study group
Investigator	Multiple investigators
Theoretical	Tests of magnitude of loss hypothesis and two rival hypotheses: self-efficacy and social support
Methodological	Multiple statistical techniques
	Analysis of structured interview data

major hypothesis that effects of loss are proportional to their magnitude, and two rival hypotheses of mediating effects of stress on health, social support and self-efficacy. In methodological triangulation, multiple statistical techniques were used to demonstrate the independence of linked pairs of bereaved participants and to test the magnitude of loss hypothesis, and interview data were analyzed to identify stressors and mediators of stressors.

THE CONTROVERSY, WITH AUTHOR COMMENTARY

Curious about how we tend to talk past one another, and finding nursing's progress toward better understandings of opposing views slow at best, I will present two polarized points of view about research triangulation, with special attention to how they do and don't speak to each other. For the reader who strives to arrive at a personal judgment concerning the wisdom or the legitimacy of combining qualitative and quantitative research approaches, this discussion of opposing views may help to clarify what is at stake as well as the differences and difficulties in these arguments.

Moccia's (1988) argument against combining research approaches is selected to represent this stance because it is such a cogent explication and because it serves to complement the careful grounding for qualitative research laid out in Chapters 1 through 3. Gortner's (1990) argument for a philosophy of nursing science that clearly consigns qualitative researchers to an ancillary role in the discipline is also selected for two reasons. First, it too is such a cogent explication of a view that dismisses qualitative research as a misdirected, otherwise worthy, endeavor. Second, few articles have appeared in the preceding decade that pointedly, and publicly, articulated the concerns and criticisms of many nurse researchers and students of nursing research. Each of these scholars' arguments will be described, accompanied by the author's commentary. It is hoped that the commentary will be successful in extending the necessary ongoing dialogue in this controversy.

Moccia (1988) argued against "appeasement and compromise" in decisions concerning whether and when to use qualitative or quantitative methods or a combination of the two. She cited four problems in the compromise approach:

1. The reality of limited resources of time, energy, and expertise in any given study or for any given researcher;
2. The flawed assumption that nursing research questions are atheoretical, lending themselves to a variety of methodological options;
3. A denial of the significance of the influence of philosophies of science in research and theory development;
4. The avoidance of commentary on the political function of research traditions (p. 2).

In arguing for a reframing of the debate about methods in nursing research, Moccia offered the clarification that we are faced with a very fundamental choice about what nursing is to become: the choice of methods is really about the choice of continuing to develop knowledge that is aimed at prediction and control of people and their problems, or of aligning ourselves with methods that serve recipients of nursing care, methods that assist people with understanding their experiences. But, this equates research with practice: every situation presents a research project; and surely, Moccia is not arguing that qualitative research findings do not constitute knowledge that can somehow be used to assist others outside of the situation that produced the findings.

Qualitative research produces a certain *kind* of knowledge. It produces knowledge of the range of possibilities, given shared historicity, which does offer a degree of predictability in health care situations. Qualitative research also contributes to what is understood about the nature of being human. It serves to relate us to one another, opening up a new sense of community with others, which, in turn, is linked to behaving more humanely with one another. Qualitative research thus has a sensitizing effect in the nurse–patient relationship that has valuable, "good" outcomes for people in nursing.

Nursing necessarily uses many knowledges in order to practice holistically, in recognition that multiple perspectives constitute truth. It has chosen to strive for holism in its orientation, its intending, toward the practice world. Because truth is a matrix of perspectives, because being scientific in the positivist tradition is one of those perspectives, and because a view of the person as object yields a perspective as nearly true as any other, nurses need to synthesize multiple perspectives to accomplish their practice aims. If nursing scholars fail to interpret the relevance of research findings to practice in terms of a synthesis that admits multiple perspectives, it is not likely that practice will achieve an art–science coherence, a holistic orientation, or a distinctive character that renders nursing with an identity in the health care field.

As Moccia indicated, the question of combining research approaches pivots on the consequences of choice for nursing morally, ideologically, and politically. The kinds of questions posed as research questions, the kinds of data admitted as research data, and the processes used to generate the data all contribute to the definition of nursing and ultimately to practice activities themselves. But nursing does use other sciences, and this confuses the issue. If one accepts the notion that there is (or could be) a unique body of knowledge in nursing, or a unique application of knowledge, this is to say that nursing has boundaries and a perspective that distinguish it from other disciplines. For some qualitative researchers, the qualitative approach focuses our attention on certain kinds of phenomena from a particular perspective that is congruent with nursing intentions, but also clearly contrary to the positivist tradition in research. The relevance of qualitative methods for them has more to do with defining and creating nursing than with the methods per se. As Moccia (1988) stated,

> *The research activity contributes to the emergence of a world or reality that was not there before the research. Through such research the knowledge created is logically characterized by the same attributes that identify human phenomena, e.g., the rational and the emotional, the objective and the subjective, and the passionate and the controlled. Logically, then, such characteristics also describe the science created through such an approach to research. (p. 3)*

The idea of creating knowledge rather than discovering it is a unique feature of at least some interpretations of qualitative research. Through interview, for example, the researcheds' reflection on and presentation of their experiences in language form create certain meanings that might not otherwise appear for them. Still, as research that produces knowledge, it must be understood as just one possible mode of awareness. Although it strives to give voice to human experiences, it is just one perspective on those experiences. Qualitative research cannot claim to have an exclusive corner on truth. Qualitative research findings are holistic only in the sense of meaning and coherence within the perspective of research participants. They are not holistic in the sense of disclosing all possible perspectives, nor is this generally the aim of qualitative studies. This distinction from the sense of the term "holistic" when used to describe nursing care is important.

In Moccia's view, the methods debate concerns a distinction "among research activities that serve nurses and nursing, those that serve patients and the public's health, and those that serve both" (1988, p. 6). She argued against the effort to predict and control based on both the resistance of holistic human phenomena to prediction and control, and nurses' interest in their patients as autonomous, self-determining subjects rather than objects. Yet, to recall the kinds of knowledge that qualitative research produces, knowledge of *some* of the possibilities and even of probabilities does not have to be applied so as to cut off other possibilities, choice, and uniqueness. It seems to go without saying that nurses need to be able to predict (in a general way) such human experiences as pain and suffering, grieving, birthing, and so on, in order to anticipate and deliver needed care. This does not mean, for example, that a nurse can or should be able to predict precisely how John Doe will respond, but nurses do need to predict that he is likely to have pain, that his cultural history and identification may influence his response in certain ways, or that the meaning of his diagnosis to him is likely to be influenced by sociocultural meanings in certain ways. Being human does mean something; we do share a common world of objects; we share multiple capacities, a common stock of everyday knowledge, and a common range of human possibilities within the contexts of the various worlds in which we find ourselves. This commonality includes those perspectives, among others, that are particularly focused in medical science and health care technology. In fact, it is because of our continually changing contexts that the work of qualitative research is never finished.

To be in health care situations with patients and to contribute meaningfully to those situations, nurses continue to need access to the multiple perspectives that constitute holistic assessment and intervention. If nursing is to claim the patient's experiencing as its unique focus, this claim will be furthered by such access. Why do qualitative research if not to disclose shared humanness and human possibility? We cannot, should not, close off our scientific mode of awareness. But, we should not adhere strictly to it if nursing's ambition to be expert in human experiencing of health and health care situations is to be realized.

Qualitative methods are designed to get inside the skin of the actors in these situations. However, as Gadow (1977) explained, the lived body and the object body both need to be understood to practice nursing. She stated:

> *The history of professionalism in nursing suggests that nursing has focused exclusively upon the lived body and the object body in turn. . . . Nursing can now surpass both of these extremes: the nurse, as advocate of the patient's wholeness, is committed to advocacy of neither the shattered lived body nor the duly imposed object body. Nursing can, in short, make possible for the patient an enrichment of the lived body by the object body, and an enlivening of the object body by the lived body. The nurse can assist the patient to recover the objectified body at a new level at which it is neither mute immediacy nor pure otherness, but an otherness-made-mine, a lived objectiveness. . . . The nurse assists me, the patient, to live my objectness as my own, instead of allowing it to remain alien. That unity which I achieve is more fully expressive of my totality than even the lived body was. (pp. 24–25)*

In this way, nurses are in a position to offer assistance to patients with a truly humanistic science, not merely with well-honed counseling skills, but also with substantive knowledge about human health experiences.

Gortner (1990) acknowledged the significance of nursing values and nursing philosophy in traditional ways; that is, she cited the guidance of values in nursing activities, including scientific enterprises, and suggested:

> *What well may be foundational in humanistic philosophy (concern for person and meaning) can remain as philosophy; it need not be translated into scientific strategies . . . and used to the exclusion of other options. Further, the practice of science and the scientific method, the search for explanations, regularities, and predictions about the human state should not be viewed as being incompatible with*

*professional beliefs about practice and societal and per-
sonal worth. (p. 102)*

She went on to cite the foundational nature of humanistic philosophy in Scandinavian nursing research as evidence of the potential
for an intimate link between nursing philosophy and nursing research, noting that the "renewed interest in humanism and history
has infused us with an appreciation for and sensitivity to the human condition, in the links between objective measures of reality
and personal subjective ones" (1990, p. 103). What Gortner accomplished with this statement was reinforcement of an essentially di-
chotomous split between our humanism and our science—one that
was reaffirmed in Gortner's proposal for a nursing science philosophy. In this proposal, she established that human understanding,
arising from interpretations of phenomena from the patient's perspective, is a basic premise in nursing science, but then went on to
reaffirm the positivist tradition with its emphasis on measurement,
causal inference, and knowledge that allows for prescriptions for
practice (pp. 103–105).

Despite the respect accorded to qualitative methods as an aid
to the linkage between philosophy and research, they are not included in nursing science, which Gortner defined as public
knowledge, meaning, in turn, intersubjective consensus among
scholars. In so doing, Gortner neglected to attend to strategic
points about the irreconcilability of the philosophical frameworks that support two research traditions in a variety of disciplines, and to the claims of intersubjectivity as an essential feature in the qualitative paradigm. However, she credited the idea
of grounding quantitative research formally and practically in a
body of knowledge generated through qualitative research, and
this was a promising overture of compromise in its most positive
sense. Recognizing qualitative research as truly foundational to
quantitative efforts in the field would be facilitated doubtlessly by
a comprehensive inclusion of the former in nursing science. To do
so requires, as Moccia stated, redefinition of science and the profession. To arrive at this, there must be continuing attention,
specifically, to the nature of reality, truth, and human experience. Though not all nursing scholars may be inclined to ponder

such philosophical questions, their importance is brought into relief by the neglected discussion of these premises by those who either oppose qualitative methods altogether or who regard them as merely a collection of techniques that may be applied to quantitative purposes.

Gortner's essay represented the kind of appeasement and compromise position that Moccia criticized. On the surface, considerable appreciation was expressed for qualitative researchers whose interest resides in "human understanding," which, for Gortner, was a worthy endeavor in nursing philosophy, but distinct from scientific activities. The problem in this stance is the failure to include qualitative research as part of legitimate science, which will prevent adequacy in the body of knowledge that nursing produces. The idea that values and meanings determine our research behavior as well as our practice behavior is not recognized as a tangible and practical feature of qualitative research activity. Values are dismissed as if they had no practical consequences on public knowledge, as if there really were an absolute truth awaiting discovery. There is a seductiveness in Gortner's essay in its appeal to a desire for orderliness in the discipline, with clear separation of nursing science from other nursing activities despite a weakly described linkage among them. The reaffirmation of the positivist tradition in the point of view represented by Gortner's proposal is perhaps an expression of the preference to continue in the mainstream of scientific endeavors in health care and a reluctance to confront the fact of choices before us.

To wait out the death of the debate is to refuse choice. It is not enough to say values and philosophy are nice, and of course there is interaction between nursing philosophy and nursing research. Consciousness has been raised, and, increasingly, researchers are recognizing that their use of research techniques has consequences for research participants and for the evolution of nursing practice in health care. When viewed as merely a collection of techniques, qualitative research methods can easily be triangulated in studies, as illustrated by the applications described earlier in the chapter. Goodwin and Goodwin (1984), for example, lay out this view directly: "The qualitative–quantitative distinction is primarily one of methods of data collection, analysis, and interpretation" (p. 378). Inattentiveness to the philosophical framework for qualitative research, or rejection of it, allows this.

An alternative basis for triangulated research can be located in an understanding of nursing phenomena from a practice perspective such as that explicated by Gadow (1977). The kinds of questions about these phenomena—in fact, the very emergence of phenomena as nursing phenomena—should be grounded in nursing philosophy if that philosophy really means something about nursing or for nursing. Clarity in identity and purpose will go far in guiding researchers in what they attend to, how they proceed with attending to it, and their use of the information produced by the research effort. Phenomenologically, what is argued is a need to establish a phenomenological baseline for our concepts, our theories, and our subsequent science. Other disciplines and other schools of thought within the nursing discipline might refer to this baseline to do science in the positivist tradition, and such science, in turn, will continue to become a part of our worlds, transforming human experience and creating new possibilities. In this sense, the work of establishing a phenomenological baseline is continuous. We have witnessed, for example, modification in theories of grieving as more is learned about how grieving is lived through by people. We have come to understand that the timetable for grieving varies considerably; that the meaning of loss is open to a range of possibilities; that living through loss is highly contextual, highly embodied, highly enmeshed in a range of possible perspectives; and clearly intersubjective.

Duffy (1987) has provided a discussion of benefits of triangulation that focuses the potentially complementary and supplementary relation of qualitative and quantitative methods (p. 132). Springing from a view of differences between these two approaches as differences in not only techniques but also perspectives, she suggested that each perspective has limitations and, thus, the overriding purpose of triangulation is to counterbalance the weakness of one perspective with the strength of the other. When one's attention is drawn to the world of nursing practice, various practical concerns surface, notably, the need of nurses for concepts and theories to guide practice in the hectically paced world of health care. There has been unquestionably insufficient knowledge for them to use to size up situations quickly; to recognize who among their patients needs and chooses to explore and to determine their experiences; to know not only how to guide, but where; to know when and how to apply information in health-producing ways; to determine coherence in health care situations that are intimidatingly complicated with multiple participants and multiple perspectives. Nurses cannot be expected to approach each patient care situation without such knowledge; that is to say, without such generalizations about possibilities and probabilities. We do need science, and science is concerned with regularities, but also with possibilities.

There is an appeal to the idea that nursing would define itself as being, by choice, concerned with particular aspects of truth that are addressed by the qualitative research paradigm. As noted in Chapters 1 through 3, this kind of explicit acknowledgment of the discipline's interest and concern needs to avoid the trap of discounting the presence and import of the positivist perspective in the world. This perspective along with others are "real" and a part of the world to which nurses and patients belong, and thus cannot be discounted in the chosen perspective of human experiencing of the world. Consensus about a nursing perspective, however, does not seem to be imminent.

Practically speaking, then, nursing research is likely to continue to house two schools of thought. (Parenthetically, there is a third school of thought, but one hears little about it in the literature these days; that is, little from positivists who see no merit or authenticity in the arguments of the qualitative paradigm.) The first school adheres carefully to the qualitative paradigm, inclusive of its particular view of the nature of being human and of reality, the nature of nursing practice, and the kind of knowledge that serves the intentions of such a nursing worldview. Researchers who subscribe to this worldview will not triangulate their studies, in part because the introduction of measurement in their relationship with participants would alter the nature of that relationship and interfere with the data-generating dialogue of mutual benefit to researcher and researched. But, they would not deny the positivist worldview that is such a prominent part of health care situations.

The second school of thought concerns itself less with world-views, accepts positivist premises as practical at the least, and makes use of qualitative research strategies as needed or desired to broaden understanding of those phenomena selected for research attention. Studies that flow from this way of regarding methodological options might be essentially qualitative or quantitative and might reflect the researcher's selective commitment to one or the other research paradigms. Unfortunately, this second school of thought, as currently practiced in research, does not recognize what is intended in the use of qualitative research to produce a phenomenological baseline; that is, the juxtaposition of quantitative research in a secondary role.

As Gortner and others who promote triangulation have pointed out, the interests and concerns of qualitative researchers are not irrelevant to quantitative researchers. There can be productive dialogue between the two. Neither school of thought necessarily need block the other; multiple paradigms within a single discipline are characteristic of our world anyway. We can live with blatant conflicts in ways of thinking about the discipline, and might profit from it. In the meantime, researchers who locate a rationale in the purposes of triangulation explicated in the literature should be welcomed to the discipline's exploration of research methodologies. Appeasement and compromise are among our possibilities as is the purist approach to qualitative research. The only danger at this point is a patronizing ear for the minority voice of the qualitative tradition, with the expectation that this too will pass.

REFERENCES

Campbell, J. (1989). A test of two explanatory models of women's responses to battering. *Nursing Research, 38*(1), 18–24.

Denzin, N. (1978). *The research act: A theoretical introduction to sociological methods* (2nd ed.) New York: McGraw-Hill.

Duffy, M. (1987). Methodological triangulation: A vehicle for merging quantitative and qualitative research methods. *Image: The Journal of Nursing Scholarship, 19*(3), 130–133.

Fielding, N., & Fielding, J. (1986). *Linking data.* Beverly Hills, CA: Sage.

Gadow, S. (1977). Existential advocacy: Philosophical foundation of nursing. Presented to Four State Consortium on Nursing and the

Humanities, Phase I Conference, *Nursing the humanities: A public dialogue*, Farmington, CT.

Goodwin, L., & Goodwin, H. (1984). Qualitative vs. quantitative research or qualitative and quantitative research? *Nursing Research, 33*(6), 378-380.

Gortner, S. (1990). Nursing values and science: Toward a science philosophy. *Image: The Journal of Nursing Scholarship, 22*(2), 101-105.

Knafl, K., & Breitmayer, B. (1991). Triangulation in qualitative research: Issues of conceptual clarity and purpose. In J. Morse (Ed.), *Qualitative nursing research: A contemporary dialogue* (pp. 209-220). Newbury Park, CA: Sage.

Moccia, P. (1988). A critique of compromise: Beyond the methods debate. *Advances in Nursing Science, 10*(4), 1-9.

Murphy, S. (1989). Multiple triangulation: Applications in a program of nursing research. *Nursing Research, 38*(5), 294-297.

ADDITIONAL REFERENCES

Allen, D. (1985). Nursing research and social control: Alternative models of science that emphasize understanding and emancipation. *Image: The Journal of Nursing Scholarship, 17*(2), 58-64.

Jick, T. (1983). Mixing qualitative and quantitative methods: Triangulation in action. In M. van Manen (Ed.), *Qualitative methodology* (pp. 135-148). Beverly Hills, CA: Sage.

Lather, P. (1986). Research as praxis. *Harvard Educational Review, 56*(3), 257-277.

Mitchell, E. (1986). Multiple triangulation: A methodology for nursing science. *Advances in Nursing Science, 8*(4), 18-26.

Munhall, P. (1986). Methodological issues in nursing research: Beyond a wax apple. *Advances in Nursing Science, 8*(3), 1-5.

Powers, B. (1987). Taking sides: A response to Goodwin and Goodwin. *Nursing Research, 36*(2), 122-126.

Schultz, P. (1987). Toward holistic inquiry in nursing: A proposal for synthesis of patterns and methods. *Scholarly Inquiry for Nursing Practice, 1*(2), 135-146.

Smith, J. (1983). Quantitative versus qualitative research: An attempt to clarify the issue. *Educational Researcher, 12*(3), 6-13.

Tinkle, M., & Beaton, J. (1983). Toward a new view of science: Implications for nursing research. *Advances in Nursing Science, 5*(2), 27-36.

18

Evaluating
Qualitative Research

Marlene Zichi Cohen
Kathleen A. Knafl

Q ualitative researchers have a long-standing interest in promoting excellence in qualitative inquiry. This interest is reflected in a considerable body of literature addressing "quality control" issues and standards in qualitative research. Much of this literature is directed to providing investigators with guidelines for enhancing the overall quality of their research. For example, Sandelowski (1986) presented strategies qualitative researchers can use to make their work more rigorous without compromising its relevance. Her discussion drew heavily on Guba and Lincoln's (1981) earlier presentation of standards of rigor for qualitative research. Other authors across a variety of disciplines have identified strategies for ensuring the quality of qualitative investigations (Kirk &

Miller, 1986; Le Compte & Goetz, 1982; Patton, 1990; Woods & Cantanzaro, 1988). In a similar vein, Sandelowski, Davis, and Harris (1989) identified strategies for writing qualitative research proposals that communicate the assumptions and rigor underlying qualitative inquiry. Other authors have provided guidelines for reporting qualitative research (Field & Morse, 1985; Knafl & Howard, 1984; Wolcott, 1990).

In addition to developing guidelines for ensuring quality in the design, conduct, and reporting of their investigations, qualitative researchers have recognized the need to explicate evaluative guidelines so that the products of their research efforts can be judged appropriately. Concerns about the use of appropriate criteria for evaluating qualitative research are not new to nurse researchers. In an early article published in *Nursing Research,* Glaser and Strauss (1966) questioned "the applicability of the canons of quantitative research as criteria for judging the credibility of qualitative research and analysis" (p. 56). They argued in favor of using criteria "based on generic elements of qualitative methods for collecting, analyzing, and presenting data" (p. 56). Since that time, other qualitative researchers in nursing have developed frameworks for judging the merit of qualitative investigations (Aamodt, 1983; Burns, 1989; Cobb & Hagemaster, 1987; Morse, 1991; Parse, Coyne, & Smith, 1985). Our intent in this chapter is to provide an overview of these existing evaluative schemes. In addition, we describe several projects undertaken by the Qualitative Special Interest Group of the Midwest Nursing Research Society (SIG/Qual) to develop evaluative criteria and explore how reviewers judge the strengths and weaknesses of qualitative research.

FRAMEWORKS FOR EVALUATING QUALITATIVE RESEARCH

Table 18-1 provides an overview of several general frameworks put forth by nurse researchers for evaluating qualitative research. The frameworks are general in the sense that none is linked to a specific qualitative approach such as grounded theory or phenomenology. As shown in Table 18-1, there are several overlapping

Table 18-1
Frameworks for Evaluating Qualitative Research

Aamodt (1983)	Parse, Coyne, & Smith (1985)	Cobb & Hagemaster (1987)	Burns (1989)	Leininger (1990)	Morse (1991)
Discovery	Substance	Context	Descriptive vividness	Meaning-in-context	Emergent design
Assumptions	Clarity	Importance	Heuristic relevance	Transferability	Investigator competence
Context	Integration	Expertise	Analytical preciseness	Confirmability	Creativity
Contribution		Problem	Methodological congruence	Credibility	Qualitative grounding
		Purpose	Theoretical connectedness	Recurrent patterning	Explicitness
		Literature		Saturation	
		Sample			
		Data collection			
		Data analysis			
		Human subjects			

criteria. Aamodt (1983), Cobb and Hagemaster (1987), Burns (1989), and Leininger (1990) agreed that qualitative studies should be judged in part based on their significance (i.e., contribution, importance, relevance, transferability).

Regarding the importance of context in evaluating qualitative studies, Aamodt (1983) emphasized the importance of conveying the context in which the verbal or behavioral actions of interest occur, and Cobb and Hagemaster (1987) discussed the importance of understanding the investigator's role in the research setting. Burns (1989) noted the responsibility of the investigator to present a full description of the research site and subjects as well as a description of the actual process of doing the research. She pointed out that, because "all data are context specific, the evaluator of a study must understand the context of that study" (p. 48).

Consistent with their focus on evaluating qualitative proposals, Cobb and Hagemaster (1987) and Morse (1991) identified the competence of the investigator as a key criterion. Morse argued that, for major grant applications, "evaluation of the investigator is critical and should be weighted most heavily" (1991, p. 149). Finally, Cobb and Hagemaster (1987) and Burns (1989) identified the importance of evaluating the clarity and specificity of the analytic activities that lead to or are intended to lead to the study results. In particular, they pointed out the need to indicate the processes and decisions underlying the final organization and presentation of the data.

Beyond these overlapping criteria, there is considerable variation in both the overall focus of these evaluative schemes and the specific criteria cited. Cobb and Hagemaster's (1987) categories reflect standard evaluative criteria. Acknowledging this, they pointed out that "the questions forming the content of each category address concerns unique to qualitative research" (p. 139). Thus, each criterion is followed by a list of questions linking it to qualitative inquiry. For example, the following questions come under the "Sample" criterion:

1. Are the unique issues of sampling in a qualitative study adequately addressed?
2. Are the potential characteristics of the sample outlined?

This framework provides a clearly articulated useful set of questions for reviewers to use in evaluating qualitative proposals.

On the other hand, Morse's (1991) criteria suggested much broader expectations for qualitative proposals. She directed the reviewer to look for evidence of an emergent design, an experienced qualitative investigator, creative thinking and building on existing work in the field, recognition of the distinct nature of qualitative research, and explicit examples of how the work of the proposed study will be carried out. Morse argued that it is the responsibility of the investigator to write a proposal that "excites and intrigues the reviewers, to stimulate their interest in your ideas and your topic" (1991, p. 150). Taken together, these two frameworks complement one another by providing both a set of general expectations (Morse, 1991) and specific criteria (Cobb & Hagemaster, 1987) for evaluating qualitative proposals.

The four remaining authors also provided varying degrees of specificity in the evaluative frameworks they put forth. Aamodt (1983) described the four factors she lists as dimensions of qualitative research which "suggest a beginning for a set of criteria for evaluating qualitative research" (p. 398). She summarized the importance of these dimensions:

> *The issues grounding a distinctive criteria for qualitative methodologies include, in part, discovering, describing, and labeling an idea, conceptualizing assumptions to bracket a territory for study, recognizing the reflex activity of the researcher and the object of study, developing detailed descriptions of contextual settings necessary to data in qualitative research, and showing the usefulness of the substantive or theoretical data to nursing practice, research, or theory.* (p. 400)

In contrast, Burns (1989), Leininger (1990), and Parse et al. (1985) included considerable elaboration of the evaluative criteria they put forth. Burns's criteria followed a discussion of the nature of qualitative research and research reports. Her discussion of each of her five standards included threats to achieving the standard of which the reviewer needs to be aware. In addition to the three previously discussed dimensions—descriptive vividness, heuristic relevance, and analytical preciseness—Burns cited methodological congruence and theoretical connectedness as important evaluative criteria. According to Burns, methodological congruence requires the reviewer to assess both the metatheory or underlying assumptions and specific qualitative approach that guide the research. Methodological congruence includes rigor in documentation, procedural rigor, ethical rigor, and auditability. Documentation of the rigor of the study refers to specifying both the philosophical and methodological underpinnings of the study. Procedural rigor requires the investigator to demonstrate the accuracy and representativeness of the data. Ethical rigor directs the researcher to demonstrate that the subjects' rights were protected during the research, and auditability addresses the documentation of the process by which the results of the study emerged from the data. The standard of theoretical connectedness "requires that the theoretical schema developed from the study be clearly expressed, logically consistent, reflective of the data and compatible with the knowledge base of nursing" (Burns, 1989, p. 50).

Interestingly, Burns also discussed skills that she believes are needed to critique qualitative research effectively. These included context flexibility or the ability to see things from different perspectives, skills in inductive reasoning and conceptual thinking, and the ability to transform ideas across levels of abstraction.

Drawing heavily on the work of Lincoln and Guba (1985), Leininger (1990) spoke to the importance of the investigator's demonstrating that data have been reaffirmed through a sustained process of observation and informant interviewing (confirmability). Leininger also believes that qualitative studies should be evaluated in terms of the investigator's ability to support their credibility, to identify recurrent patterns of behavior, and to collect data until there is a redundancy of information (saturation).

Citing the work of both Batey (1977) and Kaplan (1964), Parse et al. (1985) identified three broad evaluative criteria: substance, clarity, and integration. Substance refers to the adequacy of the ideas underlying the research. Clarity includes the logical development of ideas as well as the effective communication of those ideas. Integration is the coherent linking of the various aspects of the study. These three standards are applied across four dimensions of the research process: conceptual, ethical, methodological, and interpretive. Like Cobb and Hagemaster's (1987) framework, this one includes a series of specific questions the reviewer can use in applying each of the three criteria or standards to each of the four research domains.

These schemes, which vary in both their purpose and level of specificity, provide the reviewer with considerable choice in selecting an evaluative framework. Cobb and Hagemaster (1987) and Morse (1991) linked their criteria to evaluating qualitative proposals; the other authors discussed the evaluation of qualitative research reports. Each of the frameworks contributes to setting reasonable expectations and appropriate standards for reviewers of qualitative research to follow and the selection of one over the other rests on the purpose of review and the reviewer's preference for general guidelines as opposed to more detailed criteria.

EVALUATING QUALITATIVE RESEARCH USING DIFFERENT APPROACHES

Although the frameworks discussed in the previous section provide useful guidelines for evaluating qualitative research, they fail to take into account important differences among specific qualitative approaches. These differences across approaches can have important implications for the evaluation of qualitative research. Sandelowski (1986) noted that "the term qualitative inquiry is a very imprecise and often misleading label referring to many widely divergent research methods. . . . Each of these methods has its own rules concerning aims, evidence, inference, and verification" (pp. 27–28). Recognizing the importance of these differences and the confusion sometimes surrounding the evaluation of qualitative research, the Qualitative Special Interest Group of the Midwest Nursing Research Society (SIG/Qual), in 1987, prepared guidelines that are available from the authors for reviewing qualitative research reports based on some of the major qualitative approaches.

These detailed guidelines highlight both similarities and differences across the four approaches included in the SIG/Qual document (description grounded theory, phenomenology, critical research). All these approaches emphasize the importance of presenting a rich, contextual understanding of the subject matter. Further, investigators using these methods typically rely heavily on intensive interviewing and/or participant observation for data collection. At the same time, studies based on these approaches reflect different underlying purposes, procedures, and styles of presentation. For example, grounded theorists focus on the identification and conceptualization of basic social processes that explain human behavior, and phenomenologists aim to understand the lived experiences of their subjects. Investigators using each approach use different interview strategies and different data reduction and analysis techniques. Moreover, there often are differences *within* the major qualitative approaches, and the reviewer may need to take them into account. For example, ethnographers working from different cultural theories and phenomenologists reflecting different philosophical traditions will address different kinds of research questions and use different data collection and analysis methods. Thus, in addition to being knowledgeable of the general frameworks for evaluating qualitative research described in the previous section, reviewers also need to be aware of differences across qualitative approaches and to take these difference into account when reviewing a manuscript. The additional readings provided at the end of this chapter include useful information for evaluating research using a specific qualitative approach. It is especially important that researchers identify and reviewers recognize the purpose of the study and its relationship to the qualitative approach chosen and the overall design of the research.

In addition to delineating appropriate criteria for evaluating qualitative research, it also is instructive to understand the kinds of criteria reviewers actually apply to qualitative research. In the following section, we describe another project undertaken by SIG/Qual to identify what reviewers see as the unique strengths and weakness of qualitative research.

A REVIEW OF REVIEWS

Criteria for evaluating qualitative research grant proposals have been developed. A variety of helpful publications focus on grant writing (e.g., Tornquist & Funk, 1990), and several focus on qualitative grant writing (Marshall & Rosman, 1989; Sandelowski et al., 1989; Tripp-Reimer & Cohen, 1989). Although these criteria exist, qualitative researchers continue to have concerns about whether appropriate criteria are used to evaluate qualitative research grant proposals. Discussions among members of SIG/Qual led three members to seek summary statements ("pink sheets") from researchers who had written qualitative research grant proposals. The analysis of the reviews of the 20 pink sheets received is reported more completely in Cohen, Knafl, and Dzurec (1993, in press).

The review of these pink sheets to find common themes was coupled with the literature on criteria for evaluating grants and federal grant review criteria in order to better understand criteria actually used to evaluate qualitative research proposals. The reviewers of these proposals did indeed identify common strengths and weaknesses.

Qualitative researchers generally did a good job of establishing the scientific contribution of the research. It was important to show that the research was likely to yield new information and that the topic to be studied was one of significance. The parts of the proposal need to fit together in a coherent and consistent manner. The literature review needs to lead logically to the specific aims by showing what is known and how the study will expand this knowledge. The importance of the knowledge to the nursing profession should be shown. Grant writers who choose to base their research on a theory need to organize the literature review in such a way, to show why the approach chosen is the most appropriate in the context of that theory. If a particular theory is not used as a context for the proposed research, justification is needed.

Those proposals with higher priority scores (i.e., less favorable reviews) most often had comments about difficulties with the methods section. The investigator needs to show that the method proposed is sound for the stage of research being proposed and that the method will achieve the aims specified. Congruence of purpose, aims, and research design need to be made apparent by the writers. Furthermore, the stated research questions must be consistent with the stated specific aims.

Proposal reviewers indicated that investigators need to describe clearly the details of the proposed research methods. The critiques showed the importance of describing the method in detail. Preliminary work, pilot projects, and previous related research can help the grant writer be clear about the details of the approach. For example, this early work can demonstrate how research assistants will be trained and can clarify the appropriate questions and probes that will be used in interviews because these are the most commonly used "instruments." Preliminary work can also clarify whether persons with appropriate experiences to serve as informants are available and willing to devote the time required by the proposed design.

Discussion of preliminary research also can illustrate how data will be analyzed to answer the research question(s). Methods for qualitative analysis are less well known and standardized than are quantitative analysis procedures. A clear description (as appropriate) of a systematic plan for data organization, interviews, data processing, analysis, and sample feasibility is needed.

Qualifications of the principal investigation (PI) and the research team were carefully scrutinized by reviewers. This was an area that was most often a strength in these qualitative proposals. Letters of support, appropriateness of consultants, and the PI's record of research and professional experience were all critiqued by reviewers of the proposals studied.

Because researchers have so much invested in the success of their proposals, many have strong emotional responses to the reviews. Some researchers feel angry and misunderstood when their work is reviewed. However, researchers can choose to use the help of the reviewers to revise the work and resubmit it, or they can submit it elsewhere. Given the page constraints of most proposals, the reviewers' comments can help the writer focus on the most essential details to include. The review may also raise important points that the researcher had not considered.

The reviews analyzed showed that, contrary to common belief, qualitative methods do not generally leave researchers at a disadvantage for competitive funding. A well-written qualitative grant proposal, according to this analysis, is one in which the writer thoroughly develops a statement of a relevant, significant problem for nursing, and addresses that problem using appropriate methods or combinations of methods. The problem presented in the proposal should be based on an appropriate literature review, and the research methods should be discussed clearly, thoroughly, and succinctly. Providing a rationale for methods used in qualitative studies was viewed by reviewers as useful, as is writers' acknowledgment of how the study can be interpreted as valid and reliable.

Having knowledgeable, appropriate, and qualified reviewers is clearly important. Although Cohen et al. (1993, in press) analyzed only the reviews and not the grant applications, the reviews were consistent and the feedback they provided was helpful and appropriate. The comments of the reviewers addressed similar issues across proposals and guided the researchers to discuss or elaborate on important areas. No reviews asked researchers to include areas that were inappropriate to the method. For example, phenomenological studies were not criticized for not using a theory to guide analysis.

The well-written proposal tells a story. If the story is disjointed, confusing, inconsistent, inaccurate, or of little significance, reviewers will not support it. On the other hand, if the story captures the reviewers and holds the reviewers' attention from start to finish, without introducing annoying problems that interrupt the flow and obscure the writers' intent, it will gain support from the reviewers.

The wise grant writer anticipates differences between qualitative and quantitative methods—for example, in terms of sample size, validity/reliability vs. truth value/accuracy—and speaks to those issues in the body of the proposal. According to our review, the wise grant writer will demonstrate a knowledgeable, systematic approach. After the review, the wise grant writer reaps the benefits of feedback and funding.

Although persons doing qualitative research may feel that their methods put them at a disadvantage for competitive funding, analysis of the 20 summary statements from grant proposals suggested that reviewers are cognizant of salient issues and are able to respond appropriately to those issues. Proposals that are clearly written, internally consistent, meaningful, and have potential impact for the discipline of nursing are, indeed, well-received by reviewers.

NON-FEDERAL GRANT REVIEW CRITERIA

Members of SIG/Qual also discussed the need to better understand how research is evaluated by non-federal funding sources. Although the criteria used by federal funding sources are widely available, this is less consistently true with smaller agencies. Four members of SIG/Qual sought review criteria from a number of non-federal funding sources. (These members were Marlene Zichi Cohen, Laura Dzurec, Kathy Knafl, and Kathryn Murphy.)

Not all agencies contacted were willing to share their criteria, but evaluation varied tremendously among those who did send criteria. (Because agencies did not give permission to share their criteria, only a summary is included here.) Some groups are guided less by evaluation of the scientific aspects of the research proposed than by how the research fits the mission of the organization providing the funds.

A comprehensive compilation of all the criteria we collected showed that, although some agencies used many specific criteria, some used only a few. Some of the language used in the criteria suggest quantitative studies, but the ideas can be reframed by qualitative researchers and those who evaluate the proposals. For example, the terms validity and reliability carry connotations that are not appropriate to many qualitative methods, but these can easily be addressed as issues of accuracy. Issues of accuracy are indeed appropriate and important in all qualitative research methods. This indicates the need for reviewers who understand the method proposed. Only knowledgeable reviewers will be able to apply the review criteria appropriately.

We compared criteria used by federal agencies, general nursing organizations, and specialty nursing organizations, in order to better understand how they apply to qualitative research.

The criteria used by the Division of Research Grants (DRG) at the National Institutes of Health (NIH) for study section reviews of all grant proposals are appropriate to qualitative methods. These criteria are: significance and originality from a scientific and technical standpoint; adequacy of the methodology to carry out the research; qualifications and experience of the principal investigator and staff; reasonable availability of resources; reasonableness of the proposed budget and duration; other factors: human subjects, animal welfare, biohazards, and so on.

The criteria used by nursing organizations were sometimes more detailed than these federal criteria. However, some nursing organizations had less detailed criteria than the federal criteria. Despite these differences, there were some common criteria.

Most agencies evaluate the budget for appropriateness and adequacy of justification. All the agencies that sent us criteria also evaluated specific aims, hypotheses, or problem statements for clarity, and most evaluated appropriate and logical consistency among purpose, aims, and hypotheses. Most had criteria about the project's significance and some evaluated the proposal's relevance to agency concerns.

All agencies evaluated the literature and theoretical or conceptual framework. All had criteria about the appropriateness of the literature cited. Most evaluated the strength and currency of the literature cited and the relationships identified among the literature and the variables under study.

Most groups evaluated the adequacy of the sampling of subjects in some way. All evaluated the appropriateness of the design. Most also looked at reliability and validity of any measurement instruments. Most agencies have criteria related to an appropriate plan for data analysis. Institutional review board approval and an appropriate time frame for the proposed research were evaluated by most agencies. All agencies evaluated the adequacy of facilities and equipment available for the research.

Because the criteria used to evaluate proposals vary widely, the most helpful approach for the proposal writer may be to contact a specific agency and request review criteria prior to writing a proposal.

CONCLUDING REMARKS

Downs (1990, p. 325) recently called for a "refined and tightened up" review process. The criteria used are, of course, only appropriate if reviewers understand how they apply to qualitative research. This leads to several responsibilities for qualitative researchers. Experienced researchers must take the responsibility to seek roles as reviewers for journals and for funding agencies. Enlisting peers for these roles is also important.

Once these roles are held, reviewers have the responsibility to determine where their skills are sufficient or insufficient for conducting reviews. For example, a grounded theorist may not be able to fairly evaluate phenomenological research. Being clear about what we can and cannot review is important.

It is also important to evaluate the merits of a proposal or manuscript with appropriate standards that are not too rigid. Many philosophers of science have described how research methods evolve and have indicated that this very evolution leads to the most important findings. Our criteria need to allow room for researchers who "break the rules" in creative and appropriate ways to obtain information that will be useful to advance nursing science and practice.

REFERENCES

Aamodt, A. (1983). Problems in doing nursing research: Developing criteria for evaluating qualitative research. *Western Journal of Nursing Research, 5,* 398–402.

Batey, M. (1977). Conceptualization: Knowledge and logic guiding the research process, *Nursing Research, 26,* 324–329.

Burns, R. (1989). Standards for qualitative research. *Nursing Science Quarterly, 2,* 44–52.

Cobb, A., & Hagemaster, J. (1987). Ten Criteria for evaluating qualitative research proposals. *Journal of Nursing Education, 26,* 138–143.

Cohen, M. Z., Knafl, K., & Dzurec, L. C. (1993, in press). Grant writing for qualitative research: Analysis of reviewers' comments. *Image: The Journal of Nursing Scholarship.*

Downs, F. (1990). Words from a Dutch aunt. *Nursing Research, 39*(6), 325.

Field, P., & Morse, J. (1985). *Nursing research: The application of qualitative approaches.* London: Crown Helm.

Glaser, B., & Strauss, A. (1966). The purpose and credibility of qualitative research. *Nursing Research, 15,* 56-61.

Guba, E., & Lincoln, Y. (1981). *Effective evaluation.* San Francisco: Jossey Bass.

Kaplan, A. (1964). *The conduct of inquiry: Methodology for behavioral science.* Scranton, PA: Chandler.

Kirk, J., & Miller, M. (1986). *Reliability and validity in qualitative research.* Beverly Hills, CA: Sage.

Knafl, K., & Howard, M. (1984). Interpreting and reporting qualitative research. *Research in Nursing and Health, 7,* 17-24.

Le Compte, M., & Goetz, J. (1982). Problems of reliability and validity in ethnographic research. *Review of Educational Research, 52,* 31-60.

Leininger, M. (1990). Ethnomethods: The philosophic and epistemic bases to explicate transcultural nursing knowledge. *Journal of Transcultural Nursing, 1,* 40-51.

Lincoln, Y., & Guba, E. (1985). *Naturalistic Inquiry.* Beverly Hills, CA: Sage.

Marshall, C., & Rosman, G. (1989). *Designing qualitative research.* Newbury Park, CA: Sage.

Morse, J. (1991). On the evaluation of qualitative proposals. *Qualitative Health Research, 1,* 147-151.

Parse, R., Coyne, A., & Smith, M. (1985). *Nursing research: Qualitative methods.* Bowie, MD: Brady.

Patton, M. (1990). *Qualitative evaluation and research methods* (2nd ed.). Newbury Park, CA: Sage.

Sandelowski, M. (1986). The problem of rigor in qualitative research. *Advances in Nursing Research, 8*(3), 27-37.

Sandelowski, M., Davis, D., & Harris, B. (1989). Artful design: Writing the proposal for research in the naturalistic paradigm. *Research in Nursing and Health, 12,* 77-84.

Tornquist, E., & Funk, S. (1990). *How to write a research grant proposal. Image, The Journal of Nursing Scholarship, 22,* 44-51.

Tripp-Reimer, T., & Cohen, M. Z. (1989). Funding strategies for qualitative research. In J. M. Morse (Ed.), *Qualitative nursing research: A contemporary dialogue* (pp. 225-238). Rockvill, MD: Aspen.

Wolcott, H. (1990). *Writing up qualitative research.* Newbury Park, CA: Sage.

Woods, N., & Catanzaro, M. (1988). *Nursing research: Theory and practice.* St. Louis: Mosby.

ADDITIONAL READINGS

Grounded Theory

Bowers, B. (1988). Grounded theory. In B. Sarter (Ed.), *Paths to knowledge: Innovative research methods for nursing* (pp. 33-59). New York: National League for Nursing.

Chenitz, W. C., & Swanson, J. M. (1986). *From practice to grounded theory: Qualitative research in nursing.* Menlo Park, CA: Addison-Wesley.

Glaser, B., & Strauss, A. (1967). *The discovery of grounded theory: Strategies for qualitative research.* New York: Aldine.

Phenomenology

Cohen, M. Z. (1987). A historical overview of the phenomenologic movement. *Image: The Journal of Nursing Scholarship, 19,* 31-34.

Lynch-Sauer, J. (1985). Using phenomenological research to study nursing phenomena. In M. Leininger (Ed.), *Qualitative research methods in nursing* (pp. 93-107). Orlando, FL: Grune & Stratton.

Omery, A. (1983). Phenomenology: A method for nursing research. *Advances in Nursing Science, 5*(2), 49-63.

Ethnography

Fetterman, D. (1989). *Ethnography step by step.* Newbury Park, CA: Sage.

Leininger, M. (1985). Ethnography and ethnonursing: Models and modes of qualitative data analysis. In M. Leininger (Ed.), *Qualitative research methods in nursing* (pp. 33-71). Orlando, FL: Grune & Stratton.

Robinson, M., & Boyle, J. (1984). Ethnography: Contributions to nursing research. *Journal of Advanced Nursing, 9,* 43-49.

Critical Research

Bunting, S., & Campbell, C. (1990). Feminism and nursing: Historical perspectives. *Advances in Nursing Science, 12*(4), 11-24.

Duffy, M. E. (1985). The critique of research: A feminist perspective. *Health Care for Women International, 6,* 341-352.

Hall, J., & Stevens, P. E. (1991). Rigor in feminist research. *Advances in Nursing Science, 13*(3), 16-29.

Index

Other Books of Interest from NLN Press